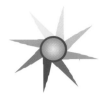

W9-BMZ-606

Perspective Press

The
PHARMACY TECHNICIAN

Morton Publishing Company
www.morton-pub.com

Morton Publishing

First Edition
Copyright © 1999 by Morton Publishing Company

Printed in the United States of America.

Morton Publishing Company
925 West Kenyon Avenue, Unit 12
Englewood, CO 80110
phone: 1-303-761-4805
fax: 1-303-762-9923

International Standard Book Number
0-89582-472-8

01 02 03 / 9 8 7 6 5 4 3

THE PHARMACY TECHNICIAN
TABLE OF CONTENTS

TABLE OF CONTENTS

TABLE OF CONTENTS

ACKNOWLEDGEMENTS

CONTRIBUTORS

I'd like to thank the following people for their contributions to this book. They have done a great job in drafting material, making suggestions, and providing general assistance which has made this the book it is.

Robert P. Shrewsbury, Associate Professor of Pharmaceutics, University of North Carolina-Chapel Hill
> *Bob developed the material for chapters 4, 7, 8, 9, 10, 11 and the Appendix on Drug Classifications. His involvement in this book has been invaluable.*

Brenda Hanneson Vonderau, B.Sc. (Pharm.), and Peter Vonderau, R.Ph.
> *Brenda and Peter developed the chapter on Prescriptions.*

Joseph Medina, R.Ph., Director of Pharmacy Technician Program, Arapahoe Community College
> *Joe developed the Calculations chapter as well as the end of chapter multiple choice questions.*

Cindy Johnson, R.PH., MSW
> *Cindy developed the Information chapter.*

Andrew Cordiale, CPhT, Hospital Inventory Technician/Buyer
> *Andrew developed material for the Inventory chapter and provided valuable input as well as photographs that have been used in the art program.*

Mary F. Powers, Ph.D., R.Ph., Coordinator, Pharmacy Technology, Mercy College of Northwest Ohio, Toledo OH
> *Mary developed the Financial Issues chapter.*

Betsy A. Gilman, Pharm.D.
> *Betsy developed the material on Community Pharmacy and helped in getting valuable photography that has been transformed into art in this book.*

Pamela Nicoski, Pharm.D., and Elizabeth Dodds, Pharm.D.
> *Pam and Libby developed the Institutional Pharmacy chapter.*

EVERYONE ELSE

I'd also like to specially thank the following individuals for their valuable input and assistance:
> Samuel Blackman, MD, University of Illinois at Chicago Circle, College of Medicine
>
> Janet Wakelin, Director, Pharmacy Technology Program, Cuyahoga Community College, Cleveland OH
>
> Jack Arthur, R.Ph., for advice and photography.
>
> Ami Teague Deaton and Lori Coleman of UNC-Chapel Hill, for their photography.
>
> Lynette De Rosa for photography.
>
> Robin Cavallo, Pottstown Memorial Medical Center, for photography.

I'd also like to thank three great artists for their assistance: Tammy Newnam, Claudette Barjoud, and Anna Veltfort; and Doug Morton, whose sponsorship makes this book possible. Finally, I'd like to thank my family whose support and patience is essential and deeply appreciated: Joan, Hannah, Joan, Wilma Jean, and Jimmy.

Dennis Hogan, Publisher

How To Use This Book

This book has been specially designed and developed to make learning easier and more productive. Besides the extensive use of illustrations to both provide information and reinforce text discussion, the text uses a distinctive facing page design that makes it easier to identify important points and to make connections between concepts. Illustrations are never a page or two away from the text. Topics are presented in perspective. Information is easy to find and understand. Some of the other key features of this design are:

➡ A **running glossary** represented by the symbol at right is presented throughout the text to emphasize important vocabulary.

➡ We have used the **Rx symbol** to indicate points of emphasis and suggestion because these are a recipe for success.

➡ End of chapter **Reviews** that provide:

    ✔ a checklist of the **Key Concepts** in the chapter,

    ✔ a **Match the Terms** section that tests knowledge of the terminology.

    ✔ **Multiple Choice** questions in the *choose the best answer* format.

We think you'll find this book a useful guide to understanding the principles, career concepts, and pharmacy skills you'll need to be a successful pharmacy technician. We also hope that you find this to be one of the best texts you will use.

AMERICAN PHARMACEUTICAL ASSOCIATION
BASIC PHARMACY AND PHARMACOLOGY SERIES

Dear Student or Instructor,

The American Pharmaceutical Association (APhA), the national professional society of pharmacists in the United States, and Morton Publishing Company, a publisher of educational texts and training materials in healthcare, are pleased to present this outstanding textbook, *The Pharmacy Technician*. It is one of a series of distinctive texts and training materials for basic pharmacy and pharmacology training published under this banner: *American Pharmaceutical Association Basic Pharmacy and Pharmacology Series*.

Each book in the series is oriented toward developing an understanding of fundamental concepts. In addition, each text presents applied and practical information on the skills necessary to function effectively in positions such as technicians and medical assistants who work with medications below the prescriber level and whose role in healthcare is increasingly important. Each of the books in the series uses a visual design to enhance understanding and ease of use and is accompanied by various instructional support materials. We think you will find them valuable training tools.

The American Pharmaceutical Association and Morton Publishing thank you for using this book and invite you to look at other titles in this series, which are listed below.

John A. Gans, PharmD
Executive Vice President
American Pharmaceutical Association

Douglas N. Morton
President
Morton Publishing Company

TITLES IN THIS SERIES:

The Pharmacy Technician
Pharmacy Technician Workbook and Certification Review
Basic Pharmacology
Drug Card Workbook

The
Pharmacy Technician

ORIGINS

In earliest times, medicine was based in magic and religion.

Like many ancient peoples, Sumerians living between the Tigris and Euphrates rivers around 4,000 B.C. believed that demons were the cause of illness. They studied the stars and the intestines of animals for clues to the supernatural causes of man's condition and fate. In many cultures, physicians were priests, and sometimes considered gods or demi-gods. The Egyptian Imhotep, for example, born around 3,000 B.C., was a priest and adviser to pharaohs and was the first physician known by name. After his death, he was named a demi-god and eventually a god: the Egyptian God of medicine.

The supernatural approach to treating illness gradually gave way to a more scientific approach, based on observation and experimentation.

Around 400 B.C., the Greek physician Hippocrates developed a more scientific approach which has guided western medicine for much of the time since. He promoted the idea of diagnosing illness based on careful observation of the patient's condition, not supernatural or other external elements. He also wrote the oath which physicians recited for centuries and still honor today: the Hippocratic Oath. From Hippocrates and others following in his footsteps, an approach to medicine in which natural causes were examined scientifically gradually grew to become the dominant approach to treating human illness.

 synthetic with chemicals, combining simpler chemicals into more complex compounds, creating a new chemical not found in nature as a result.

The God of Medicine

The ancient Greek Aesculapius was said to have been such an extraordinary physician that he could keep his patients from dying and even raise the dead. This skill angered Pluto, the god of the underworld, because it reduced the number of his subjects. At Pluto's request, Zeus killed Aesculapius with a lightning bolt, then named him the God of medicine. Aesculapius's daughter, Panacea, became the Goddess of medicinal herbs.

MEDICAL MYTH

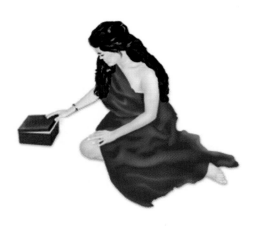

Pandora's Box

As punishment for Prometheus's theft of fire for mankind, the Greek God Zeus created Pandora and had her collect "gifts" for man from the gods. These gifts were really punishments that included disease and pestilence. They were released upon the world when Pandora opened her box.

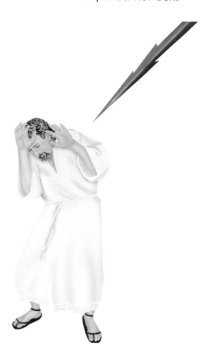

NATURE'S MEDICINE

A Treatment for Malaria

Malaria had long been one of the most deadly diseases in world history, until medicine made from the bark of a Peruvian tree, the Cinchona, was discovered. The medicine was **quinine,** popularly called "Jesuit's powder" for the Spanish priests that sent it to Europe from the New World. Its use along with preventive measures aimed at eradicating the cause of malaria brought the deadly disease under control.

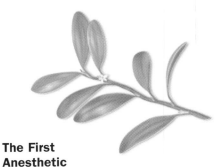

The First Anesthetic

Long before Spanish explorers noticed it, the Indians of the Andes chewed coca leaves for their medicinal effects, which included increased endurance. The active ingredient in the leaves was **cocaine,** which in 1884 was shown to be the first effective local anesthetic by Carl Koller, a Viennese surgeon. This discovery revolutionized surgery and dentistry, since previously anesthesia was administered on a general basis—that is, to the whole body. Eventually, because of its harmful properties when abused, a man-made substitute was developed, called **procain** or **novocain.**

Besides looking to the supernatural, ancient man also looked to the natural world for medical answers.

Early man understood that plants and other natural materials had the power to treat or relieve illness. The ancient Sumerians used about 250 natural medicines derived from plants, many of which are still used today. Around 3000 B.C., the Chinese Emperor Shen Nung is said to have begun eating plants and other natural materials to determine which were poisonous and which were beneficial. One of the first known practitioners of "trial and error" drug testing, he is believed to have established 365 "herbs" that could be used in health treatments. Over the centuries, this number was gradually expanded by various Chinese physicians into the thousands. Herbal medicine remains a major component of Chinese medicine today.

Through the ages, people have used drugs to treat illnesses and other physical conditions.

Ancient cultures around the world used medicines made from natural sources, many of which contained drugs that we still use today. Over the past two centuries, however, science found ways to create *synthetic* drugs, which often have advantages in cost, effect, and availability. Some of these man-made drugs replaced natural drugs and others were for entirely new uses. Today, while we still rely on many drugs derived from natural sources, we use more than twice as many synthetically produced drugs as naturally produced ones. As a result, the number of illnesses and physical conditions that can be treated with drugs is constantly increasing.

Nature's Aspirin

The ancient Greek physicians Hippocrates and Dioscorides both wrote about the pain relieving ability of the bark of a white willow tree that grew in the Mediterranean. In the 1800's, more than 2,000 years after Hippocrates' time, the active ingredient in the willow bark, **salicylic acid**, was derived by chemists. However, because of difficulties in taking salicylic acid internally, **acetylsalicylic acid**, popularly known as **aspirin**, was developed and it eventually became the most widely used drug in the world.

MEDICINE THROUGH THE AGES

— A Timeline —

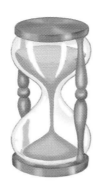

3000 B.C.

The **Egyptian Imhotep,** born around 3,000 B.C., was a priest and adviser to pharaohs and the first physician known by name. After his death, he was named a demi-god and eventually a god: the Egyptian God of medicine.

4000 B.C.

Ancient **Sumerians** studied the stars and animal intestines to divine man's fate and physical condition.

500 B.C.

The **Greek Alcmaeon,** a student of Pythagorus, saw diseases as a result of a loss of the body's natural equilibrium, rather than the work of the gods.

| 4000 B.C. | 3000 B.C. | 2000 B.C. | 1000 B.C. | 500 B.C. | 250 B.C. |

3000 B.C.

The **Chinese Emperor Shen Nung** is said to have begun tasting plants and other natural materials to determine which were poisonous and which were beneficial. One of the first known practitioners of "trial and error" drug testing, he is credited with establishing hundreds of herbal medicines.

600 B.C.

A cult following **Aesculapius, the Greek God of Medicine,** established centers where medicine was practiced. These early clinics became training grounds for the great Greek physicians of later years.

400 B.C.

A number of medical documents are written by different Greek physicians under the name **Hippocrates.** The works avoid the supernatural and religious and represent an approach to medicine that is grounded in scientific reasoning and close observation of the patient. They contain writings about the conduct of physicians, including the famous Hippocratic oath.

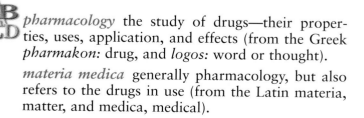

pharmacology the study of drugs—their properties, uses, application, and effects (from the Greek *pharmakon*: drug, and *logos*: word or thought).

materia medica generally pharmacology, but also refers to the drugs in use (from the Latin materia, matter, and medica, medical).

100 B.C.

King Mithridates of Pontos practiced an early form of immunization by taking small amounts of poisons so that he could build his tolerance of them. It is said that he was so successful at this that when he eventually decided to kill himself through poisoning, he was unable to, and had to be killed by someone else. The potion Mithridates developed, Mithridaticum, was believed to be good at promoting health and was used for fifteen hundred years.

77 B.C.

Dioscorides, a Greek physician working in the Roman Legion, wrote the **De Materia Medica**, five books that described over 600 plants and their healing properties. His work was the main influence for Western pharmaceutics for over sixteen hundred years. One of the remedies he described was made from the bark of a type of willow tree, the active ingredient of which was salicylic acid, the natural drug on which acetylsalicylic acid (aspirin) is based. He also described how to get opium from poppies.

162 A.D.

The Greek physician **Galen** went to Rome and became the greatest name in Western medicine since Hippocrates both through his practice and extensive writings, nearly 100 of which survive. He believed there were four "humours" in man which needed to be in balance for good health, and he advocated "bleeding" to assist that balance. He also believed in the vigorous application of a scientific approach to medicine and his emphasis on education, observation, and logic formed the cornerstone for Western medicine.

| 200 B.C. | 100 B.C. | 1 A.D. | 100 A.D. | 200 A.D. |

200 B.C.

The first official Chinese "herbal," the **Shen Nung Pen Tsao**, listing 365 herbs for use in health treatments, is believed to have been published. This can be considered an early Chinese forerunner to the FDA approved drug list..

100 A.D.

The **Indian physician Charaka** wrote the **Charaka Samhita**, the first great book of Indian medicine, which among other things described over 500 herbal drugs that had been known and used in India for many centuries.

 Note: since the use of drugs goes so far back in history, we use many terms based on Greek or Latin words.

 pharmacopeia an authoritative listing of drugs and issues related to their use.

pharmaceutical of or about drugs; also, a drug product.

panacea a cure-all (from the Greek *panakeia*, same meaning).

MEDICINE THROUGH THE AGES
— A Timeline —

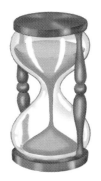

900 A.D.

The **Persian Rhazes** wrote one of the most popular textbooks of medicine in the Middle Ages, the **Book of Medicine Dedicated to Mansur**. A man of science, Rhazes was also an **alchemist** who believed he could turn lesser metal into gold. When he failed to do this, the Caliph ordered him beaten over the head with his own chemistry book until either his head or the book broke. Apparently, it was a tie. Rhazes lost sight in one eye but lived to continue his work.

1500 A.D.

When the Spanish found them, the **Indians of Mexico** had a well established pharmacology that included more than 1,200 drugs and was clearly the result of many hundreds of years of medical practice. One plant, the sarsaparilla, became very popular in Europe for its use on kidney and bladder ailments and can be found to this day in many medicinal teas.

1580 A.D.

In China, **Li Shi Zhen** completed the **Pen Tsao Kang Mu**, a compilation of nearly 2,000 drugs for use in treating illness and other conditions.

1630 A.D.

Jesuits sent **quinine** back to Europe in the early sixteen hundreds. Also called Jesuit's powder, it was the first drug to be used successfully in the treatment of the dreaded disease malaria.

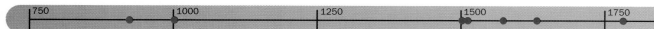

1000 A.D.

Perhaps the greatest Islamic physician was **Avicenna**. His writings dominated medical thinking in Europe for centuries. He wrote a five volume encyclopedia, one of which was devoted to natural medications and another to compounding drugs from individual medications.

1500 A.D.

In the early fifteen hundreds, a Swiss alchemist who went by the name of **Paracelsus** rejected the "humoural" philosophy of Galen and all previous medical teaching other than Hippocrates. Though he had many critics, he is generally credited with firmly establishing the use of chemistry to create medicinal drugs. Included in his work is the first published recipe for the addictive drug laudanum, which became a popular though tragically abused drug for the next three hundred years.

1785 A.D.

The **British Physician, William Withering**, publishes his study of the **foxglove** plant and the drug it contained, **digitalis**, which became widely used in treating heart disease. Foxglove had been used since ancient times in various remedies but Withering described a process for creating the drug from the dried leaves of the plant and established a dosage approach.

ABCD *antitoxin* a substance that acts against a toxin in the body; also, a vaccine containing antitoxins, used to fight disease.

antibiotic a substance which harms or kills microorganisms like bacteria and fungi.

1803

The German pharmacist **Frederich Serturner** extracts morphine from opium.

1846

In Boston, the first publicized operation using **general anesthesia** is performed. Ether is the anaesthetic.

1890

Effective **antitoxins** are developed for diptheria and tetanus, giving a major boost to the development of medicines that fight infectious disease.

1899

Acetylsalicylic acid, popularly known as **aspirin,** is developed because of difficulties in using salicylic acid, a drug contained in certain willow trees that had long been used in the external treatment of various conditions.

1928

In Britain, **Alexander Fleming** discovers a fungus which produces a chemical that kills bacteria. He names the chemical, **penicillin.** It is the first antibiotic drug.

1943

Russell Marker is able to create the **hormone progesterone,** the first reliable birth control drug, from a species of Mexican yam.

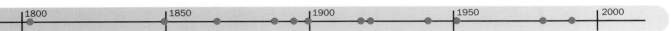

| 1800 | 1850 | 1900 | 1950 | 2000 |

1864

Louis Pasteur's experiments show that microorganisms cause food spoilage, and that heat can be used to kill them and preserve the food. Though others had proposed principles of **"germ theory"** previously, Pasteur's work is instrumental in it becoming widely accepted.

1884

In 1884, **Carl Koller,** a Viennese surgeon, discovers that cocaine, the active ingredient in coca leaves, was useful as a local anesthetic in eye surgery, and cocaine is established as the **first local anesthetic**.

1921

In Toronto, Canada, **Frederick Banting** and **Charles Best** show that an extract of the hormone, **insulin,** will lower blood sugar in dogs and so may be useful in the treatment of the terrible disease diabetes. The biochemist James B. Collip then develops an extract of insulin pure enough to test on humans. The first human trial in January, 1922 proves successful and dramatically changes the prospects for all diabetics.

1951

James Watson and **Francis Crick** identify the structure of **DNA**, the basic component within the cell that contains the organism's genetic code.

1981

First documented cases of **AIDS.**

1988

The **Human Genome Project** is begun with the goal of mapping the entire DNA sequence in the human genome, This information will provide a better understanding of hereditary diseases and allow the development of new treatments for them.

 hormone chemicals produced by the body that regulate body functions and processes.

human genome the complete set of genetic material contained in a human cell.

THE 20TH CENTURY

The average life span in the United States increased by over twenty years in the Twentieth Century.

At the beginning of the century, the average American lived only into their early fifties. By 1995, the average life expectancy at birth in the United States had risen to 75.8 years. Similar changes were seen throughout the industrialized world and to a lesser extent in developing countries. The growth of hospitals, advances in the treatment of disease, improved medical technology, better understanding of nutrition and health, and the rapid increase in the number of effective drugs and vaccines have all contributed to this profound change in improved life experience.

A major factor in the increased health and life expectancy seen in this century was the dramatic growth in pharmaceutical medicine.

Since the eighteenth century, there was a growing interest and success in creating man-made or synthetic medicines. The creation of aspirin in 1899 was followed by more pharmaceutical research and discoveries that spurred the growth of a worldwide industry committed to creating medicines for virtually every illness and condition. The discovery of the antibiotic penicillin was followed shortly by a World War in which its mass production was seen as critical to Allied success. This and other war related drug needs stimulated the U.S. pharmaceutical industry to dramatically boost its capacity and production. Ever since, pharmaceutical research and development in the U.S. has grown substantially and continually, making it the world's leading producer of medical pharmaceuticals with more than $100 billion in annual worldwide sales.

LIVING LONGER

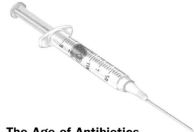

The Age of Antibiotics

In World War I, more soldiers died from infections than the wounds themselves. Although penicillin was discovered as an antibiotic in 1928, it was difficult to produce and for years not much was made of the discovery. With the start of World War II, however, British scientists looked again at penicillin and established that it was effective in fighting infections. Already under attack from Germany and unable to develop mass production methods for penicillin, the British sought help in the United States. In 1942, the Pfizer pharmaceutical company was able to develop a method for mass production of the drug, and by D-Day the Allied army was well stocked with it. Its use saved many thousands of lives during the war and revolutionized the pharmaceutical industry. A period of intense research and discovery in the field of antibiotics began, and many new antibiotics were developed which have dramatically contributed to improved health and increased life expectancy.

Living Longer

Improved pharmaceutical products have had a major effect on the life span of Americans and others in the twentieth century. In the U.S., the life span has increased over 50% in the last century, with much of the increase due to the discovery and use of disease fighting drugs.

source: National Center of Health Statistics

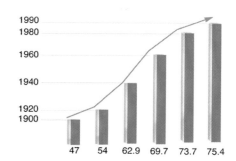

THE DRUG INDUSTRY

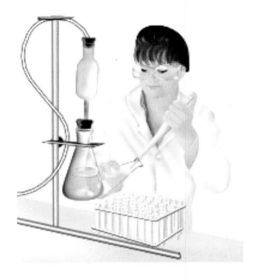

Patenting Discoveries

As with other scientific and technological areas, patenting new discoveries is an important part of the pharmaceutical development process since it protects against illegal copying of the discovery. The company holding the patent is then able to control the marketing of the product and use this as a way to recover their original investment. Since patenting generally occurs long before a drug is approved, however, a company generally has only about ten years of patent protection left in which to market their product without competition from direct copies called "generic" versions.

With the increasing availability of powerful drugs, their regulation became more important than ever.

Leaders and governments have long sought to regulate the use of medicinal drugs because of their effect on the population's health. The explosive growth of pharmaceuticals in the twentieth century made governments throughout the world keenly aware of the importance of setting and maintaining standards for their distribution and use.

In the United States, drug regulation is performed by the Food and Drug Administration.

FDA activity is a major factor in the nation's public health and safety. Before a drug can be marketed, it must be shown through testing that it is safe and effective for its intended use. Once marketed, the FDA monitors drugs to make sure they work as intended, and that there are no serious negative (adverse) effects from their use. If drugs that are marketed are found to have adverse effects, the FDA can recall them (take them off the market).

The discovery of new drugs requires a major investment of time, research, and development.

The pharmaceutical industry employs thousands of scientists and devotes about one-sixth of its income to research and development. Bringing a new drug to market is a long and difficult process in which the vast majority of research does not produce a successful drug. Thousands of chemical combinations must be tried in order to find one that might work as hoped. Once a potentially useful drug is created, it must undergo an extensive testing and approval process before it can be made available to the public. In the United States, the length of time from the beginning of development through testing and to ultimate FDA approval is often more than ten years.

It's in the Genes

One of the most exciting areas of pharmaceutical research is performed by molecular biologists studying human genes. While antibiotics are the answer for many infectious diseases, many other diseases which seemed based on heredity are effectively untreatable. The study of the human genome has shown that many diseases are related to genetic defects. This has led to the creation of new drugs that can successfully treat many diseases previously considered untreatable. As a result, the field of biotechnology has become the most dynamic area of pharmaceutical research and development.

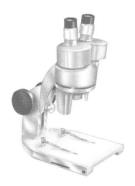

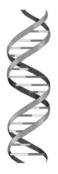

PHARMACY TODAY

A "prescription" drug is one that has been ordered or "prescribed" by a physician or other licensed prescriber to treat a patient. Though physicians occasionally give patients the actual medication, in most cases the individual who dispenses the prescribed medication to the patient is a pharmacist. Pharmacists at the more than 50,000 community pharmacies account for approximately half of the distribution of prescription drugs in the United States. The rest reach consumers primarily through hospitals, mass merchandisers, food stores, mail order pharmacies, clinics, and nursing homes-- all of which employ pharmacists for the dispensing of medications.

The pharmacist has consistently been rated as the professional most trusted by the public, even more than members of the clergy.

The sheer number of available drugs, their different names and costs, multiple prescriptions from different physicians, and the involvement of third-party insurers are among the many factors which make using prescription drugs a complex area for consumers. As a result, they rely on pharmacists to provide information and advice on prescription and over-the-counter medications in easy to understand language. They also routinely ask the pharmacist to make recommendations about less expensive generic substitutes for a prescribed drug.

In 1990, the U.S. Congress required pharmacists to provide consulting services to Medicaid patients in the Omnibus Budget Reconciliation Act (OBRA).

Since then, a number of states have begun requiring this for all patients, and it is generally considered a fundamental service for pharmacists to provide.

To help with this increasing complex environment, pharmacists use powerful computerized tools and specially trained assistants.

Computers put customer profiles, product, inventory, pricing, and other essential information within easy access. Assistants in the form of **pharmacy technicians** perform many tasks that pharmacists once performed. As a result, pharmacists dispense more prescriptions and advice than ever before.

THE PHARMACIST

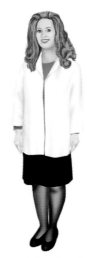

A Trusted Profession

In December, 1997, pharmacists received the highest "honesty and ethics" rating from Americans for the ninth straight year in Gallup polls.

1. pharmacists
2. clergy
3. medical doctors
4. college teachers
5. dentists

Education

To become a pharmacist, an individual must graduate from an accredited college of pharmacy (of which there are about 80 in the U.S.), pass a state licensing exam, and perform an internship working under a licensed pharmacist. Once licensed, the pharmacist must receive continuing education to maintain their license. Pharmacists seeking to teach, do research, or work in hospitals often must have an advanced Doctor of Pharmacy degree (Pharm.D.). Three out of five pharmacists work in community pharmacies; one out of four in hospitals.

PHARMACY SETTINGS

Most pharmacists and pharmacy technicians work in either a community pharmacy or hospital setting, with community pharmacy being the area of greatest employment (about half of all pharmacists and technicians). However, there are a number of other environments where significant employment can be found. The primary environments for pharmacist and technician employment are:

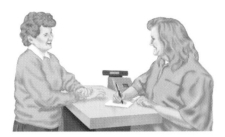

➡ **community pharmacies:** the area of greatest employment

➡ **hospitals:** the next greatest area of employment

➡ **mail order operations:** pharmacy businesses that provide drugs by mail to patients—a fast growing area.

➡ **long-term care:** residence facilities that provide care on a long-term rather than acute or short-term basis.

➡ **managed care:** care that is managed by an insurer.

➡ **home care:** care provided to patients in their home, often by a hospital or by a home care agency working with a home care pharmacy.

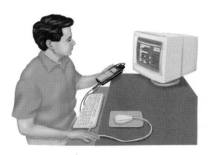

ECONOMIC TRENDS

In thirty years, the cost of health care in the United States rose over 2,500 percent! As a result, there have been increasing efforts by government, industry, and consumers to find ways to control the costs of care. Though drugs represent only a small fraction of overall health care expenses, they have also been included in these efforts.

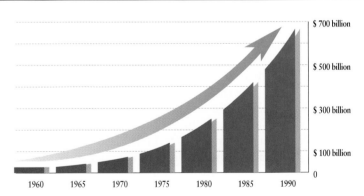

➡ A result of the **managed care** movement is that the majority of prescriptions are now paid by private third parties such as HMO's and other insurance companies, instead of directly by consumers.

➡ Along with this is a trend toward the use of closed "formularies," lists of drugs which are approved for use. These lists rely substantially on substituting generic drugs in place of more expensive brands that may be prescribed by the physician. By 1996, the use of generics had doubled in ten years to 40% of dispensed prescriptions.*

➡ Another cost cutting trend is the increasing use of "therapeutic substitution" in which a chemically different drug that performs a similar function is substituted, usually because it is less expensive.

source for text: Pharmaceutical Research and Manufacturers of America;
source for illustration: U.S. Statistical Abstract

COMPUTERS IN PHARMACY

Pharmacies use powerful computerized tools that help productivity.

Computerized pharmacy management systems put customer profiles, product, inventory, pricing, and other essential information within easy access. They also automate elements like label printing, inventory management, stock reordering, and billing. As a result, pharmacies and pharmacists dispense more prescriptions and information than ever before.

Pharmacy computer systems may be developed by the user to meet specific needs, purchased ready-made, or provided by a drug wholesaler.

Wholesalers provide inventory management systems to their customers as part of their service. The wholesaler actually owns the system. It is primarily designed for placing orders with the wholesaler, though it may also contain various other elements. Large pharmacy chains have the business volume to justify the expense of developing comprehensive systems that are tailored to their needs. Smaller operations usually buy a commercially available system. Whatever the operation, a computerized pharmacy management system is an indispensable productivity tool.

Although each pharmacy computer system has its own specific features, many general principles of computer usage apply to all systems.

The most important element is stated in the classic computer axiom: garbage in, garbage out. That is, the information produced by the computer is only as good as the information that is entered into it. This means special care has to be taken when entering information (generally called data) to make sure it is correct. A simple mistake in data entry can result in the wrong medication being given to the wrong patient or in any number of other serious problems.

R **keyboard skills:** Considering how much data entry is required, being able to type at least forty five words per minute is an important skill.

computer knowledge: Many systems use personal computers or similar custom hardware, so familiarity with using computers is important.

A SAMPLE SYSTEM

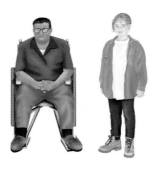

Patient Profile

Allows complete patient profiles, including prescribers, insurer, and medication history; identifies drug interactions for patients taking multiple medications.

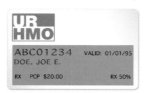

UR HMO
ABC01234   VALID: 01/01/95
DOE, JOE E.
RX   PCP $20.00   RX 50%

Billing

Checks policies of third parties such as HMOs and insurers; authorizes third party transactions and credit cards electronically.

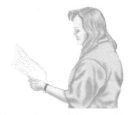

Management Reporting

Forecasting, financial analysis.

data What information that is entered into and stored in a computer system is called.

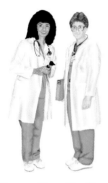

Prescriber Profile

Allows prescriber profiles, including state identification numbers, and affiliations with facilities and insurers.

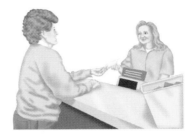

Education/Counseling

Patient information about drugs, usage, interactions, allergies, etc.

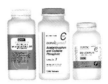

Product

Locates items by various means– brand name, generic name, product code, category, supplier, etc.

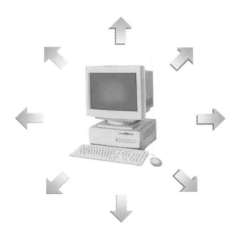

Pharmacy computer systems generally offer most or all of these features, as well as a number of others.

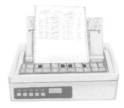

Inventory

Adjusts inventory as prescriptions are filled; analyzes turnover; produces status reports; automatically re-orders based on inventory levels, generates purchase orders.

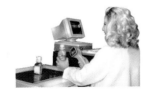

Pricing

Provides prices for medications and possible substitutes; automatically updates prices; scans prices from bar codes.

Security

Password protection restricts access to authorized users for different features.

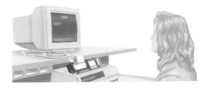

Labeling

Creates label, receipt, customer information and usage instructions.

REVIEW

KEY CONCEPTS

- ✔ People have used drugs derived from plants to treat illnesses and other physical conditions for thousands of years.
- ✔ The ancient Greeks used the bark of a white willow tree to relieve pain. The bark contained salicylic acid, the natural forerunner of the active ingredient in aspirin.
- ✔ Cocaine was the first effective local anesthetic.
- ✔ The foxglove plant contains the drug digitalis, which has been widely used in treating heart disease.
- ✔ Louis Pasteur's experiments show that microorganisms cause food spoilage, and that heat can be used to kill them and preserve the food.
- ✔ Frederick Banting and Charles Best showed that an extract of the hormone, insulin, lowered blood sugar in dogs and might be useful in the treatment of diabetes.
- ✔ Alexander Fleming discovered the antibiotic chemical, penicillin.
- ✔ The Human Genome Project is an attempt to map the entire DNA sequence in the human genome. This information will provide a better understanding of hereditary diseases and how to treat them.
- ✔ The average life span in the United States increased by over twenty years in the Twentieth Century.
- ✔ In World War I, more soldiers died from infections than the wounds themselves.
- ✔ To become a pharmacist in the United States, an individual must graduate from an accredited college of pharmacy, pass a state licensing exam, and perform an internship working under a licensed pharmacist.
- ✔ Once licensed, the pharmacist must receive continuing education to maintain their license.
- ✔ Increasing costs of health care have brought increased efforts to control the cost of prescription drugs, on aspect of which is the use of closed "formularies" that rely substantially on substituting generic drugs in place of more expensive brands.
- ✔ Computerized pharmacy management systems put customer profiles, product, inventory, pricing, and other essential information within easy access. One result has been that pharmacies and pharmacists dispense more prescriptions and information than ever before.

SELF TEST

MATCH THE TERMS.   *answers can be checked in the glossary*

antibiotic	combining simpler chemicals into more complex ones, creating a new chemical not found in nature.
antitoxin	an authoritative listing of drugs and issues related to their use.
hormone	of or about drugs; also, a drug product.
human genome	a cure-all.
materia medica	the study of drugs—their properties, uses, application, and effects.
panacea	generally pharmacology, but also refers to the drugs in use.
pharmaceutical	a substance that acts against a toxin in the body
pharmacology	a substance which harms or kills microorganisms like bacteria and fungi.
pharmacopeia	chemicals produced by the body that regulate body functions and processes.
synthetic	the complete set of genetic material contained in a human cell.

CHOOSE THE BEST ANSWER.   *answers are in the back of the book*

1. Derived from the bark of the Peruvian tree, "Jesuit's Powder," use along with preventive measures, help keep this disease under control.
   a. smallpox
   b. malaria
   c. polio
   d. tuberculosis

2. In most cases the individual who dispenses the prescribed medication to the patient is the
   a. prescribing physician
   b. nurse
   c. medical office assistant
   d. pharmacist

3. As for employment opportunities, the Pharmacy Technician may find the greatest opportunity in
   a. the hospital setting
   b. the community setting
   c. home health care
   d. mail order operations

4. The FDA is required to
   a. ensure that a drug is safe and effective for its intended use.
   b. to monitor a drug after it is marketed to ensure it works as intended.
   c. to monitor a drug for any adverse effects.
   d. all of the above.

PHARMACY TECHNICIAN

In health care, "technicians" are individuals who are given a basic level of training designed to help them perform specific tasks.

This training often is provided at community and technical colleges or even on the job. By comparison, health care "professionals" such as physicians and pharmacists receive more extensive and advanced levels of education.

To perform their duties, pharmacists today rely upon the assistance of trained support staff called pharmacy technicians.

Technicians perform essential tasks that do not require the pharmacist's skill or expertise. They work under the direct supervision of a licensed pharmacist who is legally responsible for their performance.

Pharmacy technicians perform such tasks as filling prescriptions, packaging doses, performing inventory control, and keeping records.

Having technicians perform these tasks gives the pharmacist more time for activities which require a greater level of expertise, such as consulting with patients. As the job of the pharmacist has become more complex, the need for pharmacy technicians has increased. As a result, pharmacy technician is a rapidly growing occupation offering many opportunities.

Like pharmacists, most pharmacy technicians are employed in community pharmacies and hospitals. However, they are also employed in clinics, home care, long term care, mail order prescription pharmacies, and various other settings. Depending upon the specific setting and job, they may perform at different levels of specialization and skill. An introductory level technician job at a pharmacy requires general skills. In various hospital and other environments, there are specialized technician jobs which require more advanced skills developed from additional education, training and experience. Compensation for these specialized positions is greater than it is for entry level positions.

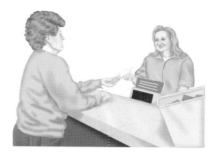
receiving prescriptions

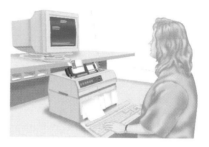
using computers

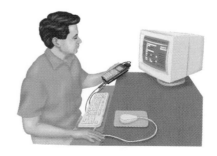
inventory control

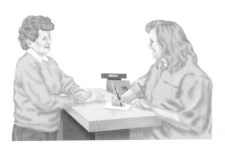

taking patient information

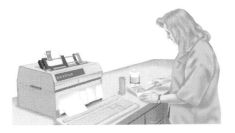

filling prescriptions

The Pharmacy Technician

The activities on these pages may be part of a pharmacy technician's job responsibilities. However, **specific responsibilities and tasks for pharmacy technicians differ by setting and are described in writing by each employer** through job descriptions, policy and procedure manuals, and other documents. What individuals may and may not do in their jobs is often referred to as their "scope of practice." The pharmacist's scope of practice is of course much greater than the technician's. As part of their job requirement, all technicians are required to know specifically what tasks they may and may not perform, as well as which tasks must be performed by the pharmacist.

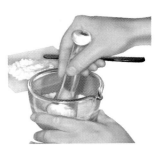

compounding

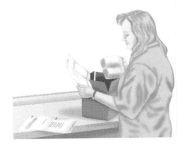

ordering

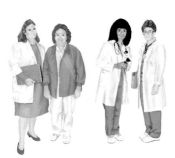

working with a team of health care professionals

PERSONAL STANDARDS

There are personal standards for pharmacy technicians.

Employers may specify these standards as part of the job requirement. Many, though not all, are outlined on these pages. There are standards for behavior, skill, health, hygiene and appearance. Anyone seeking to become a pharmacy technician should consider how they compare in each of these areas and what they must do to excel in them.

The pharmacy technician is a member of a team, the patient's health care team.

For this team to succeed, all its members, including the technician, must work together for the welfare of the patient. If a member of the team fails to perform as required, including the technician, there can be serious consequences for the patient. Anyone wishing to become a pharmacy technician must be able to work cooperatively with others, communicate effectively, perform as expected, and act responsibly. The patient's welfare depends upon it.

inventory to make an accounting of items on hand; also, with people, to assess characteristics, skills, qualities, etc.

confidentiality the requirement of health care providers to keep all patient information private among the patient, the patient's insurer, and the providers directly involved in the patient's care.

Technicians should have these personal qualities:

✔ **Dependable**

The patient, the pharmacist, and the patient's health care team will depend upon you performing your job as required. You must do what you are required to do, whether anyone is observing you or not.

✔ **Detail Oriented**

Patients must receive medications exactly as they have been prescribed. Drugs, whether prescription or over the counter, can be dangerous if misused, and mistakes by pharmacy technicians can be life-threatening.

✔ **Trustworthy**

You will be entrusted with confidential patient information, dangerous substances, and perishable products. In addition, many drugs are very expensive and you will be trusted to handle them appropriately.

Respect for the Patient

The patient's welfare is the most important consideration in health care. To ensure this, there are various government laws and professional standards which guarantee basic **patient rights** and require health care providers to explain these rights to each patient.

Specific patient rights may differ somewhat from setting to setting. Technicians must know and honor the patient's rights for the setting in which they work. Among others, patients are generally guaranteed the right to **privacy, confidentiality, the information necessary for informed consent, and the freedom to refuse treatment.**

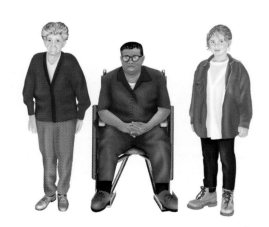

THE TECHNICIAN: A PERSONAL INVENTORY

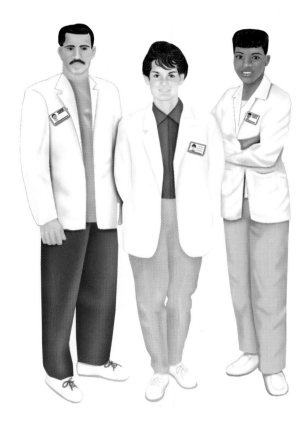

Technicians must be capable and competent in the following skill areas:

✔ Mathematics And Problem Solving

You will routinely use perform mathematical calculations in filling prescriptions and other activities.

✔ Language and Terminology

You must learn the specific pharmaceutical terminology that will be used on your job.

✔ Computer Skills

You will regularly use computers for entering patient information, maintaining inventory, filling prescriptions, and so on.

✔ Interpersonal Skills

You will interact with patients/customers, your supervisor, co-workers, physicians, and others. You must be able to communicate, cooperate, and work effectively.

Technicians must follow these personal guidelines:

✔ Health

You must maintain good physical and mental health. If you become physically or mentally run-down, you increase the chance of making serious mistakes.

✔ Hygiene

Practice good hygiene. You will interact closely with others. Poor hygiene may hurt your ability to be effective. You will also be expected to perform in infection free conditions and poor hygiene can violate this requirement.

✔ Appearance

Your uniform and personal clothing should be neat, clean, and functional. Shoes should be comfortable. Clothes should allow the freedom of movement necessary to perform your duties. Hair should be well-groomed and pulled back if long. Fingernails should be neat and trim.

 There are legal aspects to many of these standards. Failing to follow them can hurt your job performance and result in legal violations.

TRAINING & COMPETENCY

Training and competency requirements for pharmacy technicians differ from setting to setting.

Technician training is generally based on job requirements for the specific workplace, particular skills involved, any applicable professional standards, and state regulations. There are no federal requirements. In many settings, training is provided **on-the job**. Technician candidates must have a high school diploma or GED.

An example of a model curriculum for technician training is that of The American Society of Health-system Pharmacists (ASHP).

The ASHP is the leading association for pharmacists practicing in hospitals, and other health care systems. Their curriculum provides a national standard for developing technician competency. It can be adapted to different pharmacy settings and the specific needs of an individual training program. Training programs that meet ASHP standards can receive accreditation from it in recognition of having done so. The ASHP curriculum is also endorsed by the **Pharmacy Technician Educator's Council (PTEC).**

Your training program will prepare you to do your job.

Training programs may be found at community, technical, and career colleges as well as in on-the-job settings such as community pharmacies, hospitals and other institutional settings. Training generally covers pharmaceutical terminology, drug action, dosing, calculations, law, compounding, inventory control, computer skills, interpersonal skills, and various aspects of pharmacy practice.

Your employer will monitor and document your competency.

Your employer is legally responsible for your performance and therefore your competency. In addition to monitoring this on a daily basis, you will receive regularly scheduled performance reviews. The frequency of performance reviews will vary by employer and setting and be indicated in your job description or other employee information. Through these reviews and other means, your employer will document your competency to perform your job.

TRAINING

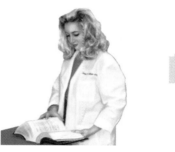

Training Program

Depending upon your setting, you will receive training in some or all of the following areas:

- drug laws
- terminology
- prescriptions
- calculations
- drug routes and forms
- drug dosage and activity
- infection control
- compounding
- preparing IV admixtures
- biopharmaceutics
- drug classifications
- inventory management
- pharmacy literature

An important part of training is exposure to actual workplace settings. Many technicians receive this in the form of **on-the-job** training from their employer or as internships for students at community colleges and other training programs

competent being qualified and capable.

COMPETENCY

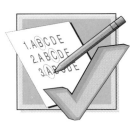

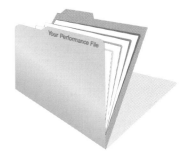

Testing

Demonstration of competency during training will generally be through written tests and practical demonstrations. In on-the-job training or internships, your performance will be directly judged by the supervising pharmacist.

Performance

After you have qualified as competent, your employer will continue to monitor and document your performance and competency throughout your employment. These files may include:

➡ performance reviews

➡ complaints

➡ comments by your supervisor and and other appropriate personnel.

Continuing Education

Pharmacy is a dynamic field that changes constantly. There are always new drugs, treatments, methods and other developments. As a result, continuing education is a critical element in maintaining competency for pharmacy technicians. In order to perform your job as required, you must continually learn new information. Ultimately, this will make your job more interesting and you more effective.

℞ For information regarding ASHP accredited programs, contact:
The American Society of Health-system Pharmacists
7272 Wisconsin Ave.
Bethesda, MD 20814
301-657-3000

CERTIFICATION

Since there is no federal standard for training or competency, a valuable career step for pharmacy technicians is getting national *certification*.

In the United States, pharmacy technician certification is performed by the **Pharmacy Technician Certification Board (PTCB)**. To receive certification, technicians must pass a standardized national examination which tests their knowledge and competency in basic pharmacy function and activity areas.

Certification is a mark of achievement that employers, colleagues, and others will recognize.

If you pass the examination, you will receive a certificate and wallet card indicating this and you will be able to use the **CPhT** designation after your name. This designation stands for Certified Pharmacy Technician and is good for two years. Beyond verifying your competence as a technician, this indicates that you have a high level of knowledge and skill and can be given greater responsibilities. This in turn means that you may earn more.

Certification must be renewed every two years.

Because pharmacy is a constantly changing field, maintaining skills and competence requires continuing education. In order to renew their certification every two years, CPhTs must meet requirements of 20 contact hours of pharmacy-related continuing education, including at least one hour in pharmacy law. Up to ten contact hours of continuing education can occur at the CPhT's practice site under the supervision of a registered pharmacist, and these hours can be customized to fit the specific needs of the CPhT.

 certification a legal proof or document that an individual meets certain objective standards, usually provided by a neutral professional organization.

 Technician certification information can be obtained by calling the Pharmacy Technician Certification Board at 202-429-7576 or through the mail at this address: PTCB, 2215 Constitution Avenue, N.W., Washington, DC 20037.

THE EXAMINATION

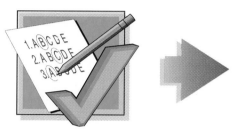

The certification exam tests these areas:

- ➡ assisting the pharmacist in serving patients;
- ➡ medication distribution and inventory control systems;
- ➡ pharmacy operations.

Other facts about the exam:

- ➡ It contains 125 multiple choice questions for which the best answer must be chosen.
- ➡ Exams last three hours and are conducted by the Professional Examination Service, a non-profit company which performs national certification and licensure examinations.
- ➡ To take the exam, candidates must have a high school diploma or GED. To pass, they must have a score of at least 650 on the exam's scoring system which ranges from 300-900.

Sample Exam Questions

The sample questions below reflect the "choose the best answer"
format of the exam. This type of question requires careful reading
and judgment. In some cases, there may be more than one answer
that is at least partially correct. However, there will only be one
correct answer that is the best and most complete answer.

1. Pharmacies located in hospitals are required to follow regulations of this organization:

1. ASHP
2. USP
3. ASCP
4. JCAHO

2. Of the following schedules of drugs, which is for drugs with no accepted medical use in the United States?

1. Schedule I
2. Schedule II
3. Schedule III
4. Schedule IV

3. Of the following needles, which size is the most likely to cause coring?

1. 13 G
2. 16 G
3. 20 G
4. 23 G

4. A solution of Halperidol (Haldol®) contains 2mg/ml of active ingredient. How many grams would be in 473 ml of this solution?

1. 9.46 gm
2. 0.946 gm
3. 0.0946 gm
4. 0.00946 gm

5. You have a 70% solution of Dextrose 1000ml. How many Kg of Dextrose is in 400 ml of this solution?

1. 280 Kg
2. 28 Kg
3. 2.8 Kg
4. 0.28 Kg

6. Which is the largest capsule size?

1. size 5
2. size 3
3. size 1
4. size 0

answers:
1. 4
2. 1
3. 1
4. 2
5. 4
6. 4

REVIEW

KEY CONCEPTS

✔ Pharmacy technicians perform essential tasks that do not require the pharmacist's skill or expertise.

✔ Pharmacy technicians work under the direct supervision of a licensed pharmacist who is legally responsible for their performance.

✔ The specific responsibilities and tasks for pharmacy technicians differ by setting and are described in writing by each employer through job descriptions, policy and procedure manuals, and other documents.

✔ Having technicians perform these tasks gives the pharmacist more time for activities which require a greater level of expertise, such as consulting with patients.

✔ What individuals may and may not do in their jobs is often referred to as their "scope of practice."

✔ Like pharmacists, most pharmacy technicians are employed in community pharmacies and hospitals.

✔ However, they are also employed in clinics, home care, long term care, mail order prescription pharmacies, and various other settings.

✔ In various hospital and other environments, there are specialized technician jobs which require more advanced skills developed from additional education, training and experience.

✔ Pharmacy technicians are entrusted with confidential patient information, dangerous substances, and perishable products.

✔ Drugs, whether prescription or over the counter, can be dangerous if misused, and mistakes by pharmacy technicians can be life-threatening.

✔ Pharmacy technicians routinely use perform mathematical calculations in filling prescriptions and other activities.

✔ Pharmacy technicians must learn the specific pharmaceutical terminology that will be used on the job.

✔ Pharmacy technicians must be able to communicate, cooperate, and work effectively with others.

✔ There is no federal standard for pharmacy technician training or competency.

✔ In the United States, a valuable career step for pharmacy technicians is getting national certification by the Pharmacy Technician Certification Board (PTCB).

✔ The CPhT designation, Certified Pharmacy Technician, is good for two years. It verifies an individual's competence as a technician, and indicates a high level of knowledge and skill.

SELF TEST

MATCH THE TERMS. *answers can be checked in the glossary*

certification

competent

confidentiality

personal inventory

professionals

scope of practice

technicians

what individuals may and may not do in their jobs.

to make an accounting of items on hand; also, with people, to assess characteristics, skills, qualities, etc.

the requirement of health care providers to keep all patient information private among the patient, the patient's insurer, and the providers directly involved in the patient's care.

being qualified and capable to perform a task or job.

a legal proof or document that an individual meets certain objective standards, usually provided by a neutral professional organization.

individuals who are given a basic level of training designed to help them perform specific tasks.

individuals who receive extensive and advanced levels of education before being allowed to practice, such as physicians and pharmacists.

CHOOSE THE BEST ANSWER. *answers are in the back of the book*

1. The pharmacy technician can do the following functions except:
   a. take patient information
   b. fill prescription orders
   c. compound prescription orders
   d. advise patients on medications

2. Pharmacy Technician certification and re-certification is the responsibility of this organization:
   a. ASHP
   b. PTEC
   c. PTCB
   d. ACPE

3. In the pharmacy setting, any procedure involving professional discretion or judgement is the responsibility of the
   a. pharmacy technician
   b. lead pharmacy technician
   c. store manager
   d. pharmacist

4. After passing the Pharmacy Technician National Certification exam, pharmacy technicians may use the following designation after their name:
   a. PT
   b. RPhT
   c. CPhT
   d. none of the above

DRUG REGULATION

— A TIMELINE —

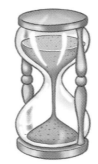

There are many laws in the United States concerning the safety and effectiveness of food, drugs, medical devices and cosmetics. Regardless of whether a product is produced in the United States or is imported, it must meet the requirements of these laws. The leading enforcement agency at the federal level for these regulations is the Food and Drug Administration. On these pages are brief descriptions of U.S. federal laws and their significance.

Food and Drug Act of 1906

Prohibited interstate commerce in adulterated or misbranded food, drinks, and drugs. Government pre-approval of drugs is required.

1927 Food, Drug and Insecticide Administration

The law enforcement agency is formed that would be renamed in 1930 as the Food and Drug Administration.

1950 Alberty Food Products v. U.S.

The United States Court of Appeals rules that the purpose for which a drug is to be used must be included on the label.

1900   1910   1920   1930   1940   1950

1911 Sherley Amendment

This law was enacted in response to the Supreme Court's interpretation that the 1906 Food and Drugs Act only applied to misleading information about the ingredients of a drug, as opposed to its effects. It prohibits false and misleading claims about the **therapeutic** effects of a drug.

1938 Food, Drug and Cosmetic (FDC) Act

In response to the fatal poisoning of 107 people, primarily children, by an untested sulfanilamide concoction, this comprehensive law requires new drugs be shown to be safe before marketing.

1951 Durham-Humphrey Amendment

This law defines what drugs require a prescription by a licensed practitioner and requires them to include this **legend** on the label: "Caution: Federal Law prohibits dispensing without a prescription."

therapeutic serving to cure or heal.

legend drug any drug which requires a prescription and either of these "legends" on the label: "Caution: Federal law prohibits dispensing without a prescription," or "Rx only."

1962 Kefauver-Harris Amendments

Requires drug manufacturers to provide proof of both safety and effectiveness before marketing the drug.

1966 Fair Packaging and Labeling Act

This requires all consumer products in interstate commerce to be honestly and informatively labeled.

1970 Controlled Substances Act (CSA)

The CSA classifies drugs that may be easily abused and restricts their distribution. It is enforced by the Drug Enforcement Administration (DEA) within the Justice Department.

1983 Orphan Drug Act

Provides incentives to promote research, approval and marketing of drugs needed for the treatment of rare diseases.

1987 Prescription Drug Marketing Act

Restricts distribution of prescription drugs to legitimate commercial channels and requires drug wholesalers to be licensed by the states.

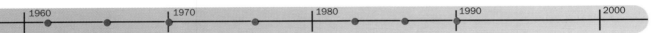

1960 1970 1980 1990 2000

1970 Poison Prevention Packaging Act

Requires child-proof packaging on all controlled and most prescription drugs dispensed by pharmacies. Non-child-proof containers may only be used if the prescriber or patient request one.

1976 Medical Device Amendment

Requires pre-market approval for safety and effectiveness of life-sustaining and life-supporting medical devices.

1990 Omnibus Budget Reconciliation Act (OBRA)

Among other things, this act required pharmacists to offer counseling to Medicaid patients regarding medications.

1997 FDA Modernization Act

Changed the legend requirement to "**Rx only**," with a phase in period until February, 2003.

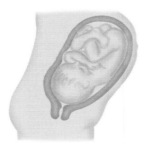

The Thalidomide Lesson

In 1962, a new sleeping pill containing the drug, thalidomide, was found to cause severe birth defects when used by pregnant women. This included lost limbs and other major deformities that affected thousands of children in Europe, where the drug had been widely used. In the United States, the drug was not yet approved for marketing and was only being used in tests, so it affected a small number of children. However, the nature of the defects and the number of children affected created a public demand in the U.S. for tighter drug regulation that resulted in the Kefauver-Harris Amendments. From then on, drugs would have to be shown to be both safe and effective before they could be marketed in the United States.

NEW DRUG APPROVAL

All new drugs, whether made domestically or imported, require FDA approval before they can be marketed in the United States. A new drug is any drug proposed for marketing after 1938 that was not already recognized as safe and effective. This represents the vast majority of drugs on the market.

Before it will be approved, a new drug must be shown to be both safe and effective and that its benefits substantially outweigh its risks.

It is the responsibility of the drug manufacturer (not the FDA) to provide proof of this to the FDA's **Center for Drug Evaluation and Research (CDER).** The proof is based on extensive testing which begins in the laboratory, where chemical analysis is performed, and moves on to animal testing and then clinical trials with people. The FDA estimates that the testing process currently takes 8.5 years.

"Clinical trials" involve testing the drug on people.

Clinical tests begin with small numbers of participants over a short period of time and eventually expand into large groups of participants over long periods. Trial participants must give their informed consent. Among other things, it means the person must be told of the risks of the treatment along with other treatment options in language they can understand. Participants are also free to leave the trial at any time they wish.

ABCD *placebo* an inactive substance given in place of a medication.

pediatric having to do with the treatment of children.

TESTING

Animal Testing

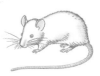

Once laboratory testing of a proposed new drug is finished, the drug is tested on animals before it will be tested on humans. Drug companies try to use as few animals and to treat them as humanely as possible. Since different species often react differently, more than one species is usually tested. Drug absorption into the bloodstream is monitored carefully. Only a fraction of a percent of drugs tested on animals are ever tested on humans.

Placebos

Placebos are inactive substances, not real medications, that are administered to give the patient the impression he or she is receiving a potentially effective medication. This provides a valuable comparison against patients who receive a test drug. Patients in trials must freely agree to the possibility that they may be given a placebo. They must also be informed of an effective treatment if one is available.

Testing Children

Children are not included in trials until a drug has been fully tested on adults. Drugs which have not been tested on children generally state on the label that their safety and effectiveness has not been established for children. Some drugs, however, may carry label information for pediatric use that is based on studies of adults and other pediatric treatment information.

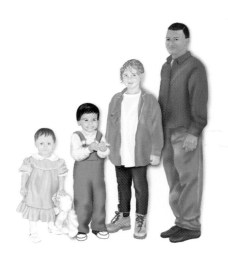

Testing Phases in Humans

There are **three phases** of testing a new drug in humans. Testing begins with a small number of participants for a short time and this gradually increases to a large number of participants over long periods of time. The goals of each phase also change from indicating a minimal level of safety to ultimately verifying the safety, effectiveness and dosage for widespread use. Only about 25% of drugs tested in phase 1 successfully complete phase 3.

phase 1

- ➥ **20-100 patients**
- ➥ **time: several months**
- ➥ **purpose: mainly safety**

phase 2

- ➥ **up to several hundred patients**
- ➥ **time: several months to two years**
- ➥ **purpose: short-term safety but mainly effectiveness**

phase 3

- ➥ **several hundred to several thousand patients**
- ➥ **time: one to four years**
- ➥ **purpose: safety, dosage, and effectiveness**

source: Food and Drug Administration

During the trial phase, a proposed new drug is called an investigational new drug (IND).

It is available for use only within the trial groups unless granted a special "treatment" status which is sometimes given to provide relief to critically ill patients outside of clinical trials. An example of this is AZT, which was used on thousands of AIDS patients who were not part of a clinical trial prior to the drug receiving FDA approval. It is worth noting, however, that such drugs are extremely expensive and are excluded from coverage by most insurers and HMOs.

Tests are "controlled" by comparing the effect of a proposed drug on one group of patients with the effect of a different treatment on other patients.

Patients have the same condition and similar characteristics and are placed in control groups at random to make sure the groups have essentially the same characteristics. The different treatment may be no drug at all, a placebo, a drug known to be effective, or a different dose of the same drug.

The patients in a trial are always "blind" to the treatment.

They are not told which control group they are in. In a "double-blind" test, neither the patients nor the physicians know what the medication is. So patients or their physicians may not be influenced into imagining effects one way or the other. Medical results alone determine the drug's effectiveness and its safety.

Medical Products Other Than Drugs

Medical devices and biological products such as insulin and vaccines must also meet FDA testing and approval requirements. The **Center for Devices and Radiological Health (CDRH)** is responsible for devices. The **Center for Biologics Evaluation and Research (CBER)** is responsible for biological products made from living organisms.

MARKETED DRUGS

A patent for a new drug gives its manufacturer an exclusive right to market the drug for a specific period of time under a brand name. During this time, the manufacturer attempts to recover the costs of the drug's research and development. A drug patent is in effect for 17 years from the date of the drug's discovery. Since the testing and approval process takes years to complete, for many years drugs reached the market with only half their patent time left. To compensate for this, the Hatch-Waxman Act of 1984 provided for up to five year extensions of patent protection to the patent holders to make up for time lost while products went through the FDA approval process.

Once a patent for a brand drug expires, other manufacturers may copy the drug and release it under its pharmaceutical or "generic" name.

Manufacturers of generic drugs do not need to perform the safety and effectiveness testing required of new drugs. However, they need to demonstrate that the drug is **pharmaceutically equivalent** to the proprietary (patented brand) drug—that it has same active ingredients, same dosage form, same route of administration, and same strength, and that it is **therapeutically equivalent**—that the body's use of the drug is the same. This is measured by the rate and extent to which the active ingredients are absorbed into the bloodstream.

Over-The-Counter (OTC) drugs are drugs which do not require a prescription.

They can be used upon the judgment of the consumer. There are over 100,000 OTC drugs in 80 therapeutic categories marketed. The FDA publishes acceptable ingredients for OTC drugs in "Drug Monographs." The manufacturer of an OTC drug must follow monograph requirements to be able to market their drug without undergoing the FDA new drug approval process. Though some OTC drugs were available before FDA approval was required, the FDA has been reviewing them under the "OTC Drug Review Program," and all new OTC drugs require FDA approval.

ABCD *labeling* important associated information that is not on the label of a drug product itself, but is provided with the product in the form of an insert, brochure, or other document.

LABELS AND LABELING

While all drugs are required to have clear and accurate information for all labels, inserts, packaging, and so on, there are different information requirements for various categories of drugs. Information requirements for OTC drugs are designed to enable consumers to use them without medical advice. Manufacturers of prescription drugs do not have to include directions for use on their labels since such directions must be supplied by the prescriber and dispenser. In many cases, important associated information may not fit on the label itself, and it will be provided in the form of an insert, brochure, or other document that is referred to as **labeling**. We'll look at labels and label information requirements on these next few pages.

Look Alike, Sound Alike

Federal laws require that a drug and/or its container not be imitative of another drug so that the consumer will be misled. Nevertheless, there are many drugs with similar sounding names in similar looking packages. It is therefore essential for pharmacy technicians to pay close attention to the details of drug names and packaging. Using the wrong drug can have very serious consequences.

OTC LABELS

Over-the-counter medications do not require a prescription but sometimes prescriptions are written for them for insurance or other reasons. In addition, patients often seek counseling regarding the use of over-the-counter medications. As a result, the pharmacy technician will deal with OTC medications regularly and should be familiar both with their label information and how to handle inquiries about them. **Since OTC medications are not without risks, all patients requesting information on them should be referred to the pharmacist.**

The following information should be contained on the labels of over-the counter-medications.

- product name
- name and address of manufacturer or distributor
- list of all active and other ingredients
- amount of contents
- adequate warnings
- adequate directions for use

Many over-the-counter products have labels that are difficult to read, understand, or both. At right is a label format proposed by the FDA to make it easier to read and understand the information currently contained on over-the-counter medication labels. Note that this format is not a requirement.

a proposed FDA label format
for OTC medications

Active Ingredient (In Each Tablet)	Purpose
Chlorpheniramine Maleate 4 mg...Antihistamine	

Uses: for the temporary relief of these symptoms of hay fever
- ► sneezing   ► runny nose   ► itchy, watery eyes

Warnings

Ask a Doctor Before Use
 If You Have:

- ► glaucoma
- ► a breathing problem such as emphysema or chronic bronchitis
- ► difficulty in urination due to enlargement of the prostate gland

 If You Are:

- ► taking sedatives or tranquilizers

When Using This Product:

- ► marked drowsiness may occur
- ► alcohol, sedatives, and tranquilizers may increase the drowsiness effect
- ► avoid alcoholic beverages
- ► use caution when driving a motor vehicle or operating machinery
- ► excitability may occur, especially in children

If pregnant or breast-feeding, ask a health professional before use.
Keep out of reach of children. In case of overdose, get medical help right away.

Directions:

Adults and children over 12 years:	Take 1 tablet every 4 to 6 hours as needed. Do not take more than 6 tablets in 24 hours.
Children 6 to under 12 years:	Take 1/2 tablet every 4 to 6 hours as needed. Do not take more than 3 tablets in 24 hours.
Children under 6 years:	Ask a doctor.

SAMPLE LABELS

MANUFACTURER STOCK LABEL

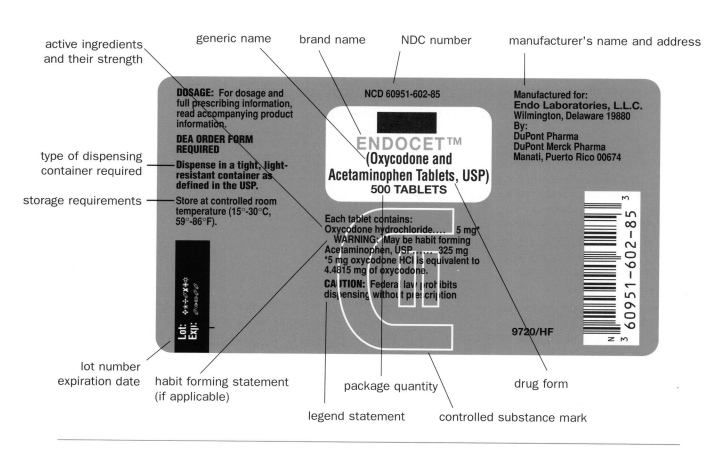

active ingredients and their strength

generic name

brand name

NDC number

manufacturer's name and address

type of dispensing container required

storage requirements

lot number
expiration date

habit forming statement (if applicable)

package quantity

drug form

legend statement

controlled substance mark

DOSAGE: For dosage and full prescribing information, read accompanying product information.

DEA ORDER FORM REQUIRED

Dispense in a tight, light-resistant container as defined in the USP.

Store at controlled room temperature (15°-30°C, 59°-86°F).

NCD 60951-602-85

ENDOCET™
(Oxycodone and Acetaminophen Tablets, USP)
500 TABLETS

Each tablet contains:
Oxycodone hydrochloride.... 5 mg*
WARNING: May be habit forming
Acetaminophen, USP...... 325 mg
*5 mg oxycodone HCl is equivalent to 4.4815 mg of oxycodone.

CAUTION: Federal law prohibits dispensing without prescription

9720/HF

Manufactured for:
Endo Laboratories, L.L.C.
Wilmington, Delaware 19880
By:
DuPont Pharma
DuPont Merck Pharma
Manati, Puerto Rico 00674

Lot:
Exp:

Labeling

In addition to a container label, manufacturer prescription drugs must also be accompanied by labeling which includes information on the following: clinical pharmacology, indications and usage, contraindications, warnings, precautions, adverse reactions, drug abuse and dependence, dosage, and packaging. This information is designed to inform both the prescriber and the dispenser regarding the drug.

ABCD *NDC (National Drug Code) number* the number assigned by the manufacturer. The first five digits indicate the manufacturer. The next four indicate the medication, its strength, and dosage form. The last two indicate the package size.
controlled substance mark the mark (CII-CV) which indicates the control category of a drug with a potential for abuse. See pages 34-35.

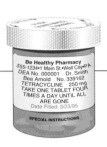

DISPENSED PRESCRIPTION DRUG LABEL

Minimum requirements on prescription labels for most drugs generally are as follows:

    ✔ name and address of dispenser

    ✔ prescription serial number.

    ✔ date of prescription or filling

    ✔ name of prescriber

And any of the following that are stated in the prescription:

    ✔ name of patient

    ✔ directions for use

    ✔ cautionary statements

Certain drugs have greater requirements, and many states impose greater requirements.

Typical elements on a prescription label:

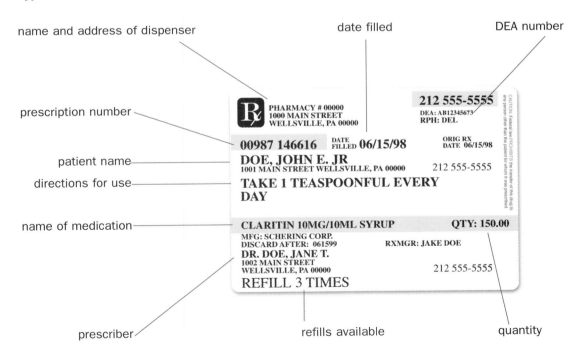

CONTROLLED SUBSTANCES

The government tightly controls the use of drugs that can be easily abused.

The 1970 Controlled Substances Act (CSA) identified five groups or schedules of such drugs as **controlled substances** and put strict guidelines on their distribution. It required manufacturers, distributors, or dispensers of controlled substances to register with the Drug Enforcement Administration (DEA) of the Justice Department. This created a "closed system" in which only registered parties can distribute these drugs.

The five control schedules are as follows*:

Schedule I:

➥ Each drug has a high potential for abuse and no accepted medical use in the United States. It may not be prescribed. Heroin, various opium derivatives, and hallucinogenic substances are included on this schedule.

Schedule II:

➥ Each drug has a high potential for abuse and may lead to physical or psychological dependence, but also has a currently accepted medical use in the United States. Amphetamines, opium, cocaine, methadone, and various opiates are included on this schedule.

Schedule III:

➥ Each drug's potential for abuse is less than those in Schedules I and II and there is a currently accepted medical use in the U.S., but abuse may lead to moderate or low physical dependence or high psychological dependence. Anabolic steroids and various compounds containing limited quantities of narcotic substances such as codeine are included on this schedule.

Schedule IV:

➥ Each drug has a low potential for abuse relative to Schedule III drugs and there is a current accepted medical use in the U.S., but abuse may lead to limited physical dependence or psychological dependence. Phenobarbital, the sedative chloral hydrate, and the anesthetic methohexital are included in this group.

Schedule V:

➥ Each drug has a low potential for abuse relative to Schedule IV drugs and there is a current accepted medical use in the U.S., but abuse may lead to limited physical dependence or psychological dependence. Compounds containing limited amounts of a narcotic such as codeine are included in this group.

*21 USC Sec. 812 as of 1/96. Note: these schedules are revised periodically. It is important to refer to the most current schedule.

REGULATIONS

Labels

Manufacturers must clearly label controlled drugs with their control classification.

Record keeping

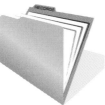

Distributors are required to maintain accurate records of all controlled substance activity. This includes accurate records of inventory as well as drugs dispensed. Schedule-II prescription records must be kept separate from non-controlled drug records, though they may be kept with other controlled drug records.

Security for Controlled Drugs

Schedule II drugs must be stored in a locked tamper-proof narcotics cabinet that is usually secured to the floor or wall. Schedule III, IV, and V drugs may be kept openly on storage shelves in retail and hospital settings.

Joint responsibility

By law, both the prescriber and the dispenser of the prescription have joint responsibility for the legitimate medical purpose of the prescription. This is primarily intended to ensure that controlled substances not be prescribed for inappropriate reasons.

DEA Number

All prescribers of controlled substances must be authorized by the DEA. They are assigned a DEA number which must be used on all controlled drug prescriptions.

SAMPLE LABELS AND ORDER FORM

Manufacturer containers and labels for C-II, C-III, and C-IV controlled drug products . Note that the control substance marks are prominent.

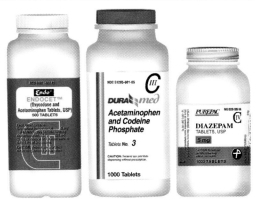

A sample C-I and C-II order form. It must be signed by a registered person, in triplicate. Note that C-III-C-V don't require federal order forms. Because of the lower potential for abuse they are controlled by the record keeping requirements for all controlled substances.

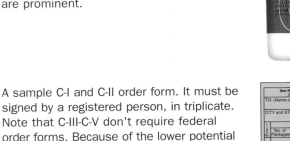

CONTROLLED SUBSTANCE PRESCRIPTIONS

Controlled-Substance Prescriptions

Controlled-substance prescriptions have greater requirements at both federal and state levels than other prescriptions, particularly Schedule II drugs. On controlled substance prescriptions, the DEA number must appear on the form and the patient's full street address must be entered.

On Schedule II prescriptions, the form must be signed by the prescriber (no phoned or faxed prescriptions allowed). In many states, there are specific time limits that require Schedule II prescriptions be promptly filled. Quantities are limited and no refills are allowed. When the prescription is filled, the pharmacist draws a line across it indicating it has been filled.

Federal requirements for Schedules III-V are less stringent than for Schedule II. Refills and faxed prescriptions are allowed, for example. However, state and other regulations may be stricter than federal requirements, so it is necessary to know the requirements for your specific job setting.

DEA Numbers

DEA numbers are required by federal law but administered by the states. They have two letters followed by seven single-digit numbers, e.g., AB1234563. **The following should always be true of a DEA number on a prescription form:** if the sum of the first, third and fifth digits is added to twice the sum of the second, fourth, and sixth digits, the total should be a number whose last digit is the same as the last digit of the DEA number.

PUBLIC SAFETY

Though the FDA approval process is quite thorough, it is impossible to fully prove that a drug is safe for use.

No matter how many people participate in the clinical trials, the number is always just a fraction of how many will use a drug once it is approved. So there is always the risk that the drug may produce adverse side effects when used on a larger population. To monitor this, the FDA maintains a reporting program called **MedWatch** which encourages health care professionals to report adverse effects that occur from the use of an approved drug or other medical product. MedWatch does not monitor vaccines. That is performed by the Vaccine Adverse Event Reporting System.

The FDA has several options if it determines that a marketed drug presents a risk of illness, injury, or gross consumer deception.

It may seek an *injunction* that prevents the manufacturer from distributing the drug; it may seize the drug; or it may issue a *recall*. Of these, recalls are considered the most effective, largely because they involve the cooperation of the manufacturer, which after all is the only party that knows where the drugs have been distributed. As a result, recalls are the FDA's preferred means of removing dangerous drugs from the market.

adverse effect an unintended side affect of a medication that is negative or in some way injurious to a patient's health.

injunction a court order preventing a specific action, such as the distribution of a potentially dangerous drug.

recall the action taken to remove a drug from the market and have it returned to the manufacturer.

A Manufacturer Recall

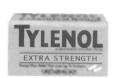

When someone tampered with a small number of Tylenol capsule packages and fatally poisoned seven people, Johnson & Johnson immediately recalled the capsules from the market. This swift and responsible action resulted in a highly favorable public response and increased popularity for Tylenol—and Johnson & Johnson.

RECALLS

Recalls are, with a few exceptions, voluntary on the part of the manufacturer. However, once the FDA requests a manufacturer recall a product, the pressure to do so is substantial. The negative publicity from not recalling would significantly damage a company's reputation, and the FDA would probably take the manufacturer to court, where criminal penalties could be imposed. The FDA can also require recalls in certain instances with infant formulas, biological products, and devices that pose a serious health hazard. Manufacturers may of course recall drugs on their own and do so from time to time for any number of reasons.

Recall Classifications

There are three classes of recalls:

Class I

Where there is a strong likelihood that the product will cause serious adverse effects or death.

Class II

Where a product may cause temporary but reversible adverse effects, or in which there is little likelihood of serious adverse effects.

Class III

Where a product is not likely to cause adverse effects.

How an FDA requested recall works:

Reports of adverse effects

The FDA receives enough reports of adverse effects or misbranding that it decides the product is a threat to the public health. It contacts the manufacturer and recommends a recall.

Manufacturer agrees to recall

If the manufacturer agrees to a recall, they must establish a recall strategy with the FDA that addresses the depth of the recall, the extent of public warnings, and a means for checking the effectiveness of the recall. The depth of the recall is identified by wholesale, retail, or consumer levels. The effectiveness may require anything from no follow-up to a complete follow-up check of everyone who should have been notified of the recall. Checks can be made by personal visit, phone calls, or letters.

Customers contacted

Once the strategy is finalized, the manufacturer contacts its customers by telegram, mailgram, or first-class letters with the following information:

- ✔ the product name, size, lot number, code or serial number, and any other important identifying information.
- ✔ reason for the recall and the hazard involved.
- ✔ instructions on what to do with the product, beginning with ceasing distribution.

Recalls listed publicly

Recalls are listed in the weekly FDA Enforcement Report.

LAW AND
THE TECHNICIAN

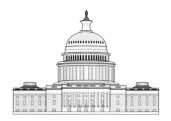 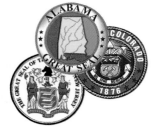

FEDERAL LAW

Federal laws provide a foundation for the state laws which govern pharmacy practice in every state. In addition to the specific drug laws enforced by the FDA and DEA, there are federal laws regulating the treatment of patients (especially in nursing homes) that apply to various aspects of pharmacy practice. These laws also guarantee certain patient rights which must be observed by all. These rights include: privacy and confidentiality, right to file complaints, information necessary for informed consent, and the right to refuse treatment. It is necessary for all health care workers, including pharmacy technicians, to know the specific patient rights that apply to their workplace.

STATE LAW

In each state, there is a **state board of pharmacy** responsible for licensing all prescribers and dispensers. State boards also administer state regulations for the practice of pharmacy in the state. In many cases, state regulations are stricter than federal, and the stricter state regulation must be followed. By definition, this means that the lesser Federal requirements are also being met. Therefore, following both state and federal regulations is mandatory.

Each state has specific regulations which may or may not be different from other states. For example, a few states allow pharmacists to prescribe under limited conditions. Many allow nurse practitioners and physician assistants to prescribe. When states allow non-physicians to prescribe, they limit their **scope of authority.** That is, a non-physician prescriber may only prescribe for certain conditions and must follow a strict set of rules (called a **protocol**) that determines the prescription. Non-physician prescribers include dentists, veterinarians, pharmacists, nurse practitioners, and physician assistants, among others. Since states differ on many aspects of pharmacy practice, including who may and may not prescribe, it is necessary to know and your own state's regulations.

States regulate the work of pharmacy technicians largely by holding the pharmacist supervising a technician responsible for the technician's performance. If a technician fails to observe any relevant law, the supervising pharmacist is subject to a penalty by the state board. As a result, the supervising pharmacist must explain all the regulations (federal, state, and local) that apply to the technician as part of the job description, and must work with the technician to assure **compliance** with those regulations.

compliance doing what is required.
negligence failing to do something that should or must be done.

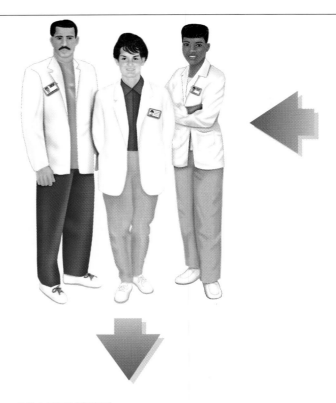

LIABILITY

Legal liability means you can be prosecuted for misconduct. This is true even if you are directed to do it by a supervisor, physician, patient, or customer. Misconduct doesn't necessarily mean you intended to do something, or even that you actively did it. You can be guilty of misconduct by simply failing to do something you should have done. This is called **negligence**, and is the most common form of misconduct. Here are some ways the pharmacy technician can be negligent:

- ➡incorrectly labeling the prescription.
- ➡failing to maintain patient confidentiality.
- ➡failing to recognize expired drugs.
- ➡calculation errors.
- ➡dispensing the wrong medication.
- ➡incorrect handling of controlled substance.
- ➡inaccurate record keeping.

OTHER STANDARDS

Besides the FDA, DEA, and the State Board of Pharmacy, there are various professional bodies and associations which set and maintain pharmacy standards. These include:

- ➡**American Society of Health-System Pharmacists**: The ASHP is a 30,000 member association for pharmacists practicing in hospitals, HMOs, long-term care facilities, home care agencies, and other health care systems. It is an accrediting organization for pharmacy residency and pharmacy technician training programs.
- ➡**United States Pharmacopeia**: The USP is a voluntary not-for-profit organization that sets standards for the manufacture and distribution of drugs and related products in the United States. These standards are directly referred to by federal and state laws and are published in the "United States Pharmacopeia and the National Formulary."
- ➡**Joint Commission on Accreditation of Health Care Organizations**: JCAHO is an independent non-profit organization that establishes standards and monitors compliance for nearly twenty thousand health care programs in the United States. JCAHO-accredited programs include hospitals, health care networks, hmos, and nursing homes, among others.
- ➡**The American Society for Consultant Pharmacists**: The ASCP sets standards for practice for pharmacists who provide medication distribution and consultant services to nursing homes.

Basic criminal and civil laws also apply to pharmacy technicians, which means that crimes like theft, discrimination, sexual harassment, fraud, etc. are punishable just as they would be outside of your job.

REVIEW

KEY CONCEPTS

✔ In the United States, the leading enforcement agency at the federal level for regulations concerning drug products is the Food and Drug Administration.

✔ The distribution of drugs that may be easily abused is controlled by the Drug Enforcement Administration (DEA) within the Justice Department.

✔ Before it is approved for marketing, a new drug must be shown to be both safe and effective and that its benefits substantially outweigh its risks.

✔ Federal law defines what drugs require a prescription by a licensed practitioner.

✔ Manufacturers' containers for prescription drugs must have this legend on the label: "Caution: Federal Law prohibits dispensing without a prescription." By 2003, it must be changed to "Rx only."

✔ Pharmacists must offer counseling to patients regarding medications.

✔ Federal law requires child-proof packaging on all controlled and most prescription drugs dispensed by pharmacies.

✔ Placebos are inactive substances, not real medications, that are used to test the effectiveness of drugs.

✔ Once a patent for a brand drug expires, other manufacturers may copy the drug and release it under its pharmaceutical or "generic" name.

✔ All drugs are required to have clear and accurate information for all labels, inserts, packaging, and so on, but there are different information requirements for various categories of drugs.

✔ The minimum requirements on prescription labels for most drugs are as follows: name and address of dispenser, prescription serial number, date of prescription or filling, name of prescriber, name of patient, directions for use, and cautionary statements.

✔ Controlled drugs have greater requirements for labeling.

✔ Manufacturers must clearly label controlled drugs with their control classification.

✔ All prescribers of controlled substances are assigned a DEA number which must be used on all controlled drug prescriptions.

✔ There is always the risk that an approved drug may produce adverse side effects when used on a larger population.

✔ Recalls are, with a few exceptions, voluntary on the part of the manufacturer.

✔ Federal laws provide a foundation for the state laws which govern pharmacy practice in every state.

✔ State boards of pharmacy are responsible for licensing all prescribers and dispensers and administering regulations for the practice of pharmacy in the state.

✔ Legal liability means you can be prosecuted for misconduct.

SELF TEST

MATCH THE TERMS.   *answers can be checked in the glossary*

adverse effect

controlled substance mark

injunction

labeling

legend drug

liability

NDC (National Drug Code)

negligence

pediatric

placebo

recall

therapeutic

a court order preventing a specific action, such as the distribution of a potentially dangerous drug.

an inactive substance given in place of a medication.

an unintended side affect of a medication that is negative or in some way injurious to a patient's health.

any drug which requires a prescription and this "legend" on the label: Rx only.

failing to do something you should have done

having to do with the treatment of children.

important associated information that is not on the label of a drug product itself.

means you can be prosecuted for misconduct.

serving to cure or heal.

the action taken to remove a drug from the market and have it returned to the manufacturer.

the mark (CII-CV) which indicates the control category of a drug with a potential for abuse.

the number on a manufacturer's label indicating the manufacturer and product information.

CHOOSE THE BEST ANSWER.   *answers are in the back of the book*

1. Pharmacies located in the health care institutions (hospitals, etc.) are required to follow regulations of this organization.
   a. ASHP
   b. USP
   c. ASCP
   d. JCAHO

2. The practice of pharmacy is influenced by federal and state laws. Which major federal law deals with the issue of safety caps?
   a. Federal Food, Drug and Cosmetic Act (FDC)
   b. The Controlled Substance Act (CSA)
   c. The Poison Prevention Packaging Act
   d. The Hazardous Substance Labeling Act

3. Of the following Schedule of drugs, which one deals with drugs that have no accepted medical use in the United States?
   a. Schedule I
   b. Schedule II
   c. Schedule III
   d. Schedule IV

4. Recalls, actions taken to remove a drug from the market, are based on different classes. Which class of Recall indicates there is a strong likelihood that the product will cause serious adverse effects or death.
   a. Class I
   b. Class II
   c. Class III
   d. Class IV

TERMINOLOGY

Root	Prefix
Suffix	C.V.

Medical dictionaries contain thousands of words that are used in medicine and pharmacy.

Many of the words don't look like words commonly used in literature or speech, and at first glance they can be quite intimidating. But the secret to learning medical science terminology is to learn that there is a system, or order, to it. The purpose of this chapter is to explain this system.

Medical science terminology is made up of a small number of root words.

Most of these root words originate from either Greek or Latin words. Words developed from the Greek language are most often used to refer to diagnosis and surgery. Words from the Latin language generally refer to the anatomy of the body.

Numerous suffixes and prefixes are attached to the root word.

The suffixes and prefixes give specifics to the meaning of the root word. The suffix is a modifier attached to the end of the root word, and the prefix is attached to the front of the root word. So each medical science term will have at least one root word and then a suffix or prefix to complete the meaning. It is not required that every root word have both a suffix and a prefix. Each root could have just one. In general, prefixes are used less frequently than suffixes.

Combining vowels are used to connect the prefix, root, or suffix parts of the term.

In some cases the combining vowel can be used to combine two root words. And there are some cases where the combining vowels are not used at all. Sometimes a combining vowel is added to make the word easier to pronounce. The most common combining vowel is the letter "o".

A B C D *nomenclature* a system of names specific to a particular field.

root word the base component of a term which gives it a meaning that may be modified by other components.

prefix a modifying component of a term located before the other components of the term.

suffix a modifying component of a term located after the other components of the term.

ROOT WORDS

The root word is the foundation of medical science terminology. Root words can immediately identify what part of the body a term relates to. For example, consider this list of common root words and the parts of the body to which they refer:

Root	Part of Body
card	heart
cyst	bladder
gastr	stomach
hemat	blood
hepat	liver
my	muscle
pector	chest
neur	nerve
pneum	lung
ocul	eye
derma	skin
ven	vein
mast	breast
oste	bone
nephr	kidney
ot	ear

If a phrase contains the word "cardiac," it is referring to the heart, since "card" is the root word of the word cardiac. The word "ocular" would refer to the eye since "ocul" is the root word of the word ocular.

 Learning the most popular roots, suffixes and prefixes will help you to understand a large amount of pharmaceutical terminology.

Medical Term

Medical and pharmaceutical nomenclature is a system made up of these four elements.

➡ **root words** ➡ **prefixes**
➡ **suffixes** ➡ **combining vowels**

PREFIXES

A prefix is added to the beginning of a root word to clarify its meaning. For example, *"derma"* is the root word for skin, or things related to the skin, and *"xero"* is a prefix used to describe things that are dry. So:

xero + derma = xeroderma

➡ *meaning:* a "dry skin" condition.

Consider another example. The root word for vision is *"opia,"* and the prefix for double is *"dipl."* So:

dipl + opia = diplopia

➡ *meaning:* double vision.

For a final example, consider the prefix *"sub"* and the root *"lingu."* "Sub" means under or beneath, and "lingu" is the root word for tongue. So:

sub + lingu = sublingu

➡ would mean "under the tongue."

However, there are few English words ending in "u," and so this combination is further modified with the typical suffix *"al"* which means "pertaining to," as in:

sub + lingu + al = sublingual

➡ *meaning:* pertaining to under the tongue.

SUFFIXES

The suffix is added to the end of a root word to clarify the meaning. Sometimes the connection is made without the aid of a connecting vowel.

Root	Suffix
gastr (stomach)	**itis** (inflammation)

➡ **gastritis**: inflammation of the stomach

Root	Suffix
neur (nerve)	**algia** (pain)

➡ **neuralgia**: a pain in the nerve

Sometimes a **combining vowel** (CV) is used to complete the connection of the different word parts.

1st Root	2ndRoot	Suffix	CV
pneum (lung)	**thorax** (chest)		**o**

➡ **pneumothorax**: area of the chest containing the lungs

1st Root	2ndRoot	Suffix	CV
card (heart)	**my** (muscle)	**pathy** (disease)	**i, o**

➡ **cardiomyopathy**: disease in the heart muscle tissue

COMBINING THE ELEMENTS

The last combination possibility is to have a prefix and a suffix attached to a root word.

Prefix	Root	Suffix
hypo (low)	**glyc** (sugar)	**emia** (blood)

➡ **hypoglycemia**: low blood sugar

Prefix	Root	Suffix
hyper (high)	**thyroid** (thyroid)	**ism** (state of)

➡ **hyperthyroidism**: too much thyroid activity

And then there is always the possibility that a combining vowel (CV) will be used within a word.

Prefix	Root	Suffix	CV
peri (around)	**dont** (teeth)	**ic** (pertaining to)	**o**

➡ **periodontic**: around the teeth

ORGAN SYSTEM TERMINOLOGY

Agood way to learn medical science terminology is to learn it based on the different organ systems in the body.

There are names for structures and parts of organ systems that form the root words used in medical science terminology. These names have to be learned. Then they can be applied to understand or to construct words.

The cardiovascular system distributes blood throughout the body using blood vessels called arteries, capillaries, and veins. Blood transports nutrients to the body's cells and carries waste products away from them. Blood is made up of red blood cells, white blood cells, platelets, and plasma. **Erythrocytes** (red blood cells) transport oxygen from the lungs to the body and carbon dioxide from the cells to the lungs. **Leukocytes** (white blood cells) fight bacterial infections by producing antibodies.

Blood is pumped through the cardiovascular system by the heart. Valves within the heart maintain the flow of blood in only one direction. Conductive tissue which is unique to the heart muscle is responsible for the heartbeat.

When blood is forced out of the heart, the increased pressure on the system is called the **systolic** phase. When blood pressure is monitored, this pressure is reported (in mm Hg) as the first number of a two number sequence. The **diastolic** phase, or relaxation phase, is the second number reported in blood pressure monitoring. Blood pressures are reported as systole/diastole, i.e., 120/80. A sphygmomanometer is used to measure blood pressure.

CARDIOVASCULAR SYSTEM

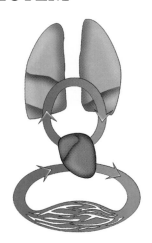

Cardiovascular Root Words

angi	vessel
aort	aorta
card	heart
oxy	oxygen
pector	chest
phleb	vein
stenosis	narrowing
thromb	clot
vas(cu)	blood vessel
ven	vein

Prefix	Root Word	Suffix	CV	Term	Meaning
hyper (high)		tension (pressure)		**hypertension**	high blood pressure.
	thromb (clot)	sis (abnormal condition)	o	**thrombosis**	condition of having blood clots in the vascular system.
	phleb (vein)	itis (inflammation)		**phlebitis**	inflammation of a vein.
	arter (artery)	sclerosis (hardening)	i, o	**arteriosclerosis**	hardening of the arteries.
	card (heart) my (muscle)	pathy (disease)	i, o	**cardiomyopathy**	disease of the heart muscle.
	my (muscle) card (heart)	ial (condition of)	o	**myocardial**	concerning heart muscle.
tachy (fast)	card (heart)	ia (condition of)		**tachycardia**	abnormally rapid heart action.

ENDOCRINE SYSTEM

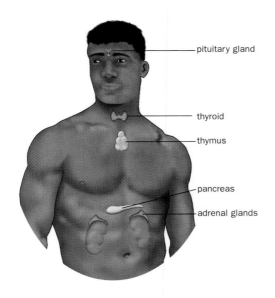

pituitary gland

thyroid

thymus

pancreas

adrenal glands

Endocrine Root Words

lipid	fat
nephr	kidney
thym	thymus
adrena	adrenal
gluc	sugar
pancreat	pancreas
somat	body

The endocrine system consists of the glands that secrete **hormones**, chemicals that assist in regulating body functions.

Several organs act as endocrine glands as well as members of other organ systems. For example, the liver, stomach, pancreas, and kidneys are members of endocrine system as well as other organ systems. Organs that belong primarily to the endocrine system include the pituitary gland, the adrenal glands, the thyroid gland, and the gonads (ovaries and testes).

The pituitary gland produces multiple hormones and is located at the base of the brain. It controls the body's growth and releases hormones into the bloodstream that control much of the activity of the other glands. The thyroid gland is located just below the larynx and releases hormones important for regulating body metabolism. There are four smaller parathyroid glands located on the thyroid gland. The thymus gland is located beneath the sternum. The pancreas is best known for its production of insulin and glucagon. The small adrenal glands are located on top of the kidneys. They produce such hormones as aldosterone, cortisol (hydrocortisone), androgens, and estrogens. The medulla region of the adrenal glands produce the catecholamines adrenaline (epinephrine) and noradrenaline (norepinephrine).

Prefix	Root Word	Suffix	CV	Term	Meaning
end (within)		crine (secrete)	o	**endocrine**	pertaining to the glands that secrete onto the bloodstream.
hyper (high)	lipid (fat)	emia (blood)		**hyperlipidemia**	increase of lipids in the blood.
hypo (low)	thyroid (thyroid gland)	ism (condition)		**hypothyroidism**	a deficiency of thyroid secretion.
	somat (body)	ic (pertaining to)		**somatic**	pertaining to the body.

 The majority of the terms in the combining tables on body system terminology are for disorders or conditions.

ORGAN SYSTEM TERMINOLOGY

GASTROINTESTINAL TRACT

The gastrointestinal (GI) tract is located in the abdomen, and is surrounded by the peritoneal lining. The GI tract contains the organs that are involved in the digestion of foods and the absorption of nutrients. These organs include the stomach, small and large intestine, gall-bladder, liver, and pancreas.

The GI tract is sometimes inappropriately referred to as the **alimentary canal.** The alimentary canal refers to the system that goes from the mouth to the anus. The alimentary canal contains organs such as lips, tongue, teeth, salivary glands, pharynx, esophagus, rectum, and anus, in addition to the GI tract.

Several organs contribute to the digestion of foods by secreting enzymes into the small intestine when food is present. Ducts carry bile from the liver (hepatic duct) and the gallbladder (cystic duct) to the duodenum. The pancreas is located behind the stomach and also contributes enzymes to the digestive process.

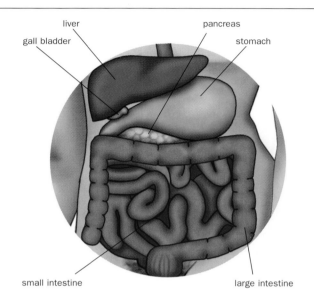

Gastrointestinal Root Words

chol	bile
col	colon
duoden	duodenum
enter	intestine
esophag	esophagus
gastr	stomach
hepat	liver
lapar	abdomen
pancreat	pancreas

Prefix	Root Word	Suffix	CV	Term	Meaning
an (no)	orexia (appetite)			**anorexia**	loss of appetite.
a (no)	phagia (swallow)			**aphagia**	inability to swallow.
	appendic (appendix)	itis (inflammation)		**appendicitis**	inflammation of the appendix.
	col (colon)	itis (inflammation)		**colitis**	inflamed or irritable colon.
dia (across, through)	rrhea (discharge)			**diarrhea**	liquid or unformed bowel movements.
	duoden (duodenum)	al (pertaining to)		**duodenal**	pertaining to the duodenum.
	hemat (blood)	emesis (vomit)		**hematemesis**	vomiting of blood.
	hepat (liver)	itis (inflammation)		**hepatitis**	inflammation of the liver from various causes.
	hepat (liver)	oma (tumor)		**hepatoma**	liver tumor.
	gastr (stomach)	itis (inflammation)		**gastritis**	inflammation of the stomach.
	gastr (stomach) } enter (abdomen) }	itis (inflammation)	o	**gastroenteritis**	inflammation of the stomach and the intestinal tract.

INTEGUMENTARY SYSTEM

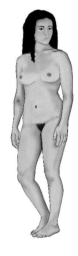

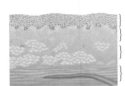

}epidermis
}dermis
}subcutaneous
}muscle

The covering of the body is referred to as the integumentary system. It is the body's first line of defense, acting as a barrier against disease and other hazards. It also helps control body temperature by releasing heat through sweat or by restricting blood vessels to act as insulation. It includes the skin, hair, and nails.

The skin is composed of the **epidermis** and **dermis.** The epidermis has no blood or nerves and is constantly discarding dead cells. The dermis, which is made of living cells, contains capillaries, nerves, and lymphatics. The dermis also contains the subcutaneous glands, sweat glands, and hair.

Hair is made of keratinized cells. Finger nails and toenails are also composed of keratin. The mammary glands, or breasts, are also considered part of the integumentary system.

The subcutaneous layer of tissue is beneath the dermis but is closely interconnected to it. It separates the skin from the other organs (the muscular system, for example, as in the illustration).

Integumentary Root Words

necr	death (cells, body)
derma	skin
cutane	skin
mast	breast
onych	nail

Prefix	Root Word	Suffix	CV	Term	Meaning
	derma (skin)	itis (inflammation)		**dermatitis**	skin inflammation.
erythro (red)	derma (skin)			**erythroderma**	abnormal redness of skin.
	lact (milk)	tation (act of secreting)		**lactation**	secretion of milk.
	mast (breast)	ectomy (removal)		**mastectomy**	surgical removal of breast.
	onych (nail)	mycosis (fungal infection)	o	**onychomycosis**	fungal infection of nails.
pach (thick)	derma (skin)		y	**pachyderma**	abnormal thickness of skin.
sub (under)	cutane (skin)	ous (pertaining to)		**subcutaneous**	beneath the skin.
trans (through)	derma (skin)	al (pertaining to)		**transdermal**	through the skin.

ORGAN SYSTEM TERMINOLOGY

LYMPHATIC SYSTEM

The lymphatic system is responsible for collecting plasma water that leaves the blood vessels, filtering it for impurities through its lymph nodes, and returning the lymph fluid back to the general circulation. The lymphatic system is the center of the body's immune system.

The largest organ in the system is the spleen. It is responsible for removing old red blood cells from the circulation. It is also a storage organ for **lymphocytes,** a type of white blood cell that attacks bacteria and disease cells. Lymphocytes release antibodies that destroy disease cells and provide immunity against them.

The thymus, tonsils, spleen, and adenoids are lymphoid organs outside the network of the lymphatic system.

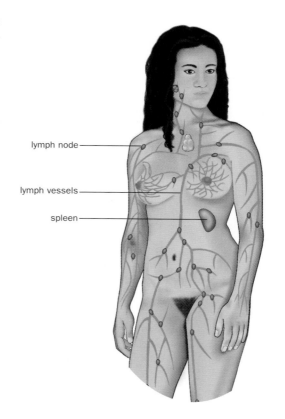

lymph node

lymph vessels

spleen

Lymphatic Root Words

aden	gland
cyt	cell
hemo, hemat	blood
lymph	lymph
splen	spleen

Prefix	Root Word	Suffix	CV	Term	Meaning
	aden (gland)	pathy (disease)	o	**adenopathy**	lymph node disease.
	hemat (blood)	oma (tumor)		**hematoma**	a collection of blood, often clotted.
	hemo (blood)	philia (attraction)		**hemophilia**	a disease in which the blood does not clot normally.
	lymph (lymph tissue)	oma (tumor)		**lymphoma**	lymphatic system tumor.
leuk (white)		emia (blood condition)		**leukemia**	a disease of blood forming tissues.
	thym (thymus)	oma (tumor)		**thymoma**	tumor of the thymus.

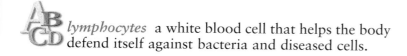

lymphocytes a white blood cell that helps the body defend itself against bacteria and diseased cells.

MUSCULAR SYSTEM

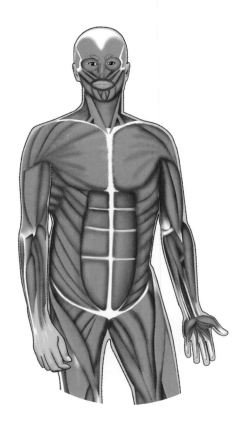

The word muscle comes from the Latin *mus* (mouse) and *cle* (little) because muscle movements resemble a mouse moving under a cover.

The body contains more than 600 muscles which give shape and movement to it. The skeletal muscles are attached to the bones by tendons. The muscles themselves are striated, i.e., made up of fibers.

The action of most muscles is called voluntary, because it is controlled consciously. Involuntary muscles operate automatically and are found in the heart, the stomach, or in walls of blood vessels.

Some muscles produce an outward or **flexor** movement and these are called agonist muscles. Antagonist muscles are the ones that contract or bring the limb back to the original position.

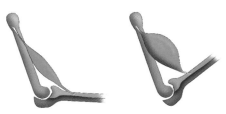

expansion and contraction of muscles

Root Words

my	muscle
fibr	fiber
tendin	tendon

Prefix	Root Word	Suffix	CV	Term	Meaning
	fibr (fiber) my (muscle)	algia (pain)	o	**fibromyalgia**	chronic pain in the muscles.
	my (muscle)	plasty (repair)	o	**myoplasty**	plastic surgery of muscle tissue.
	tendin (tendon)	itis (inflammation)		**tendinitis**	inflammation of a tendon.

 flexor movement an expansion or outward movement by muscles.

ORGAN SYSTEM TERMINOLOGY

NERVOUS SYSTEM

The most complex of the body organ systems is the nervous system, the body's system of communication. The **neuron** (nerve cell) is the basic functional unit in this system. There are over 100 billion neurons in the brain alone. Neurons also transmit information from the brain to the entire body.

The primary parts of this system are the brain and the spinal cord, called the central nervous system (CNS). The peripheral nervous system is composed of nerves that branch out from the spinal cord.

There are subdivisions of the peripheral nervous system called the autonomic nervous system and the somatic nervous system. The autonomic nervous system controls the automatic functions of the body, e.g., breathing, digestion, etc.

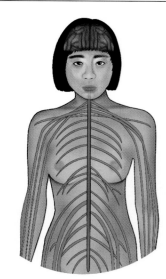

central and peripheral nervous systems

Nervous System Root Words

cerebr	cerebrum
encephal	brain
mening	meninges
myel	spinal cord
neur	nerve

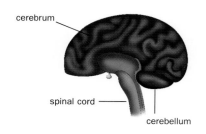

brain and spinal cord

Prefix	Root Word	Suffix	CV	Term	Meaning
	encephal (brain)	itis (inflammation)		**encephalitis**	inflammation of the brain.
	neur (nerve)	algia (pain)		**neuralgia**	severe pain in a nerve.
	neur (nerve)	oma (tumor)		**neuroma**	tumor of nerve cells.

SKELETAL SYSTEM

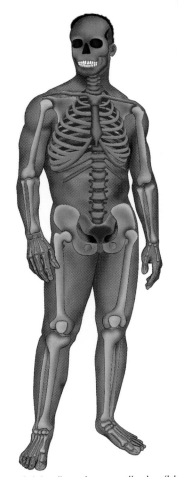

axial (red) and appendicular (blue) skeleton

The skeletal system protects soft organs and provides structure and support for the body's organ systems. Made up largely of hard **osseus** tissue, it is a living system that undergoes dynamic changes throughout life.

The system's 206 bones are called **axial** (skull and spinal column) or **appendicular** (arms, legs, and connecting bones). They are held together at joints by connective tissue called ligaments and cartilage. Joints range from rigid to those allowing full motion (e.g., the ball and socket joints of the hips and shoulders).

Skeletal System Root Words

arthr	joint
calcane	heel bone
carp	wrist
crani	cranium
dactyl	finger or toe
femor	thigh bone
fibul	small, outer lower leg bone
humer	humerus
myel	bone marrow, spinal cord
oste	bone
patell	kneecap
ped, pod	foot
pelv	pelvis
phalang	bones of fingers and toes
rachi	spinal cord, vertebrae
spondy	backbone, vertebrae
stern	sternum, breastbone
tibi	large lower leg bone
vertebr	backbone, vertebrae

Prefix	Root Word	Suffix	CV	Term	Meaning
	arthr (joint)	algia (pain)		**arthralgia**	joint pain.
	arthr (joint)	itis (inflammation)		**arthritis**	inflammation of a joint.
	carp (wrist)	al (pertaining to)		**carpal**	pertaining to the carpus in the wrist.
	crani (cranium)	malacia (softening)	o	**craniomalacia**	softening of the skull.
	oste (bone) arthr (joint)	itis (inflammation)	o	**osteoarthritis**	chronic disease of bones and joints.
	oste (bone) carcin (cancer)	oma (tumor)	o	**osteocarcinoma**	cancerous bone tumor.
	rachi (vertebrae)	itis (inflammation)		**rachitis**	inflammation of the spine.

ORGAN SYSTEM TERMINOLOGY

FEMALE REPRODUCTIVE SYSTEM

The female reproductive system produces hormones (**estrogen, progesterone**), controls menstruation, and provides for childbearing. The system contains the vagina, uterus, fallopian tubes, ovaries, and the external genitalia.

There are also two gland organs associated with the system: Bartholin's glands and mammary glands (located in breast tissue). The mammary glands produce and secrete milk at childbirth.

The vagina is a muscular tube that leads from an external opening to the cervix and uterus. The uterus is a hollow, pear-shaped organ that is the normal location for pregnancy. The fallopian tubes transport eggs from the ovary to the uterus. The ovaries are located on each side of the uterus. In sexually mature females, the uterus is prepared for the possibility of fertilization and pregnancy each month.

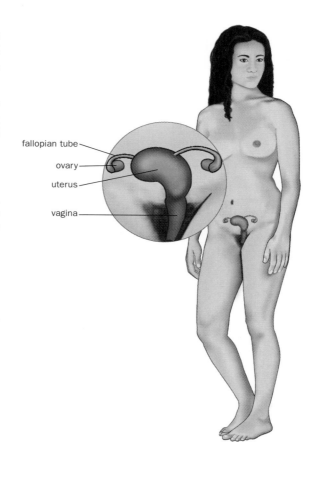

fallopian tube
ovary
uterus
vagina

Root Words

gynec	woman
hyster	uterus
lact	milk
mamm	breast
mast	breast
metr	uterus
ovari	ovary
salping	fallopian tube
toc	birth
uter	uterine

Prefix	Root Word	Suffix	CV	Term	Meaning
a (no)	men (menstrual)	orrhea (discharge)		**amenorrhea**	absence of menstruation.
dys (difficult)	men (menstrual)	orrhea (discharge)		**dysmenorrhea**	menstrual pain.
dys (difficult)	toc (birth)	ia (condition of)		**dystocia**	difficult labor.
end (within)	metri (uterus)	sis (abnormal)	o	**endometriosis**	abnormal growth of uteral tissue within the pelvis.
	gynec (woman)	logy (study of)	o	**gynecology**	the study of the female reproductive organs.
	mast (breast)	itis (inflammation)		**mastitis**	inflammation of the breast.
	salping (fallopian)	cyesis (pregnancy)	o	**salpingocyesis**	fetal development in the fallopian tube.
	vagin (vagina)	itis (inflammation)		**vaginitis**	inflammation of the vagina.

MALE REPRODUCTIVE SYSTEM

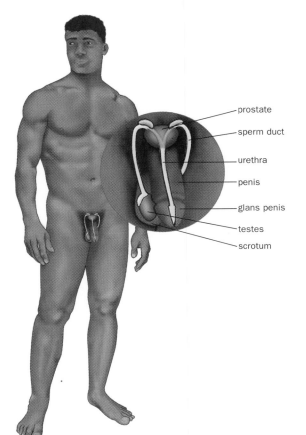

prostate
sperm duct
urethra
penis
glans penis
testes
scrotum

The male reproductive system produces sperm and secretes the hormone testosterone. The primary male sex organs are the testicles. They are the oval shaped organs enclosed in the scrotum.

The seminal glands, located at the base of the bladder, produce part of the seminal fluid. They have ducts that lead into sperm ducts called the vas deferens which carry the sperm from the testes. The prostate gland is located at the upper end of the urethra. The penis (glans penis) is the external organ for urination and sexual intercourse. The tip of the penis is covered by the prepuce (foreskin). The urethra, by which urine and semen leave the body, is inside the penis.

Root Words

andr	male
balan	glans penis
orchid, test	testis, testicle
prostat	prostate gland
sperm	sperm
vas	vessel, duct
vesicul	seminal vescles

Prefix	Root Word	Suffix	CV	Term	Meaning
a (no)	sperm (sperm)	ia (condition of)		**aspermia**	inability to produce semen.
	balan (glans penis)	itis (inflammation)		**balanitis**	inflammation of the glans penis.
crypt (hidden)	orchid (testis)	ism (state of)		**cryptorchidism**	failure of testes to drop into the scrotum.
	prostat (prostate)	itis		**prostatitis**	inflammation of prostate.
	prostat (prostate)	lith (stone)	o	**prostatolith**	a prostate stone.
	semin (testis)	oma (tumor)		**seminoma**	tumor of the testes.

ORGAN SYSTEM TERMINOLOGY

RESPIRATORY SYSTEM

The respiratory system brings oxygen into the body through inhalation and expels carbon dioxide gas through exhalation. It produces sound for speaking and helps cool the body.

The lungs have specialized tissues called **alveoli** that exchange the gases between the blood and the air. Respiratory muscles (especially the diaphragm) expand the lungs automatically, causing air to be inhaled into the upper respiratory tract. As air enters through the nose, it is warmed, moistened, and filtered. The pharynx directs food into the esophagus and air into the trachea. The larynx contains the vocal cords. The trachea, or windpipe, connects to the two bronchi (bronchial tubes) that enter the lungs.

Inside the lungs, the broncial tubes branch out and lead to the alveolar sacs that are the site of gas exchange within the lungs. The pleural cavity surrounds the lungs and provides lubrication for respiration.

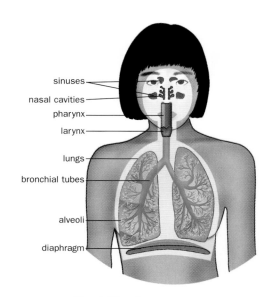

sinuses
nasal cavities
pharynx
larynx
lungs
bronchial tubes
alveoli
diaphragm

Root Words

aer	air
aero	gas
pneum	lung, air
pulmon	lung
pector	chest
nasal	nose
sinus	sinus
laryng	larynx
bronch	bronchus
ox	oxygen
capnia	carbon dioxide

Prefix	Root Word	Suffix	CV	Term	Meaning
a (no)	pnea (to breathe)			**apnea**	temporary failure to breathe.
	bronch (bronchus)	itis (inflammation)		**bronchitis**	inflammation of bronchial membranes.
cyan (blue)		sis (condition of)	o	**cyanosis**	blue discoloration of skin.
dys (difficult)	pnea (to breathe)			**dyspnea**	labored breathing.
hyper (high)	capnia (CO₂)			**hypercapnia**	excessive carbon dioxide in the blood.
hypo (low)	ox (oxygen)	ia (condition of)		**hypoxia**	abnormally low blood oxygen level.
	laryng (larynx)	itis (inflammation)		**laryngitis**	inflammation of the larynx.
para (around)	nasal (nose)			**paranasal**	near or along the nasal cavities.
	pector (chest)	algia (pain)		**pectoralgia**	chest pain.
	pneum (lung)	nia (condition of)	o	**pneumonia**	inflammation of the lungs.
	pulmon (lung)	ary (pertaining to)		**pulmonary**	pertaining to the lungs.
	sinus (sinus)	itis (inflammation)		**sinusitis**	inflammation of the sinuses.

URINARY SYSTEM

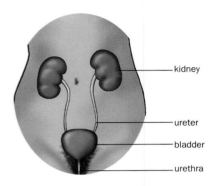

kidney

ureter

bladder

urethra

The urinary system is responsible for removing wastes from the body. The urinary system includes the kidneys, ureters, urinary bladder, and urethra.

The primary organ of the urinary system is the kidney, which filters the blood for unwanted material and makes urine. The **nephron** is the functional unit of the kidney. Plasma water from the blood passes through the nephron and through processes of reabsorption, filtration, and secretion is converted into urine.

Urine is excreted from the kidney through the ureters to the bladder. It is excreted from the bladder through the urethra.

Root Words

cyst	bladder
vesic	bladder
ren	kidney
nephr	kidney
uria	urine, urination

Prefix	Root Word	Suffix	CV	Term	Meaning
an (no)	uria (urine)			**anuria**	inability to produce urine.
	cyst (bladder)	itis (inflammation)		**cystitis**	inflammation of the bladder.
	cyst (bladder)	lith (stone)	o	**cystolith**	a bladder stone.
	nephr (kidney)	itis (inflammation)		**nephritis**	inflammation of the kidney.
poly (much)	uria (urine)			**polyuria**	excessive urination.
	ure (urine)	emia (blood condition)		**uremia**	toxic blood condition caused by kidney insufficiency or failure.

ORGAN SYSTEM TERMINOLOGY

SENSES: HEARING

The sense of hearing, as well as the maintenance of body equilibrium, is performed by the ear. The external ear consists of a funnel shaped structure which captures sound waves and channels them through an opening to the **tympanic membrane** (eardrum). The opening also contains glands that make earwax that protects the external ear.

The **middle ear** consists of three bony structures (malleus, incus, and stapes) that transmit sound from a vibrating tympanic membrane to the cochlea. The eustachian tube connects the middle ear to the nose and throat, serving to equalize the air pressure on both sides of the tympanic membrane.

The inner ear is called the **labyrinth** for obvious reasons. It consists of three areas: vestibule, cochlea, and semi-circular canals. The cochlea contains the organ of hearing. When sound waves are transmitted to it, it converts them into nerve impulses that are sent to the brain for interpretation. The semicircular canals are responsible for body equilibrium.

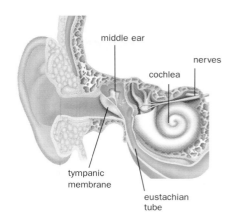

middle ear
nerves
cochlea
tympanic membrane
eustachian tube

Root Words

ot	ear
cusis	hearing condition
acous	hearing
audi	hearing
salping	eustachian tube
tympan	eardrum
myring	eardrum
cerumin	wax-like, waxy

Prefix	Root Word	Suffix	CV	Term	Meaning
	labyrinth (inner ear)	itis (inflammation)		**labyrinthitis**	inflammation of the inner ear.
	ot (ear)	algia (pain, ache)		**otalgia**	pain in the ear.
	ot (ear)	mycosis (fungal infection)	o	**otomycosis**	fungal ear infection.
	ot (ear)	orrhea (drainage)		**otorrhea**	ear infection with discharge.
para (partial)	cusis (hearing condition)			**paracusis**	hearing disorder.
	tympan (eardrum)	itis (inflammation)		**tympanitis**	inflammation of the middle ear.

SENSES: SIGHT

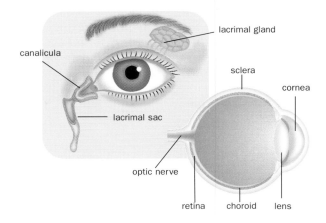

The eyes are the organs that provide sight. The eyelids protect the eye and assist in its lubrication. The conjunctiva is the blood-rich membrane between the eye and the eyelid. There are several glands that secrete fluids to protect and lubricate the eye: the **lacrimal glands** above each eye secrete tears and the meibomian glands produce sebum. Excess fluid drains into the canalicula (tear ducts).

The eye has three layers. The outer layer is composed of the sclera and the **cornea.** The sclera is the white part of the eye. The cornea is transparent so the iris (the color of the eye) and the pupil (the opening of the eye) are visible. The middle layer is called the choroid and contains blood vessels that nourish the entire eye. In the third layer, the lens focuses light rays on the **retina.** The vitreous humor (one of two fluids in the eye) lies between the retina and the lens. Rods and cones within the retina are responsible for visual reception. The **optic nerve** within the retina transmits the nerve impulses to the brain.

Root Words

blephar	eyelid
cor	pupil
dacry, lacrim	tear, tear duct
corne, kerat	cornea
retin	retina
irid, iri	iris
bi, bin	two
opia	vision

Prefix	Root Word	Suffix	CV	Term	Meaning
ambly (dull)	opia (vision)			**amblyopia**	reduction in vision.
	blephar (eyelid)	itis (inflammation)		**blepharitis**	inflammation of eyelids.
	blephar (eyelid)	optosis (dropping)		**blepharoptosis**	drooping of upper eyelid.
	conjunctiv (conjunctiva)	itis (inflammation)		**conjunctivitis**	inflammation of the conjunctiva.
end (within)	opthalm (eye)	itis (inflammation)		**endopthalmitis**	inflammation of the inside of the eye.
	irid (iris)	plegia (paralysis)	o	**iridoplegia**	paralysis of the iris.
	ocul (eye)	mycosis (fungus infection)	o	**oculomycosis**	fungal disease of the eye.
	retin (retina)	itis (inflammation)		**retinitis**	inflammation of the retina.

PHARMACY ABBREVIATIONS

Abbreviations for many medical terms are regularly used in the pharmacy.

Many of these abbreviations are from Latin words, though a number are from English. They are commonly used on prescriptions to communicate essential information on formulations, preparation, dosage regimens, and administration. The technician must know these abbreviations and their meanings.

MOST COMMON ABBREVIATIONS

Note that while it is not necessary to know the latin term from which an abbreviation comes, it has been included for reference.

	Abbreviation	Meaning	Latin term
ROUTE	a.d.	right ear	auris dexter
	a.s.	left ear	auris sinister
	a.u.	each ear	auris utro
	i.m., IM	intramuscular	
	inj.	injection	injectio
	i.v., IV	intravenous	
	i.v.p., IVP	intravenous push	
	IVPB	intravenous piggyback	
	o.d.	right eye	oculus dexter
	o.s.	left eye	oculus sinister
	o.u.	each eye	oculus utro
	p.o.	by mouth	per os
	SC, subc, subq	subcutaneously	
	top.	topically, locally	

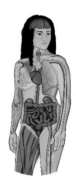

	Abbreviation	Meaning	Latin term
FORM	aq	water	aqua
	aqua. dist.	distilled water	
	caps	capsules	capsula
	DW	distilled water	
	elix.	elixir	
	liq.	liquid	liquor
	NS	normal saline	
	supp.	suppository	suppositorum
	syr.	syrup	syrupus
	tab.	tablet	tabella
	ung.	ointment	ungentum

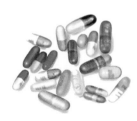

	Abbreviation	Meaning	Latin term
TIME	a.c.	before food, before meals	ante cibum
	a.m.	morning	ante meridien
	a.t.c.	around the clock	
	b.i.d.,bid	twice a day	bis in die
	h	hour, at the hour of	hora
	h.s.	at bedtime	hora somni
	p.c.	after food, after meals	post cibum
	p.r.n., prn	as needed	pro re nata
	q.i.d., qid	four times a day	quater in die
	q	each, every	quaque
	q.d.	every day	quaque die
	q.h.	every hour	quaque hora
	stat.	immediately	statim
	t.i.d., tid	three times a day	ter in die

Note that some prescribers will leave out periods in written abbreviations, and that some may use capital letters, while other may not.

	Abbreviation	Meaning	Latin term
MEASUREMENT	ī	one, ī	
	a.a. or aa	of each	ana
	ad	to, up to	ad
	aq. ad	add water up to	
	dil.	dilute	dilutus
	div.	divide	
	f, fl.	fluid	
	g., G., gm.	gram	
	gtt.	drop	guttae
	L	liter	
	mcg.	microgram	
	mEq.	milliequivalent	
	mg.	milligram	
	ml.	milliliter	
	q.s.	a sufficient quantity	quantum sufficiat
	q.s. ad	add sufficient quantity to make	quantum sufficiat ad
	ss	one-half	
	tbsp.	tablespoon	
	tsp.	teaspoon	
OTHER	c	with	cum
	d.t.d.	give of such doses	dentur tales doses
	disp.	dispense	
	f, ft.	make, let it be made	fac, fiat, fiant
	l	left	laevus
	s	without	sine
	ut dict., u.d.	as directed	ut dictum

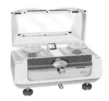

LESS COMMON ABBREVIATIONS

The following abbreviations are also used in pharmacy, though less frequently than the others on these pages.

ad lib.	at pleasure	collyr.	an eyewash	N.F.	National Formulary
add	add (thou)	comp.	compound	non.rep.	do not repeat
agit	shake, stir	cong.; C.	gallon	O.	pint
alt. h.	every other hour	c.c.	with food; with meals	occulent.	eye ointment
a.	before	d.	give (thou); let be given	o.	eye
amp.	ampule	d.	right	o.l.	left eye
ag. dest.	distilled water	dieb. alt.	every other day	o.m.	every morning
aur.; a	ear	emuls.	emulsion	p.a.a.	to be applied to affected
a.l.	left ear	et	and		part
aurist	ear-drops	e.m.p.	in the manner prescribed;	p.r.	per rectum
b.	twice		as directed	ulv.	powder
brach.	the arm	gr.	grain	s.a.	according to the art
BSA	body surface area	lin.	liniment	Sig.	write, label
c.c.	cubic centimeter	lot.	lotion	s.o.s.	if necessary
charts	powder papers; divided	min;	minum	sol.	solution
	powders	m.; M	mix	tinc.; tr.	tincture
cib.; c.	food	n.	at night	troche	lozenge
collun	a nose wash	narist.	nasal drops	tuss.	a cough
collut.	a mouthwash	neb.	a spray		

MEDICAL ABBREVIATIONS

Besides abbreviations common to pharmacy, there are abbreviations widely used in health care institutions and other environments. In addition to the abbreviations on the previous pages, these abbreviations are also important for the pharmacy technician to learn.

The following are a few of the abbreviations with medical significance that pharmacy technicians should know. Some of these abbreviations have multiple meanings. These are the most common.

Abbreviations are commonly used in hospitals and other health care settings to make record keeping easier. Note the various abbreviations on the above hospital flow sheet. Also note that these are for a specific hospital and may not be used elsewhere.

AIDS	Acquired immunodeficiency syndrome
AV	Atrial-ventricular
AMI	Acute myocardial infarction
ANS	Autonomic nervous system
BM	Bowel movement
BP	Blood pressure
CA	Cancer
COPD	Chronic obstructive pulmonary disease
CV	Cardiovascular
CVA	Cerebrovascular accident (stroke)
DI	Diabetes insipidus
DOB	Date of birth
DX	Diagnosis
ECG, EKG	Electrocardiogram
GERD	Gastroesophageal reflux disease
GI	Gastrointestinal
H	Hypodermic
HDL	High density lipoprotein
HIV	Human Immunodeficiency virus
IH	Infectious hepatitis
IO, I/O	Fluid intake and output
LDL	Low density lipoprotein
MI	Myocardial infarction
NPO	Nothing by mouth
PUD	Peptic ulcer disease
RBC	Red blood count or red blood cell
T	Temperature
TB	Tuberculosis
U	Units
VD	Venereal disease
WBC	White blood count or white blood cell
WT	Weight
XX	Female sex chromosome
XY	Male sex chromosome

DRUG CLASSIFICATIONS

The same steps in interpreting other medical science terminology can be used to interpret drug classification names.

A classification is a grouping of a number of drugs that have some properties in common.

For example, penicillin, cefoxitine, and ciprofloxacin are used to treat bacterial infections, so they are grouped in a class called anti-infectives.

Each drug has unique properties, but they all share the property of being effective against bacterial infections. So the class name "anti-infective" is created by combing "anti" and "infective" into antiinfective, meaning "against infection." Since much of drug therapy is based on opposing some physiological process in the body, many drugs classes begin with the prefix "anti" or "ant."

Root	Prefix
Suffix	C.V.

Classification names can be understood by identifying their components.

THE "AGAINST" CLASS

Some examples of the "anti" class of drugs

antacids	relieves gastritis, ulcer pain, indigestion and heartburn
antianginals	relieves heart pain
anticoagulant	dissolves or prevents blood clots
anticonvulsants	prevents seizures
antidepressants	prevents depression
antidiarrheals	stops diarrhea
antiemetics	prevents nausea and vomiting
antihistamine	blocks the effects of histamine
antihyperlipidemics	lowers high cholesterol levels
antihypertensive	reduces blood pressure
anti-inflammatory	reduces inflammation
antipruritics	prevent or relieves itching
antispasmodics	relieves intestinal cramping
antitussive	relieves coughing by inhibiting cough reflex

OTHER CLASSES

Here are examples of other classification names which can be understood by breaking down the term into its medical terminology components.

de + conges + tant	**decongestant:**	reduces nasal congestion
an + alges + ics	**analgesics:**	without pain, kills pain
hypo + glyc + emics	**hypoglycemics:**	reduce blood sugar levels
hypo + lipid + emics	**hypolipidemics:**	reduce blood lipid (cholesterol) levels
kerat + o + lytics	**keratolytics:**	destroys skin layers such as warts
contra + cep + tives	**contraceptives:**	oral contraceptives, prevent pregnancy
psych + o + tropic	**pyschotropic:**	change mental states
sperm + i + cide	**spermicide:**	formulation that destroys sperm

PREFIXES

Root	Prefix
Suffix	C.V.

Below are common prefixes used in medical and pharmaceutical science terminology.

a	without	medi	middle
ambi	both	melan	black
an	without	meso	middle
ante	before	meta	beyond, after, changing
anti	against	micro	small
bi	two or both	mid	middle
brady	slow	mono	one
chlor	green	multi	many
circum	around	neo	new
cirrh	yellow	pan	all
con	with	para	alongside or abnormal
contra	against	peri	around
cyan	blue	polio	gray
dia	across or through	poly	many
dis	separate from or apart	post	after
dys	painful, difficult	pre	before
ec	away or out	pro	before
ecto	outside	pseudo	false
end	within	purpur	purple
epi	upon	quadri	four
erythr	red	re	again or back
eu	good or normal	retro	after
exo	outside	rube	red
heter	different	semi	half
hom	same	sub	below or under
hyper	above or excessive	super	above or excessive
hypo	below or deficient	supra	above or excessive
im	not	sym	with
immun	safe, protected	syn	with
in	not	tachy	fast
infra	below or under	trans	across, through
inter	between	tri	three
intra	within	ultra	beyond or excessive
is	equal	uni	one
leuk	white	xanth	yellow
macro	large	xer	dry

SUFFIXES

PHARMACEUTICAL TERMINOLOGY

Root	Prefix
Suffix	C.V.

Below are common suffixes used in medical and pharmaceutical science terminology.

ac	pertaining to
al	pertaining to
algia	pain
ar	pertaining to
ary	pertaining to
asthenia	without strength
cele	pouching or hernia
cyesis	pregnancy
cynia	pain
eal	pertaining to
ectasis	expansion or dilation
ectomy	removal
emia	blood condition
gram	record
graph	recording instrument
graphy	recording process
ia	condition of
iasis	condition, formation of
iatry	treatment
ic	pertaining to
icle	small
ism	condition of
itis	inflammation
ium	tissue
lith	stone, calculus
logy	study of
malacia	softening
megaly	enlargement
meter	measuring instrument
metry	measuring process

oi	resembling
ole	small
oma	tumor
opia	vision
opsia	vision
osis	abnormal condition
osmia	smell
ous	pertaining to
paresis	partial paralysis
pathy	disease
penia	decrease
phagia	swallowing
phasia	speech
philia	attraction for
phobia	fear
plasia	formation
plegia	paralysis, stroke
rrhea	discharge
sclerosis	narrowing, constriction
scope	examination instrument
scopy	examination
spasm	involuntary contraction
stasis	stop or stand
tic	pertaining to
tocia	childbirth, labor
tomy	incision
toxic	poison
tropic	stimulate
ula	small
y	condition, process

REVIEW

KEY CONCEPTS

✔ Much of medical science terminology is made up of a small number of root words, suffixes and prefixes that originated from either Greek or Latin words.

✔ A prefix is added to the beginning of a root word to clarify its meaning.

✔ The suffix is added to the end of a root word to clarify the meaning.

✔ Combining vowels are used to connect the prefix, root, or suffix parts of the term.

✔ The cardiovascular system distributes blood throughout the body using blood vessels called arteries, capillaries, and veins.

✔ The endocrine system consists of the glands that secrete hormones (chemicals that assist in regulating body functions).

✔ The GI tract contains the organs that are involved in the digestion of foods and the absorption of nutrients.

✔ The integumentary system is the body's first line of defense, acting as a barrier against disease and other hazards.

✔ The lymphatic system is the center of the body's immune system.

✔ Lymphocytes release antibodies that destroy disease cells and provide immunity against them.

✔ The body contains more than 600 muscles which give shape and movement to it.

✔ The nervous system is the body's system of communication. The neuron (nerve cell) is its basic functional unit.

✔ The skeletal system protects soft organs and provides structure and support for the body's organ systems.

✔ The female reproductive system produces hormones (estrogen, progesterone), controls menstruation, and provides for childbearing.

✔ The male reproductive system produces sperm and secretes the hormone testosterone.

✔ The respiratory system brings oxygen into the body through inhalation and expels carbon dioxide gas through exhalation.

✔ The primary organ of the urinary system is the kidney, which filters the blood for unwanted material and makes urine.

✔ The sense of hearing, as well as the maintenance of body equilibrium, is performed by the ear.

SELF TEST

MATCH THE TERMS.

answers are in the back of the book

1. through the skin
2. blood tumor
3. high fat content in blood
4. brain inflammation
5. fallopian pregnancy
6. hardening of artery
7. muscle repair
8. black cell tumor
9. liver tumor
10. ointment
11. drop

a) athersclerosis
b) hyperlipidemia
c) melanocytoma
d) hepatoma
e) transdermal
f) hematoma
g) myoplasty
h) encephalitis
i) salpingocyesis
j) prn
k) gtt

12. twice a day
13. three times a day
14. four times a day
15. as needed
16. each ear
17. one-half
18. at bedtime
19. by mouth
20. topically, locally
21. every day
22. after food, after meals
23. each, every

l) tid
m) bid
n) qid
o) ss
p) au
q) ung
r) hs
s) q
t) p.c.
u) po
v) top.
w) qd

MATCH THE TERMS.

answers can be checked on page 38

1. card
2. cyst
3. derma
4. gastr
5. hemat
6. hepat
7. mast
8. my

a. bladder
b. blood
c. bone
d. breast
e. chest
f. ear
g. eye
h. heart

9. nephr
10. neur
11. ocul
12. oste
13. ot
14. pector
15. pneum
16. ven

i. vein
j. liver
k. lung
l. muscle
m. nerve
n. skin
o. stomach
p. kidney

PRESCRIPTIONS

A prescription is a written order from a practitioner for the preparation and administration of a medicine or a device.

Medical doctors (MD), dentists (DDS), veterinarians (DVM), and doctors of osteopathy (DO) are the primary practitioners allowed to write prescriptions. In some states, however, nurse practitioners, physicians assistants and/or pharmacists are also allowed limited rights to prescribe medications based on predetermined protocols (specific guidelines for practice) and in collaboration with one of the primary practitioners mentioned above.

Prescriptions are subject to many federal and state rules and regulations.

These regulations have been developed to protect the patient and to provide for certain minimum standards of practice. The rules and regulations that govern both community and hospital pharmacy practice are continually evaluated and updated as new technologies, new medications, and new protocols are developed and adopted.

Community pharmacists dispense directly to the patient and the patient is expected to administer the medication according to the pharmacist's directions.

This requires clear communication between the pharmacist and the patient. The patient receives information from the pharmacist on the prescription label and an information sheet on the medication. In addition, the pharmacist counsels the patient or the patient's representative when the prescription is purchased.

In institutional settings, nursing staff generally administer medications to patients.

As a result, the rules and regulations that govern prescription dispensing in institutional settings are quite different from those rules that apply to community practice. Labeling is quite different and many medications are packaged in individual doses.

Prescription Products

Prescriptions sometimes require the pharmaceutical preparation of a medication from ingredients (an activity called **extemporaneous compounding**). However, they are usually written for commercially available products that are specified by brand or generic name, strength, and route of administration. The pharmacist fills the prescription with that exact product or, if allowed (by the prescriber, insurer, etc.), a product that is determined to be equivalent.

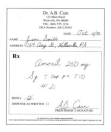

1. A prescription is written by a prescriber.

A physician/practitioner determines that a medication is necessary and communicates the details in the written form known as a prescription.

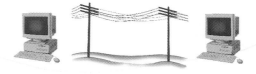

5. Prescription is processed.

The prescription is interpreted and confirmed by the system. If third party billing is involved, this is done online simultaneously.

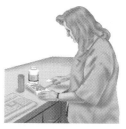

7. Prescription is prepared.

The correct product is selected and the prescribed amount of it is measured and placed into a suitable container and labeled appropriately.

The process illustrated here occurs in the community pharmacy. It is somewhat different in institutional settings where medications are administered by nursing staff, instead of the patients themselves.

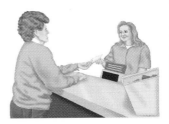

2. The written prescription is presented to the pharmacy.

The patient or a representative presents the written prescription at the pharmacy counter.

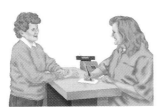

3. Prescription information is checked.

The prescription is assessed for completeness, e.g. prescriber information, drug name, strength, dosage form, directions.

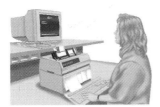

4. Patient and prescription data is entered into system.

Patient data is collected (correct spelling of name, address, insurance information, etc.) and entered into the computerized prescription system.

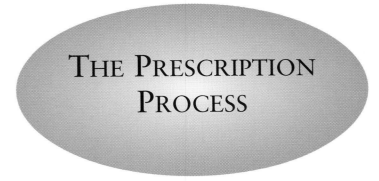

THE PRESCRIPTION PROCESS

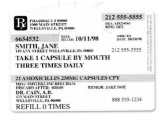

6. Label is generated.

Once the prescription and third-party billing is confirmed, the label and receipt are printed.

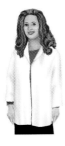

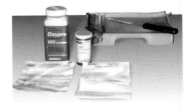

8. Prescription is checked.

If the prescription has been prepared by a technician, there is a final check by the pharmacist to make sure that it is as prescribed.

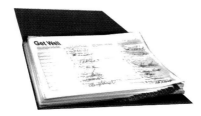

9. Patient receives the prescription.

The patient or the patient representative accepts the prescription, the sale is rung through the cash register, and the insurance log is signed.

10. Pharmacist provides counseling.

The pharmacist is called to the counter to counsel the patient or the patient representative regarding the medications as required by OBRA '90.

PRESCRIPTION INFORMATION

The modern prescription has stringent requirements designed to inform the pharmacist and protect the patient.

Today's prescription regulations vary from state to state and province to province, but generally a prescription for a community pharmacy will contain the information illustrated below.

ELEMENTS OF THE PRESCRIPTION

Prescriber information:
Name, title, office address, and telephone number

Drug Enforcement Agency (DEA) registration number of prescriber (required for all controlled substances)

Name and address of patient.

Other patient information such as age or weight is optional, but sometimes important, e.g., a child's weight.

Note: If a compound is prescribed, a list of ingredients and directions for mixing is included.

Refill instructions

DAW: Dispense As Written and/or Generic Substitution Allowed instructions (optional).

Dr. A.B. Cain
123 Main Street
Wellsville, PA 00000
TEL: (888) 555-1234
DEA Number: AB1234563

DATE *Oct 10/93*

NAME *Jane Smith*
ADDRESS *149 Any St, Wellsville, PA*

Rx

Amoxil 250 mg

Sig: ĩ cap po TID

 # 21

REFILL *Ø*
DISPENSE AS WRITTEN ☐

A.B. Cain
PRESCRIBER'S SIGNATURE

Use separate form for each controlled substance prescription.
THEFT, UNAUTHORIZED POSSESSION AND/OR USE OF THIS FORM INCLUDING ALTERATIONS OR FORGERY, ARE CRIMES PUNISHABLE BY LAW.

Date the prescription is written.

Inscription: Name (brand or generic), strength of medication and quantity.

Signa: This comes from the latin word signa, meaning "to write." It is abbreviated to **sig** and indicates what directions for use should be printed on the label.

Signature of prescriber (not required on a verbal prescription)

Note: prescriptions are written in ink, never pencil.

Additional Information

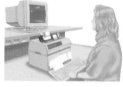

In addition to the above, the information at right must be added to the prescription in the pharmacy. This information is a product of the computerized prescription filling process. Some data are automatically assigned by the computer (e.g., prescription number), while other information is added by the pharmacist or pharmacy technician as they input the data necessary for the proper filling of the prescription (e.g., the product selected).

➡ Date the product is dispensed.
➡ Identity of the product by manufacturer and NDC (National Drug Code)—DIN (Drug Identification Number) in Canada.
➡ Prescription and/or transaction number.
➡ Insurance information for the patient.
➡ Price charged.
➡ Initials of the technician and pharmacist involved in the filling of the prescription.
➡ Signature of the pharmacist receiving the prescription if it is a verbal order.

*The prescription information on these pages applies to the community pharmacy setting. In institutions, **medication orders** are used instead of a prescription form. See chapter 16 for more information on institutional practices.*

PRESCRIPTION INFORMATION CHECKLIST

Consider these factors

➡ Is the patient's full name clear on the prescription? Has a nickname or initial been used?

➡ Is the patient's date of birth, street address, telephone number, insurance information, preference for brand or generic drugs, and allergy information already on file in the pharmacy?

➡ Is the medication for an over-the-counter product that the patient can receive without a prescription? Is the prescription for a Schedule II drug that has very special prescription requirements?

➡ When was the prescription written? How many days or weeks has it been since it was written?

➡ Is the drug available in the pharmacy in the quantity written? Does it require compounding?

➡ Is the prescription suspicious in any way? Is it written on a legitimate prescription blank and all in the same hand writing and with the same ink? Are there any signs of alteration of quantities, strength, or the name of the drug? Is this a possible drug of abuse and if so do the quantities and directions seem appropriate?

Take this action

✔ **Determine the exact name** so that multiple files are not created for one patient.

✔ **Always confirm the information on file as current.**

✔ **Check with the pharmacist on all OTC and Schedule II prescriptions.** The use of OTC medicines is not without risk. Only the pharmacist should recommend an OTC medicine.

✔ **Check with the pharmacist to determine if the prescription can be filled if it is more than a few days old.** Some prescriptions may be valid for months, but others must be verified if they are more than a few days old.

✔ **Inform the patient if there might be a delay in filling the prescription.**

✔ **Alert the pharmacist to any potential forgeries.** Let the pharmacist follow through with the patient.

---

 signa the directions for use on the prescription that must be printed on the prescription label.

R$_x$ is an abbreviation of the latin word recipe, meaning "take." Of course, the word recipe has a broader meaning in that it is a description of the amounts and steps involved in preparing a mixture of different elements. Both of these meanings can be seen in the current use of the abbreviation R$_x$.

THE FILL PROCESS

Once prescription information is finalized in the computerized prescription system, a label and receipt are printed out.

At this point, the correct medication must be selected from pharmacy stock and the prescribed amount measured or counted and packaged. If the prescription calls for a compounded product, the technician must follow pharmacy policy of its preparation.

The pharmacy technician completes the fill process by placing the correct amount of medication into an appropriate container and labeling it correctly.

This includes placing the computer-generated label on the container so it sticks firmly and is easy to read. It also includes placing the appropriate **auxiliary labels** on the container. These are the additional warning labels that are placed on filled prescription containers.

A pharmacist must check the final product and label.

When finished with preparation, the technician initials the pharmacy copy of the label and organizes the finished product, prescription order, and the stock bottle that the medication was taken from for the pharmacist to check and verify. If the prescription is correctly filled, the pharmacist initials the pharmacy copy of the label information to indicate that the prescription was correctly filled. The prescription can then be released to the patient.

Avoiding Errors

If the technician is unsure about any aspect of a prescription, he or she must ask the pharmacist for direction. Never dispense guesswork! The careful screening of prescription orders by the technician can prevent medication and other errors. Medication errors can be very serious. They include, but are not limited to the dispensing of:

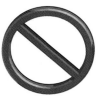

➡ the wrong medication
➡ the wrong strength, dosage form, or quantity
➡ the wrong directions
➡ the medication to the wrong patient,
➡ the dispensing of medications on the order of a forged or altered prescription.

An awareness that medication errors exist and are serious is the first step in preventing medication errors from happening.

CONSIDERATIONS

While filling the prescriptions, the technician should consider these factors:

Are the fill instructions clear and reasonable?

Do the directions, quantity, and strength fit with what is usual for this medication? Are there any opportunities for confusion e.g. is the dosing schedule q.i.d. or q.d.? Does the Sig. read: 2 hs or q hs?

Are the administration directions clear?

Are the directions clearly translated in an unambiguous fashion in order to avoid any misinterpretation by the patient e.g. does take two tablets daily mean that the patient is to take one tablet twice daily or two tablets once daily?

Are there lookalike names?

Are there any look-alike drug names that could be confused with the intended medication? For example, did the prescriber write HCTZ 50mg (hydrochlorothiazide) or HCT 250mg (hydrocortisone)? Is it Amoxicillin 875 mg or Augmentin 875 mg? Losec 20 mg or Lasix 20 mg (Canada)? Accupril 40 mg or Accutane 40 mg? Rifadin or Ritalin?

Don't add information!

Never add information that is not indicated based on what you assume the prescriber meant when writing the prescription. The prescriber has knowledge of the patient's condition that you don't. Adding directions that you assume to be correct may not be appropriate.

Pay attention to warnings!

When warning screens appear regarding potential insurance claim errors, dosing irregularities, or drug interactions, **call the pharmacist to evaluate each warning.** An ignored warning might result in the patient being over-billed, undermedicated, or hospitalized due to a severe drug-drug interaction. Only the pharmacist determines which warnings require intervention and which are for informational purposes.

THE PHARMACIST'S ROLE

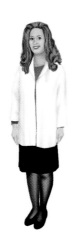

The pharmacist's role is multifaceted and includes:

✔ using his/her knowledge and expertise in order to assure that the physicians' orders are carried out accurately and safely,

✔ ensuring that the correct medication, strength and dosage form is dispensed,

✔ ensuring that the directions for the patient are clear, accurate, and unambiguous,

✔ ensuring that there are no potential problems with drug allergies, drug-drug or drug-disease interactions,

✔ ensuring that there are no misunderstandings by the patient with respect to how to take the medication,

✔ ensuring that the patient understands the beneficial effects that can be expected from the medication and the potential side effects that he/she should be cautious about while taking the medication,

✔ ensuring that the prescriber has been contacted regarding the prescription if appropriate,

✔ ensuring that the prescription has been accurately and fairly billed to the patient or the appropriate third party.

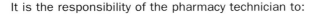

THE PHARMACY TECHNICIAN'S ROLE

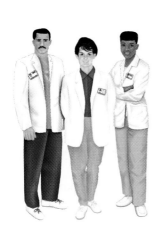

It is the responsibility of the pharmacy technician to:

✔ assist the pharmacist in the technical (non-judgment requiring) aspects of prescription filling;

✔ treat each patient, their personal information, and their medication with respect;

✔ gather all appropriate information needed in a timely, efficient, and professional manner;

✔ quickly and accurately locate the appropriate medication for dispensing, calculate quantities, and re-package medication for the prescription;

✔ quickly, accurately, and efficiently key patient data and prescription information into the computer;

✔ request the advice of the pharmacist whenever a warning screen appears during the filling of a prescription;

✔ request the advice of the pharmacist whenever judgment is required, e.g., for counseling on the use of a medications, questions regarding therapy, and so on.

Prescriptions for OTC Medications

Prescriptions may be written for over-the-counter (OTC) medications. When this happens, consult the pharmacist. The prescription is generally not filled. The pharmacist instead helps the patient locate the product on the shelf and then counsels the patient with respect to the prescriber's orders. The patient then purchases the medication as an over-the-counter product.

LABELS

The general purpose of the prescription label is to provide information to the patient regarding the dispensed medication and how to take it. Additionally, the label includes information about the pharmacy, the patient, the prescriber, and the prescription or transaction number assigned to the prescription.

As with prescriptions, requirements for prescription labels vary from state to state (and in Canada, for example, from province to province). However, a prescription label generally contains the information indicated below.

the name, address, and telephone number of the pharmacy

the date dispensed

DEA number

a prescription and/or transaction number

the name of the patient for whom the medication is dispensed

directions for use that are clear and accurate

the name, quantity, strength, manufacturer (name or NDC number), and dosage form of the medication dispensed

expiration date of the medication

the name of the prescriber

refill information.

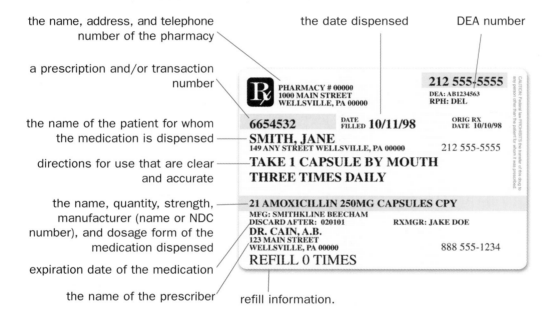

RX PHARMACY # 00000
1000 MAIN STREET
WELLSVILLE, PA 00000

212 555-5555
DEA: AB1234563
RPH: DEL

6654532 DATE FILLED 10/11/98 ORIG RX DATE 10/10/98

SMITH, JANE
149 ANY STREET WELLSVILLE, PA 00000 212 555-5555

TAKE 1 CAPSULE BY MOUTH
THREE TIMES DAILY

21 AMOXICILLIN 250MG CAPSULES CPY
MFG: SMITHKLINE BEECHAM
DISCARD AFTER: 020101 RXMGR: JAKE DOE
DR. CAIN, A.B.
123 MAIN STREET
WELLSVILLE, PA 00000 888 555-1234

REFILL 0 TIMES

CAUTION: Federal law PROHIBITS the transfer of this drug to any person other than the patient for whom it was prescribed.

DIRECTIONS FOR USE

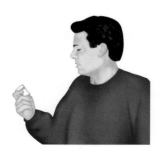

✔ **Directions should start with a verb** (take, instill, inhale, insert, apply) **and completely, clearly, and accurately describe the administration of the medication.**

✔ **Indicate the route of administration if it is not oral.** For example, use "apply to affected area", "insert rectally", etc.

✔ **Use whole words, not abbreviations.** For example, use "tablets" not "tabs."

✔ **Use familiar words, especially in measurements.** For example, use "two teaspoonsful" instead of "10 ml."

 In community pharmacy, a label that is easily understood by the patient is absolutely essential.

AUXILIARY LABELS

Additional, often colored auxiliary labels may also be applied to the prescription container in order to provide additional information to the patient (e.g. Shake Well, Keep Refrigerated, Take With Food or Milk). Many computerized prescription systems will automatically indicate which auxiliary labels to use.

Controlled substances from schedules II, III and IV must carry an auxiliary label stating:

Caution: Federal law prohibits the transfer of this drug to any person other than the patient for whom it was prescribed.

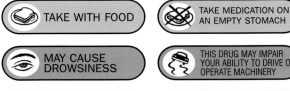
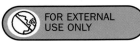
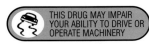
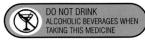
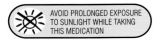
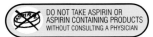

PLACING THE LABEL

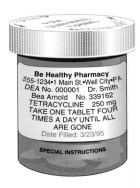

Labeling the container correctly includes:

✔ placing the computer-generated label on the container so it is parallel to the edges of the container, easy to locate, and easy to read.

✔ making sure the label sticks adequately to the container and is without creases. Some pharmacies place transparent tape over the label to protect the label from spills and prevent accidental smudging or obliteration of information.

✔ placing the appropriate auxiliary labels on the container.

INSTITUTIONAL LABELS

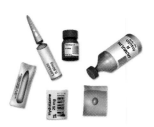

Rules for institutional pharmacy prescription labels vary by institution but often do not contain much more than the name, strength, manufacturer, expiration date, and dosage form of the medication. Since the condition of a patient in the hospital can change relatively quickly, their medication orders may be regularly updated. As a result, the nursing staff refers to the most recent physician's instructions in the patient's chart to verify prescribing information. It is also worth noting that unit dose packaging is widely used in institutional settings, and such packaging often has space for only essential identifying information about the medication.

EXAMPLES

PRESCRIPTION TO LABEL

Dr. A.B. Cain
123 Main Street
Wellsville, PA 00000
TEL: (888) 555-1234
DEA Number: AB1234563

DATE *Oct 10/98*

NAME *Jane Smith*

ADDRESS *149 Any St, Wellsville PA*

Rx

Amoxil 250 mg

Sig: ī cap po TID

 # 21

REFILL *Ø*

DISPENSE AS WRITTEN ☐

A.B. Cain
PRESCRIBER'S SIGNATURE

Use separate form for each controlled substance prescription.
THEFT, UNAUTHORIZED POSSESSION AND/OR USE OF THIS FORM INCLUDING ALTERATIONS OR FORGERY, ARE CRIMES PUNISHABLE BY LAW.

➡ Amoxil is a brand name for Amoxicillin.

➡ 250 mg is the strength.

➡ ī cap means "take one capsule."

➡ P.O. means "by mouth."

➡ TID means "three times a day."

➡ #21 means a "quantity of 21."

➡ there are no refills; generic substitution may be used.

Therefore, the prescription is for a week's supply of Amoxicillin 250mg capsules: 21 capsules, one capsule to be taken three times daily for seven days.

The label for the above prescription.

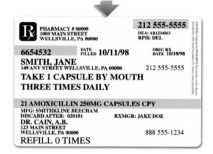

➡ The drug is Prozac.

➡ 20mg is the strength.

➡ ī cap means "take one capsule."

➡ P.O. means "by mouth."

➡ qd means "each day."

➡ #30 means a "quantity of 30."

➡ there are 2 refills; dispense as written.

Dr. A.B. Cain
123 Main Street
Wellsville, PA 00000
TEL: (888) 555-1234
DEA Number: AB1234563

DATE *Oct 6/98*

NAME *Scott Barr*

ADDRESS *345 Maple St, Wellsville PA*
D.O.B – 2/23/54

Rx

Prozac 20 mg

Sig: ī cap po qd

 # 30

REFILL *X2*

DISPENSE AS WRITTEN ☑

A.B. Cain
PRESCRIBER'S SIGNATURE

THEFT, UNAUTHORIZED POSSESSION AND/OR USE OF THIS FORM INCLUDING ALTERATIONS OR FORGERY, ARE CRIMES PUNISHABLE BY LAW.

Therefore, the prescription is for a 30 day supply of Prozac 20mg capsules: 30 capsules, one capsule to be taken each day.

℞ Note that "D.O.B." on this prescription means the date of birth. While this is optional, it is often important, and sometimes necessary, as with online adjudication of a claim.

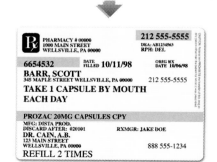

MEDICATION ORDERS

There are various formats for the medication orders used in institutional settings. Here are two samples. Note the following factors that are indicated by one or both of the examples:

➡ multiple medications are often used.

➡ abbreviations are used.

➡ orders are indicated by time of order.

➡ orders are revised to include changes in therapy.

➡ administration times are noted and signed by nursing staff.

➡ allergies are indicated.

These and other aspects of medication orders reflect the special characteristics of the institutional environment.

DOCTOR'S ORDERS	PATIENT IDENTIFICATION
	099999999 675-01
	SMITH, JOHN
	12/06/1950
	DR. P JOHNSON

DATE	TIME	DOCTOR'S ORDERS ①	DATE/TIME INITIALS	DATE/TIME INITIALS
1/31/99	2200	Admit patient to 6th floor		
		Pneumonia, Dehydration		
		All: PCN- Rash		
		Order CBC, chem-7, blood cultures stat		
		Start D5-NS @ 125 ml/hr IV q8°		
		Dr Johnson X2222		

DATE	TIME	DOCTOR'S ORDERS ②	DATE/TIME INITIALS	DATE/TIME INITIALS
2/01/99	300	Tylenol 650mg po q4-6 hrs PRN for Temp>38°C		
		Verbal Order Dr Johnson/ Jane Doe, RN		

DATE	TIME	DOCTOR'S ORDERS ③	DATE/TIME INITIALS	DATE/TIME INITIALS
2/01/99	600	Start Clarithromycin 500mg po q12°		
		Multivitamin po qd		
		Order CXR for this am		
		Dr Johnson X2222		

COMMUNITY HOSPITAL
Medication Administration Record

Room/Bed: 675-01
Patient: SMITH, JOHN
Account #: 099999999
Sex: M
Age: 48Y
Doctor: JOHNSON, P.

From 0730 on 02/01/99 to 0700 on 02/02/99

Diagnosis: PNEUMONIA; DEHYDRATION
Height: 5'11" weight: 75KG

Verified By: Susie Smith, RN

Allergies: PENICILLIN-->RASH

	0730–1530	1600–2300	2330–0700
5% DEXTROSE/0.9% SODIUM CHLORIDE 1 LITER BAG DOSE 125 ML/HR IV Q 8 HRS ORDER #2	800 JD	1600 SS	2400
MULTIVITAMIN TABLET DOSE: 11 TABLET P.O. QD ORDER #4	1000 Given @ 9AM JD		
CLARITHROMYCIN 500 MG TABLET DOSE: 500MG P.O. Q 122 HRS ORDER #5	1000 JD	2200 SS	
ACETAMINOPHEN 325 MG TABLET DOSE: 650 MG P.O. Q 4-6 HRS P.R.N. FOR TEMP>38°C ORDER # 17	1200 JD		

Init / Signature	Init / Signature
SS / Susie Smith, RN	___ / _____
JD / Jane Doe, RN	___ / _____
___ / _____	___ / _____

℞ There are rules for written information on institutional documents which generally include the requirement to use black ink.

REVIEW

KEY CONCEPTS

✔ A prescription is a written order from a practitioner for the preparation and administration of a medicine or a device.

✔ Medical doctors (MD), dentists (DDS), veterinarians (DVM), and doctors of osteopathy (DO) are the primary practitioners allowed to write prescriptions.

✔ In some states, nurse practitioners, physicians assistants and/or pharmacists are also allowed limited rights to prescribe medications.

✔ In institutional settings, "medication orders" are used instead of a prescription form.

✔ In community pharmacies, pharmacy technicians generally receive the prescription, collect patient data (correct spelling of name, address, insurance information, etc.) and enter it into a computerized prescription system.

✔ The pharmacist should be consulted on all OTC and Schedule II prescriptions.

✔ It is necessary to check with the pharmacist to determine if a prescription can be filled if it is more than a few days old.

✔ The pharmacist should be alerted to any potential forgeries.

✔ The prescription is interpreted and confirmed by the prescription system. If third party billing is involved, this is done online simultaneously.

✔ Once the prescription and third-party billing is confirmed, the label and receipt are printed and the prescription is prepared.

✔ If a prescription has been prepared by a technician, there is a final check by the pharmacist to make sure that it is as prescribed.

✔ Since the patient is expected to self-administer the medication, the pharmacist's directions for use must be clear. In addition, pharmacists are required to provide counseling to patients.

✔ In institutional settings, nursing staff generally administer medications to patients.

✔ Prescriptions may be written for over-the-counter (OTC) medications.

✔ Technicians must request the advice of the pharmacist whenever judgment is required.

✔ Computer-generated prescription labels must be placed on containers so they are easy to locate and easy to read.

✔ Many computerized prescription systems will automatically indicate which auxiliary labels to use with each drug.

✔ Controlled substances from schedules II, III and IV must carry an auxiliary label stating: "Caution: Federal law prohibits the transfer of this drug to any person other than the patient for whom it was prescribed."

SELF TEST

MATCH THE TERMS.   *answers can be checked in the glossary*

auxiliary labels

extemporaneous compounding

lookalikes

medication orders

prescription

protocols

signa, sig

a written order from a practitioner for the preparation and administration of a medicine or a device

the pharmaceutical preparation of a medication from ingredients.

specific guidelines for practice

the directions for use on a prescription that should be printed on the label.

the additional warning labels that are placed on filled prescription containers.

the form used to prescribe medications for patients in institutional settings.

drug names that have similar appearance, particularly when written.

CHOOSE THE BEST ANSWER.   *answers are in the back of the book*

The following questions are based on this information from a prescription:

Vicodin   # 15
Sig: 1 po QID prn pain
DAW   Refill prn
Dr. J Smith   AS1234563

1. Vicodin® is a Schedule III analgesic used for moderate to severe pain. Since the price of the generic version (hydrocodone/acetaminophen) is one-half the price, the patient requests the generic version. Can the generic version of this drug be dispensed to the patient?
   a.) Yes, you can request the change be made.
   b.) Yes, but the Pharmacist must make the change.
   c.) Yes, but the physician must be contacted by the Pharmacist and okay the change.
   d.) none of the above

2. If taken as directed, this prescription should last:
   a.) less than three days
   b.) less than four days
   c.) four or more days
   d.) five or more days

3. How many times can this prescription be refilled?
   a.) three times
   b.) six times
   c.) as needed
   d.) none of the above

NUMBERS

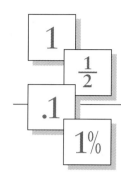

The amount of a drug in its manufactured or prescribed form is always stated numerically — that is, with numbers.

Knowing how to work with numbers is essential to the proper handling of drugs and preparation of prescriptions. This involves understanding the different number forms, measurement units, and mathematical operations that are regularly used.

ARABIC NUMBERS

The numbers we use most often are arabic numbers. Arabic numbers have different forms. They can appear as whole numbers, fractions, mixed numbers, decimals, and percentages. It is necessary to be able to multiply, divide, add, and subtract numbers of one form and to be able to convert one form of a number to another.

Whole Numbers

Whole Numbers are numbers which represent a complete unit of something, e.g., 1 can of soda, 2 quarts of milk, etc.

Fractions

Fractions are numbers which represent partial unit amounts. They are expressed as a relationship between two numbers. This relationship is called a *ratio*. One-half and seven-eighths are fractions with these relationships:

fraction		relationship
$\frac{1}{2}$	=	1 out of 2 units
$\frac{7}{8}$	=	7 out of 8 units

The top number in a fraction is called the *numerator*. The bottom is called the *denominator*. The line between represents **division by the bottom number**. This line can also be a slash (/) between two numbers on the same line, as in 1/2. The number 1/2 represents one divided by two, with one being the numerator and two being the denominator.

$$\frac{1}{2}\begin{array}{l}\text{—— numerator}\\\text{—— denominator}\end{array}$$

> Note: a colon (:) is also sometimes used in place of a slash. For example, 1:100 may be used to indicate 1/100

Mixed numbers

Mixed numbers are numbers which combine whole numbers with fractions:

$$1\tfrac{1}{2}, 2\tfrac{7}{8}, 10\tfrac{5}{6}, \text{etc.}$$

numerator the top or left number in a fraction that indicates a portion of the denominator to be used.

denominator the bottom or right number in a fraction which is divided into the numerator to give the fraction's value.

Decimals

Decimals are fractions with denominators in measures of ten, but which are expressed in a different form than the fraction. They use a **decimal point** (.) to indicate amounts less than one. Each position to the right of the decimal indicates the tenths, hundredths, thousandths, etc., that it represents:

0.1	=	one tenth
0.01	=	one hundredth
0.001	=	one thousandth.
0.0001	=	one ten-thousandth
etc.		

Percentages

Percent means by the hundred or in a hundred. Percentages are fractions in which the denominator is always 100 but which are expressed in a different form than the fraction. The **percent symbol (%)** is used to indicate percentages. It means: "out of one hundred units."

EXAMPLE:

50% means 50 units out of 100 units , or $\frac{50}{100}$, or 1/2

EXAMPLE:

$$\frac{50}{100} = 50\% \qquad \frac{25}{100} = 25\%$$

$$\frac{10}{100} = 10\% \qquad \frac{12.5}{100} = 12.5\%*$$

Note that decimals can also be combined with percentages.

Converting Numbers

Converting one number form to another is a routine element in pharmacy calculations. Solutions are given in percents. Calculators use decimals. Technicians must be competent at converting number forms.

EXAMPLE:

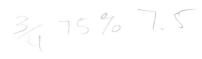

$$\frac{1}{2} = 50\% = 0.5$$

$$1 = \frac{4}{4} = 100\% = 1.0$$

$$1 = \frac{6}{4} = 150\% = 1.5$$

NUMBERS (cont'd)

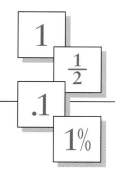

ROMAN NUMERALS

Roman numerals are letters that represent numbers. They were originally developed and used by the Roman Empire. Though arabic numbers are the primary ones used in pharmacy, Roman numerals are often used to indicate quantities in prescription or order writing. They can be capital or lower case letters, and are:

ss = $\frac{1}{2}$	L or l = 50
I or i = 1	C or c = 100
V or v = 5	D or d = 500
X or x = 10	M or m = 1000

When grouped together, these few letters can express a large range of numbers, using a simple *positional notation.* That means the position of the letters has a mathematical importance, as determined by these rules:

When the second of two letters has a value equal to or smaller than that of the first, their values are to be added.

EXAMPLE:

xx = 20	or	10 plus 10
dc = 600	or	500 plus 100
lxvi = 66	or	50 plus 10 plus 5 plus 1

When the second of two letters has a value greater than that of the first, the smaller is to be subtracted from the larger.

EXAMPLE:

iv = 4	or	1 subtracted from 5
xxxix = 39	or	30 plus (1 subtracted from 10)
xc = 90	or	10 subtracted from 100

— I V X L C D M —

positional notation the position of the number carries a mathematical significance or value.

PRACTICE PROBLEMS — CONVERTING NUMBERS

Convert these numbers to decimals:

a. $1\frac{1}{2}$ *1.5*
b. 15% *0.15*
c. $\frac{10}{100}$ *0.01*
d. $\frac{4}{4}$ *1.0*
e. 81% *0.81*
f. $\frac{6}{4}$ *1.5*
g. 6.5% *.065*

Convert these numbers to percents:

h. 1.21 *121%*
i. $\frac{6}{4}$ *150*
j. .07 *7%*
k. $\frac{6}{8}$ *75%*
l. .115 *11.5*
m. $\frac{10}{100}$ *10%*
n. .026 *2.6*

PRACTICE PROBLEMS — ROMAN NUMERALS

Write the following in Roman numerals:

a. 18 *XVIII*
b. 64 *LXIV*
c. 72 *LXXII*
d. 126 *CXXVI*
e. 100 *C*
f. 7 *VII*
g. 28 *XXVIII*

Write the following in arabic numbers:

h. xxxiii *33*
i. CX *110*
j. mc *1,100*
k. iss *1½*
l. XIX *19*
m. xxiv *24*

Interpret the quantity in each of these phrases taken from prescriptions:

n. Caps. no. xiv. *14 capsules*
o. Gtts. M. *1000 drops*
p. Tabs. no. XLVIII. *48 tabs*
q. Tabs. no. xxi *21 tabs*

 Answers for these problems can be found at the end of the text.

MEASUREMENT

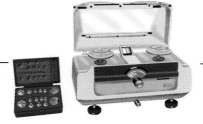

There are different systems of measurement used in pharmacy: metric, English, apothecary, and avoirdupois.

The metric system is the primary system used. Within these systems there are different measurements for weight, volume, and length, as well as for liquids and solids. It is necessary to know how to convert one type of measurement to another. There are also different measurement systems for temperature.

METRIC SYSTEM

The major system of weights and measures used in medicine is the metric system. It was developed in France in the late 18th century and is based on a decimal system. That is, **different measurement units are related by measures of ten.** Technicians need to know metric measures for both liquids and solids.

Liquids

Liquids (including lotions) are measured by **volume.** The most widely used metric volume measurements are liters or milliliters.

Unit	Symbol	Liquid Conversions
liter	L	1L = 10dl = 1000ml
deciliter	dl	1dl = 0.1L = 100ml
milliliter	ml	1ml = 0.001L = 0.01dl

Note: deciliters are rarely used in pharmacy, but are included here for reference and to illustrate the decimal relationship of these measures.

Solids

Solids (pills, granules, ointments, etc.) are measured by **weight.**

Unit	Symbol	Solid Conversions
kilogram	kg	1 kg = 1,000 g
gram	g	1 g = 0.001 kg = 1000 mg
milligram	mg	1 mg = 0.001 g = 1000 mcg
microgram	mcg or μg	1 mcg = 0.001 mg = 0.000001 g

 Milliliters are sometimes referred to as *cubic centimeters (cc)*. They are not precisely the same but are quite close and are sometimes used interchangeably. Milliliter is the preferred usage for pharmacy.

AVOIRDUPOIS SYSTEM

The Avoirdupois system is the system of weight (ounces and pounds) that we commonly use. However, one Avoirdupois unit used in pharmacy is rarely used elsewhere. It is the **grain.**

Unit	symbol	Conversions
pound	lb	1 lb = 16 oz
ounce	oz	1 oz = 437.5 gr
grain	gr	1 gr = 64.8 mg

64.8
64.8
129.6

THE GRAIN

The grain is the same weight in several different measurement systems: Apothecary, Avoirdupois, and Troy. It is said to have been established as a unit of weight in 1266 by King Henry III of England when he required the English penny to weigh the equivalent of 32 dried grains of wheat. On the metric scale, one grain equals 64.8 milligrams. However, this is often rounded to 65 milligrams and sometimes to 60 milligrams.

APOTHECARY SYSTEM

The Apothecary system is sometimes used in prescriptions, primarily with liquids. It includes the fluid ounce, pint, quart, and gallon. Although there are Apothecary weight units, they are generally not used, with the exception of the grain. The fluid ounce is a volume measure and is different than the weight ounce. It is always indicated by "fl oz."

Unit	symbol	Conversions
gallon	gal	1 gal = 4 qt
quart	qt	1 qt = 2 pt
pint	pt	1 pt = 16 fl oz
ounce	fl oz	1 fl oz = 8 fl dr
fluid dram	fl dr	1 fl dr = 60 min
minim	min or M_x	

Note: drams and minims are generally not used in pharmacy today, but are included here for reference.

 conversions the change of one unit of measure into another so that both amounts are equal.

MEASUREMENT (cont'd)

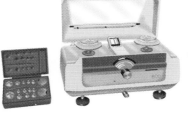

HOUSEHOLD UNITS

The teaspoon and tablespoon are common household measurement units that are regularly used in liquid prescriptions.

Unit	symbol	Conversions
teaspoon	tsp	1tsp = 5ml
tablespoon	tbs	1tbs = 3 tsp = 15ml
cup	cup	1 cup = 8 fl oz

TEMPERATURE

The **Centigrade** scale, which is also called **Celsius**, is used to measure temperature. The relationship of Centigrade (C) to Fahrenheit (F) is:

F temperature = ($1\frac{4}{5}$ times number of degrees C) + 32

EXAMPLE $212°F = 100°C$

because a) $1\frac{4}{5}$ x 100 = 180

and b) 180 + 32 = 212

C temperature = $\frac{5}{9}$ x (number of degrees F - 32)

EXAMPLE $100°C = 212°F$

because $\frac{5}{9}$ x (212-32) = $\frac{5}{9}$ x 180 = 100

Note that the temperature of water freezing is 0°C and 32°F.

CONVERSIONS

Conversions are the change of one unit of measure into another so that both amounts are equal. Following are some commonly used unit conversions.

1 L	=	33.8 fl oz	1 lb	=	453.59 g
1 pt	=	473.167 ml	1 oz	=	28.35 g
1 fl oz	=	29.57ml	1 g	=	15.43 gr
1 kg	=	2.2 lb	1 gr	=	64.8 mg

PRACTICE PROBLEMS — METRICS

Provide the abbreviation for these:

a. microgram   _Mcg_

b. Liter   _L_

c. milliliter   _ml_

d. gram   _g_

e. milligram   _mg_

f. kilogram   _Kg_

Convert these units to equivalents:

g. 1 Kg = _1,000_ g

h. 1 mg = _1000_ mcg

i. 2 gr = _130_ mg

j. 1 L   = _1000_ ml

k. 1 ml = _.001_ L

l. 1 mg = _.01_ g

PRACTICE PROBLEMS — CONVERSIONS

Convert these numbers using the conversions provided on the preceding pages as well as your knowledge of decimals:

m. 7 mg   = _7,000_ mcg

n. 3.2 g = _____ mg

o. 1 gr   = _____ g

p. 2 tbs = _____ ml

q. 0.3 L = _____ ml

r. 7 kg   = _____ g

s. 1 oz   = _____ gr

t. 0.5 kg = _____ lb

u. 10 ml = _____ tsp

v. 15 ml = _____ tbs

w. 0°C   = _____ °F

x. 250 ml = _____ L

CALCULATION SPACE

 Answers for these problems can be found at the end of the text.

EQUATIONS & VARIABLES

EQUATIONS AND VARIABLES

In the calculations of Pharmacy related problems there is often an **unknown value** that needs to be determined. To solve the unknown value involves setting up a mathematical statement between the known amounts and the unknown. This statement is called an equation. The unknown fact in an equation is called a **variable.** The variable is often indicated by the letter, x.

> **An equation is a mathematical statement in which two terms are equal.**

Equations use the equal sign (=) to indicate equivalence. The following are equations:

$$1 = \tfrac{1}{2} + \tfrac{1}{2}$$
$$1 = \tfrac{1}{2} \times 2$$

EXAMPLE

You have a prescription for 120ml of Theophylline liquid and want to know how many fluid ounces is equal to 120ml. In this case, the number of ounces is the variable x that you want to determine. Since there are 29.57 ml in each fluid ounce, one way to state this problem mathematically is the following equation:

x fl oz = (total prescribed ml) ÷ (ml/fl oz conversion rate)

or

$$x \text{ fl oz} = \frac{\text{total prescribed ml}}{\text{ml/fl oz conversion rate}}$$

$$x \text{ fl oz} = \frac{120 \text{ ml}}{29.57 \text{ ml}}$$

x fl oz = 4 (approximately)

variable an unknown value in a mathematical equation.

EXAMPLE—FILLING A CAPSULE PRESCRIPTION

You have a prescription for amoxicillin 250mg, one capsule orally, three times a day for seven days. You want to know how many doses will be needed to fill this prescription. In this case doses needed is the unknown fact or variable that you are trying to solve for.

x (doses needed) = (capsules per dose) x (doses per day) x (days)

x = (1 capsule) x (3 per day) x (7 days)

x = 21

You need 21 capsules of Amoxicillin 250mg to fill the prescription.

EXAMPLE—INTRAVENOUS SOLUTION

You are preparing an Intravenous solution (IV) that requires the addition of Potassium Chloride (KCl). You have a vial of KCl containing a concentration of 20 mEq per 10ml. How many mls of this solution should you add to the IV if the Iv should have a total of 45 mEq of KCl in it? This is made easier by first solving for the number of KCl per ml:

20 mEq divided by 10ml = 2 mEq per ml

x (mls of KCl solution) = KCl needed ÷ KCl per ml

x = (45 mEq)÷ (2mEq)

x = 22.5

You need 22.5mls of KCl solution to the IV.

RATIO & PROPORTION

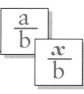

RATIO AND PROPORTION

For pharmacy technicians, perhaps the most important mathematical concepts are *ratio* and *proportion*. If you understand these concepts, you will be able to perform most of the mathematics necessary for your job.

Ratio

A ratio states **a relationship between two quantities**. The ratio of a to b can be stated as:

$$\frac{a}{b}$$

Proportion

Two equal ratios form a proportion: $\frac{a}{b} = \frac{c}{d}$

EXAMPLE

An example of this is the equation: $\frac{1}{2} = \frac{2}{4}$

$\frac{1}{2}$ and $\frac{2}{4}$ are equivalent ratios. 1 has the same relationship to 2 as 2 has to 4. Therefore, the equation is a proportion.

EXAMPLE

If one person had a box containing 5 apples and another has 3 boxes each containing 5 apples, while one may have a lot more apples than the other, they both have the same proportion of apples to boxes.

$$\frac{5 \text{ apples}}{1 \text{ box}} = \frac{15 \text{ apples}}{3 \text{ boxes}}$$

Each person has fives times as many apples as boxes. The ratios are equivalent.

EXAMPLE

A solution of 5g of a substance in 100 ml of water is equivalent to 50 g of the same substance in 1000 ml of water.

$$\frac{5g}{100ml} = \frac{50g}{1000ml}$$

Both numerators can be divided into their denominators twenty times. Therefore, the ratios are equivalent.

Solving Ratio and Proportion Problems

In a proportion equation, all four terms are related to each other and the relationship of each term to the others can be stated in different ways:

➤ $\dfrac{a}{b} = \dfrac{c}{d}$ *can be stated as* $\dfrac{b}{a} = \dfrac{d}{c}$

You can also state the equation for any one term by multiplying both sides of the equation by one of the other terms. For example:

➤ $b \times \dfrac{a}{b} = b \times \dfrac{c}{d}$ ➤ $\not{b} \times \dfrac{a}{\not{b}} = b \times \dfrac{c}{d}$

➥ *cancel out equal values*

➤ $a = \dfrac{bc}{d}$

These are also true: $b = \dfrac{ad}{c}$ $c = \dfrac{ad}{b}$ $d = \dfrac{bc}{a}$

Therefore, if three of the four terms in a proportion problem are known, an unknown fourth term (*x*) can also be calculated.

EXAMPLE

When you know the values of three of the four terms in a proportion equation, the unknown term is indicated by *x*, and the proportion equation can be written as:

$\dfrac{x}{b} = \dfrac{c}{d}$ ➡ *ratio you want = ratio you have*

Multiplying both sides of the equation by the value of b will then establish the relationship of the known terms to *x*.

$b \text{ times } \left(\dfrac{x}{b}\right) = b \text{ times } \left(\dfrac{c}{d}\right)$

⬇

$\not{b} \text{ times } \dfrac{x}{\not{b}} = b \text{ times } \dfrac{c}{d}$ ➤ $x = \dfrac{bc}{d}$

➥ *cancel out equal values*

You can then solve for the value of *x* by simple multiplication and division of the known values of b, c, and d.

x = (b times c) divided by d

RATIO & PROPORTION

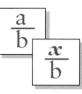

EXAMPLE

In one basket a farmer has four oranges. If every basket he has contains the same number of oranges, how many oranges does the farmer have in six baskets?

Steps

1. Define the variable and the correct ratios.

    a. define the unknown variable ➡ x (total oranges)

    b. establish the known ratio ➡ 4 oranges/1 basket

    c. establish the unknown ratio ➡ x oranges/6 baskets

2. Set up the proportion equation $\left(\frac{x}{b} = \frac{c}{d}\right)$.

$$\frac{x \text{ oranges}}{6 \text{ baskets}} = \frac{4 \text{ oranges}}{1 \text{ basket}}$$

Note that the units must the same in both the numerator and denominator:

        numerator: oranges
        denominator: baskets

3. Establish the x equation.

$$6 \text{ baskets times } \frac{x \text{ oranges}}{6 \text{ baskets}} = 6 \text{ baskets times } \frac{4 \text{ oranges}}{1 \text{ basket}}$$

$$6 \text{ baskets times } \frac{x \text{ oranges}}{6 \text{ baskets}} = 6 \text{ baskets times } \frac{4 \text{ oranges}}{1 \text{ basket}}$$

➡ *cancel out equal values and units*

$$x \text{ oranges } = 6 \text{ times } 4 \text{ oranges}$$

4. Solve for x.

$$x \text{ oranges } = 24 \text{ oranges}$$

5. Express solution in correct units.

There are **24 oranges** in the farmer's six baskets.

CONDITIONS FOR USING RATIO AND PROPORTION

1. Three of the four values must be known.

2. Numerators must have the same units.

3. Denominators must have the same units.

EXAMPLE—A PRESCRIPTION FOR TABLETS.

You receive a prescription for Zoloft® 100mg po BID x 30 days. How many tablets are needed to fill this prescription correctly?

Steps

1. Define the variable and correct ratios.

    a. define the unknown variable ➡ x = total tablets needed

    b. establish the known ratio ➡ 2 tablets / 1 day

    c. establish the unknown ratio ➡ x tablets / 30 days

2. Set-up the proportion equation.

$$\frac{x \text{ tablets}}{30 \text{ days}} = \frac{2 \text{ tablets}}{1 \text{ day}}$$

3. Establish the x equation.

$$x \text{ tablets} = 30 \text{ days times } \frac{2 \text{ tablets}}{1 \text{ day}}$$

4. Solve for x.

$$x \text{ tablets} = 30 \cancel{\text{ days}} \text{ times } \frac{2 \text{ tablets}}{1 \cancel{\text{ day}}} = 60 \text{ tablets}$$

$$x \text{ tablets} = 60 \text{ tablets}$$

5. Express solution in correct units.

60 tablets of Zoloft® 100mg are needed to fill the prescription.

RATIO & PROPORTION

$$\frac{a}{b}$$
$$\frac{x}{b}$$

EXAMPLE—A LIQUID PRESCRIPTION

You receive a prescription for Amoxicillin 75mg four times a day for ten days. You have available Amoxicillin 250 mg/5 ml 150 ml.

A. What is the correct individual dose?

1. Define the variable and correct ratios.

    a. define the unknown variable ➡ x = ml per dose

    b. establish the known ratio ➡ 5 ml / 250 mg

    c. establish the unknown ratio ➡ $x$ml / 75 mg

2. Set-up the proportion equation.

    x ml / 75 mg = 5 ml / 250 mg

3. Establish the x equation

    x ml = 75 mg times $\dfrac{5 \text{ ml}}{250 \text{ mg}}$

4. Solve.

    x ml = 75 ~~mg~~ times $\dfrac{5 \text{ ml}}{250 \text{ ~~mg~~}}$ = $\dfrac{375 \text{ ml}}{250}$ = 1.5 ml

5. Express solution in correct units.

    The dose is 1.5 ml of amoxicillin.

B. Now, how many mls of amoxicillin do you need to fill this prescription so it will last for ten full days? A simple equation can determine this. Note that it is often useful to state the equation first in words, and then restate it in numbers. Using words to describe mathematical operations helps you to visualize and better understand the mathematics involved.

Word Equation:

amount needed = (dose amount) x (doses per day) x (number of days)

    Amoxicillin needed = 1.5 ml times 4 times 10 = 60 ml

EXAMPLE—A MIXTURE DOSE

If a diarrhea mixture contains 3 ml of Paregoric in each 30 ml of mixture, how many mls of Paregoric would be contained in a teaspoonful dose of mixture?

conversion: 1 tsp = 5 ml

1. Define the variable and correct ratios.

    a.   define the unknown variable   ➡ x ml of Paregoric

    b.   establish the known ratio   ➡ 3 ml / 30 ml (mix)

    c.   establish the unknown ratio   ➡ x ml/5 ml (mix)

2. Set-up the proportion equation

x ml/ 5 ml = 3 ml / 30 ml

3. Establish the x equation

x ml= 5 ml times $\dfrac{3\ ml}{30\ ml}$

4. Solve.

x ml= 5 ~~ml~~ times $\dfrac{3\ ml}{30\ \cancel{ml}} = \dfrac{15\ ml}{30} = .5\ ml$

5. Express solution in correct units.

There are 0.5 ml of paregoric in a teaspoon.

USING CALCULATORS

Though most of these examples can be solved without the use of a calculator, the use of calculators is essential in the correct computation of many dosage calculations. Their answers are precise and provided in decimals. Since it is relatively easy to make entry mistakes on a calculator, always recheck answers. Also, use judgment. If an answer doesn't appear to make sense, check it.

RATIO & PROPORTION

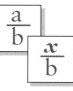

EXAMPLE—IV FLOW RATE

In the pharmacy setting, you may be asked to provide information on flow rate or **rate of administration** for an IV solution. Flow rates are calculated using ratio and proportion equations. They are generally done in ml/hour, but for pumps used to dispense IV fluids to the patient, the calculation may need to be done in ml/min.

For example, if you have an order for KCl 10mEq and K Acetate 15 mEq in D5W 1000 ml to run at 80 ml/hour, you would determine the administration rate in ml/minute as follows:

1. Define the variable and correct ratios.

    a. define the unknown variable ➡ *x* = ml

    b. establish the known ratio   ➡ 80 ml / 60 min

    c. establish the unknown ratio ➡ *x* ml/ 1 min

2. Set-up the proportion equation

    x ml / 1 min = 80 ml / 60 min

3. Establish the x equation

$$x \text{ ml} = 1 \text{ min times } \frac{80 \text{ ml}}{60 \text{ min}}$$

4. Factor and solve.

$$x \text{ ml} = 1 \cancel{\text{min}} \text{ times } \frac{80 \text{ ml}}{60 \cancel{\text{min}}} = 1.33 \text{ ml}$$

➡ *80 divided by 60 = 1.33*

5. Express solution in correct units.

The flow rate would be 1.33 ml/minute.

Note: IV Flow Rate calculations may involve *drops per ml* or *drops per minute* or involve calculating the amount of time before an IV bag will empty and require replacement. Using simple ratio and proportion equations will solve these problems.

STEPS FOR SOLVING PROPORTION PROBLEMS
1. Define the variable and correct ratios.
2. Set-up the proportion equation
3. Establish the x equation
4. Solve for x.
5. Express solution in correct units.

PRACTICE PROBLEMS — RATIO AND PROPORTION

Use the space below the problem (and the rules you've learned from the preceding pages) to work out the answer.

a. A prescription calls for 100 mg of a drug that you have in a 250mg/5ml concentration. How many ml of the liquid do you need? *2.0mL*

$x = ml$
$5ml/250mg,$
$xml/100mg.$

$xml/100mg = 5mL/250mg.$
$xml = 100mg \times \frac{5mL}{250mg.}$

$\frac{500\ mL}{250}$

b. A prescription calls for 400 mg of a drug that you have in a 50mg/ml concentration. How many ml of the liquid do you need? *8mL*

$\frac{xml}{400} \times \frac{5}{500}$

$x = mL = 500mg \times 400mg$

c. A prescription calls for 10 mg of a drug that you have in a 2mg/15ml concentration. How many ml of the liquid do you need? *75mL*

$2mg/15mL$
$XmL/10mg$

$10mg \times 15mL$

$\frac{150}{2}$

d. KCl 10 mEq and K Acetate 15mEq in D5W 1000 ml is ordered to be administered over 8 hours. What would the rate be in ml/min? *2.08ml/mn*

15 *480*

e. A prescription calls for 0.24mg of a drug that you have in a 50mcg/ml concentration. How many ml of the liquid do you need?

50mcg/ml *.24 ÷ 50* *4.8.ml*

R̥ *Answers for these problems can be found at the end of the text.*

PERCENTS & SOLUTIONS

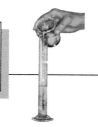

%

PERCENTS & SOLUTIONS

Percents are used to indicate the amount or **concentration** of something in a solution. Concentrations are indicated in terms of weight to volume or volume to volume.

Weight to Volume: grams per 100 milliliters ➡ **g/ml**

Volume to Volume: milliliters per 100 milliliters ➡ **ml/ml**

EXAMPLE—IV SOLUTION

If there is 50% dextrose in a 1000 ml IV bag, how many grams of dextrose are there in the bag? You can solve this by developing a proportion equation. Since 50% dextrose means there are 50 grams of dextrose in 100 ml, the equation would be:

x g divided by 1000 ml = 50 g divided by 100 ml

The x equation:

$$x \text{ g} = 1000 \text{ ml times } \frac{50 \text{ g}}{100 \text{ ml}} = 10 \text{ times } 50 \text{ g} = 500 \text{ g}$$

➡ *1000 divided by 100 = 10*

Answer: There are 500 grams of dextrose in the bag.

Another way to solve this is to **convert the percent to a decimal.** In a 50% solution, there are .5 g per ml:

50 g/100 ml = .5 g/ml

You can then multiply .5g by the total number of milliliters.

x = .5g times 1000 = 500 g

Now how many mls will give you a 10 grams of Dextrose?

The proportion equation:

x ml/10 g = 100 ml /50 g

The x equation:

$$x \text{ ml} = 10 \text{ g times } \frac{100 \text{ ml}}{50 \text{ g}} = \frac{1000 \text{ ml}}{50} = 20 \text{ ml}$$

Answer: 20 mls of 50% solution contain 10 grams of dextrose.

concentration the strength of a solution as measured by the weight-to-volume or volume-to-volume of the substance being measured.

PRACTICE PROBLEMS — PERCENTS

Convert the following fractions to percents:

    a. 60/100 = _____ %

    b. 80/100 = _____ %

    c. 12/100 = _____ %

Convert the following percents to decimals:

    d. 50% = _____

    e. 12.5% = _____

    f. 99% = _____

You have a 70% dextrose solution. How many grams in:

    g. 50 ml of solution

    h. 75ml of solution

    i. 20 ml of solution

You have a 50% dextrose solution, how many mls will give you:

    j. 25 g of dextrose

    k. 35 g

    l. 10 g

    m. You have a liquid that contains 12 mg /10 ml. What is the percent of this liquid? To solve, you will need to convert mg to g per 100ml using decimals.

℞ *Answers for these problems can be found at the end of the text.*

PERCENTS & SOLUTIONS

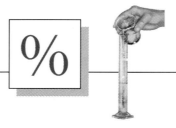

A PERCENT SOLUTION FORMULA

It is possible to set up a proportion equation specifically to convert concentrations that will be a handy tool in in converting concentrations during the preparation of **hyperalimentation** or **TPNs.**

$$\frac{x \text{ volume needed}}{\text{want \%}} = \frac{\text{volume prescribed}}{\text{have \%}}$$

EXAMPLE—A DILUTION

The physician wants a 35% solution of dextrose 1000ml. You have a 50% solution of dextrose 1000ml. How will you make up what the physician wants ?

The terms for the formula are:

volume needed	➡ x ml
want %	➡ 35% dextrose
volume prescribed	➡ 1000ml
have %	➡ 50% dextrose

The formula is:

x ml / 35% = 1000 ml / 50%

The x equation is:

$$x \text{ ml} = 35\% \text{ times } \frac{1000 \text{ ml}}{50\%} = 35 \text{ times } 20 \text{ ml} = \textbf{700 ml}$$

➡ *1000 divided by 50 = 20*

700 ml of dextrose 1000 ml will give you the 350 g of dextrose you will need in your solution. However, you will still need to add sterile water qsad until you have a total solution of 1000 ml as ordered by the physician. (qsad means quantity needed to make total volume).

Total Volume	1000 ml
Dextrose 50% Solution	-700 ml
Sterile Water (qsad)	300 ml

Answer: You need to add 300 ml of sterile water to 700 ml of 50% dextrose to create 1000 ml of 35%dextrose.

qsad the quantity needed to make a prescribed amount.

milliequivalent (mEq) the unit of measure for electrolytes in a solution.

MILLIEQUIVALENT—mEq

Electrolyte solutions are often used in hospitals. Electrolytes are substances which conduct an electrical current and are found in the body's blood, tissue fluids, and cells. Salts are electrolytes and saline solutions are a commonly used electrolyte solution.

The concentration of electrolytes in a volume of solution is measured in units called milliequivalents (mEq). They are expressed as milliequivalents per milliliter or milliequivalents per Liter.

Milliequivalents are a specific unit of measurement that cannot be converted into the metric system. A .9% solution of one electrolyte will have a different mEq value than a .9% solution of another because mEq values are different for different electrolytes. They are based on each electrolyte's atomic weight and electron properties.

If the mEq value of a solution is known, it is relatively easy to mix it with other solutions to get a different mEq volume ratio by using proportions.

EXAMPLE

A solution calls for 5 mEq of an electrolyte that you have in a 1.04 mEq / ml solution. How many ml of it do you need?

x ml/ 5 mEq = 1 ml/1.04 mEq

x ml = 5 ~~mEq~~ times $\dfrac{1 \text{ ml}}{1.04 \text{ ~~mEq~~}}$ = $\dfrac{5 \text{ ml}}{1.04}$ = 4.8ml

Answer: 4.8 ml of the solution is needed.

COMMON ELECTROLYTES:

NaCl	Sodium Chloride
MgSO4	Magnesium Sulfate
KCl	Potassium Chloride
K Acetate	Potassium Acetate
Ca Gluconate	Calcium Gluconate
Na Acetate	Sodium Acetate

 In order to calculate mEq for an electrolyte, the atomic weight and valence of the electrolyte must first be known. The weight is then divided by the valence.

PERCENTS & SOLUTIONS

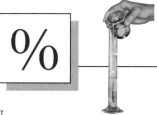

$$\boxed{\%}$$

EXAMPLE—TOTAL PARENTERAL NUTRITION

A TPN order calls for the amounts on the left (including additives) to be made from the items on the right. The total volume is to be 1000 ml. How much of each ingredient do you need to prepare this TPN ?

TPN Order	On Hand
Aminosyn 4.25%	Aminosyn 8.5% 1000 ml
Dextrose 25%	Dextrose 70% 1000 ml

Additives:

KCl 20 mEq	KCl 2mEq / ml 10 ml
MVI 10 ml	MVI 10 ml
NaCl 24 mEq	NaCl 4.4mEq / ml 20 ml

Aminosyn

Using Percent Solutions Formula:

x ml / 4.25% = 1000 ml / 8.5%

x ml = 4.25% times $\dfrac{1000\ ml}{8.5\%}$ = 1000 ml times .5

➥ *4.25 divided by 8.5 = .5*

x ml = 500 ml

500 ml of aminosyn 8.5% is needed.

Dextrose

Using Percent Solutions Formula:

x ml/ 25% = 1000 ml / 70%

x ml = 25% times $\dfrac{1000\ ml}{70\%}$ = $\dfrac{25000\ ml}{70}$

x ml = 357.14 ml dextrose ➡ 357 ml

357 ml of dextrose 70% is needed.

Note: Generally, amounts less than half are rounded down and amounts greater than half are rounded up. However, some drugs may be rounded and others may not. You will need to know when you must be precise and when you may round for each drug.

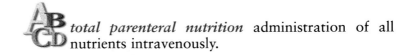

KCl

Use a proportion equation:

x ml / 20mEq = 1 ml/ 2 mEq

x ml = 20 ~~mEq~~ times $\dfrac{1\ ml}{2\ \text{mEq}}$ = 10 ml KCl

10 ml KCl are needed.

MVI

Add the 10 ml MVI on hand.

NaCl

Use a proportion equation:

x ml / 24 mEq = 1 ml / 4.4 mEq

x ml = 24 ~~mEq~~ times $\dfrac{1\ ml}{4.4\ \text{mEq}}$ = 5.45 ml

5.45 ml of NaCl is needed.

Sterile Water

Add as needed (qsad) for a volume of 1000 ml.

Word Equation:

water needed = 1000 ml minus (other ingredients)

Other ingredients:

Aminosyn	500 ml
Dextrose	357 ml
KCl	10 ml
MVI	10 ml
NaCl	5.45 ml
total	882.45 ml

water needed = 1000 minus 882.45 = 117.55

117.55 ml sterile water is needed to fill the TPN order.

PERCENTS & SOLUTIONS

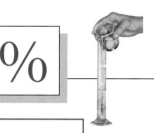

%

PERCENT SOLUTION FORMULA

$$\frac{x \text{ volume needed}}{\text{want } \%} = \frac{\text{volume prescribed}}{\text{have } \%}$$

PRACTICE PROBLEM

A TPN order calls for the amounts on the left (including additives) to be made from the items on the right. The total volume is to be 250 ml. How much of each ingredient do you need to prepare this TPN ?

TPN Order	**What you have**
Aminosyn 2.5%	Aminosyn 8.5% 500 ml
Dextrose 7. 5%	Dextrose 50% 1000 ml

Additives:

Kcl 4mEq	Kcl 2mEq/ml 10 ml
Ca Gluconate 2 mEq	Ca Gluconate 4.4mEq/ml 25 ml
Ped MVI 5 ml	Ped MVI 10 ml

Use the space to work out the answers.

    a. Aminosyn 8.5%   Answer: _____ ml

    b. Dextrose 50%   Answer:_____ ml

c. KCl 2mEq/ml   Answer: _____ ml

d. Ca Gluconate 4.4mEq/ml   Answer: _____ ml

e. Pediatric MVI 10ml   Answer: _____ ml

f. Sterile Water (qsad)   Answer: _____ ml

Answers for these problems can be found at the end of the text.

CHILDREN'S DOSES

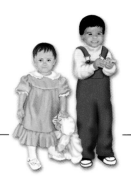

CALCULATION OF CHILDREN'S DOSES

The average doses in the U.S.P. (United States Pharmacopeia) and other drug reference sources are for adults. Doses for drugs that can be taken by a child are generally not given. When they are not, the adult dose needs to be lowered. One formula for this is:

CLARK'S RULE

$$\frac{\text{weight of child}}{\text{150 lb}} \times \text{adult dose} = \text{dose for child}$$

150 lbs is considered an average weight for an adult. This is not a very precise way to calculate pediatric doses as there are many factors besides weight which may need to be taken into account: height, age, condition, etc. Another approach is based upon multiplying the adult dose by a ratio of the child's size to that of an average adult:

BODY SURFACE AREA FORMULA

$$\frac{\text{child bsa times adult dose}}{\text{average adult bsa}} = \text{child's dose}$$

The **body surface area** of a person is based on the person's height and weight. It is always given in square meters (m²). 1.73 m² is commonly used as an average bsa for adults. A chart called a **nomogram** has been traditionally used to manually calculate bsa. Body surface area nomograms contain three columns of numbers: height, body surface, and weight. The bsa is identified by the intersection of a line drawn between the weight and height columns with the bsa column, which is in the middle. Now, bsa formulas are generally solved by computer. (There are a number that can be found on the Internet, for example.) For a comparison to the average bsa for adults (1.73 m²), a bsa for a nine year old child that was 44" tall and weighing 50 lbs would be about .92 m².

Because of the many variables, however, conversion formulas for pediatric doses are rarely used in the pharmacy. **Doses are generally given by the physician.** Children's doses are stated by kg of body weight (dose/kg). Since 1 kg = 2.2 lb, you can solve for the prescribed dose by using a proportion equation if you know the child's body weight. See the example at right.

body surface area a measure used for dosage that is calculated from the height and weight of a person and measured in square meters.

nomogram a chart showing relationships between measurements.

EXAMPLE—INFANT DOSE

An Antibiotic IV is prescribed for an infant. The dose is to be 15mg/kg twice a day. The baby weighs 12 lbs. How much drug is to be given for one dose? First you need to calculate the infant's weight in kilograms.

x kg / 12 lb = 1 kg / 2.2 lb

x kg = 12 l̶b̶ times $\dfrac{1\ kg}{2.2\ \text{l̶b̶}}$ = $\dfrac{12\ kg}{2.2}$ = 5.45 kg

You can also easily solve this with a calculator:

➡ enter   12
➡ press   divide (/) key
➡ enter   2.2
➡ press   equal (=) key
➡ answer   5.45

You can solve the next part of this problem with a proportion equation or you can set up a simple word equation.

one dose = (amount of drug) times (number of kg of infant weight)

one dose = 15 mg times 5.45

With a calculator:

➡ enter   15
➡ press   multiplication (*) key
➡ enter   5.45
➡ press   equal (=) key
➡ answer   81.75 mg

REVIEW

ROMAN NUMERALS

When the second of two letters has a value equal to or smaller than that of the first, their values are to be added.

When the second of two letters has a value equal to or smaller than that of the first, their values are to be added.

CONDITIONS FOR USING RATIO AND PROPORTION

1. Three of the four values must be known.

2. Numerators must have the same units.

3. Denominators must have the same units.

STEPS FOR SOLVING PROPORTION PROBLEMS

1. Define the variable and correct ratios.

2. Set-up the proportion equation

3. Establish the x equation

4. Solve for x.

5. Express solution in correct units.

PERCENT SOLUTION FORMULA

$$\frac{x \text{ volume needed}}{\text{want \%}} = \frac{\text{volume prescribed}}{\text{have \%}}$$

CONVERSIONS

Liquid Metric

1L	=	10dl	=	1000ml
1dl	=	.1L	=	100ml
1ml	=	.001L	=	.01dl

Solid Metric

1 kg	=	1,000 g		
1 g	=	.001 kg	=	1,000 mg
1mg	=	.001 g	=	1,000 mcg
1 mcg	=	.001 mg		

Avoirdupois

1 lb	=	16 oz
1 oz	=	437.5 gr
1 gr	=	64.8 mg (.00648 g)

Apothecary

1 gal	=	4 qt
1 qt	=	2 pt
1 pt	=	16 fl oz
1 fl oz	=	8 fl dr
1 fl dr	=	60 m

Household

1tsp	=	5ml	
1tbs	=	3 tsp	= 15ml
1 cup	=	8 fl oz	

Temperature

F temperature $= (1\frac{4}{5}$ times number of degrees C) + 32

C temperature $= \frac{5}{9}$ x (number of degrees F - 32)

Conversions Between Systems

1 L	=	33.8 fl oz	1 lb	=	453.59 g
1 pt	=	473.167 ml	1 oz	=	28.35 g
1 fl oz	=	29.57ml	1 g	=	15.43 gr
1 kg	=	2.2 lb	1 gr	=	64.8 mg

REVIEW

1. Convert the following:

A. 500 g   = _____ mg

B. 10 kg   = _____ g

C. 250 ml = _____ L

D. 325 mg = _____ g

E. 120 mcg = _____ mg

F. 102 kg = _____ lb

G. 3.56 kg = _____ g

H. 473ml   = _____ L

I. 145 lb = _____ kg

J. 30 kg   = _____ mg

2. Solve the following in the space beneath the problem:

Temperature Problem

K. Oral Polio Virus Vaccine (Poliovax®) should be stored in a temperature not to exceed 46 degrees Fahrenheit. What is this temperature in Centigrade?

Liquid Dose

L. A prescription reads for Erythromycin 150 mg every six hours for ten days. You have on hand Erythromycin 250 mg/5 ml. How much Erythromycin is needed for one dose?

Electrolyte Solution

M. You have an IV that needs MgS04 (Magnessium Sulfate) 10 mEq. You have on hand a bottle of MgS04 4 mEq/ml. How much MgS04 do you need to inject into this IV bag?

A Dilution

N. You have an order for 20% Dextrose 500ml. You have a 1000 ml bag of Dextrose 70%. How much of the Dextrose 70% do you need to use to make Dextrose 20% 500ml? How much sterile water do you need?

Rx *Answers for these problems can be found at the end of the text.*

REVIEW

3. Choose the correct answer:

O. A solution of Halperidol (Haldol®) contains 2 mg/ml of active ingredient. How many grams would be in 473 ml of this solution?

   a.) 9.46 grams
   b.) 0.946 grams
   c.) 0.0946 grams
   d.) 0.00946 grams

P. The physician orders Ferrous Sulfate 500 mg po qd x 30 days. You have on the shelf Ferrous Sulfate 220 mg/5 ml 473 ml. How many ml is required for one dose?

   a.) 5.4 ml
   b.) 8.4 ml
   c.) 11.4 ml
   d.) 13.4 ml

Q. Using the information from the previous problem, approximately how many ml are required to completely fill this prescription?

   a.) 162 ml
   b.) 252 ml
   c.) 342 ml
   d.) 402 ml

R. The infusion rate of an IV is over twelve hours. The total volume is 800 ml. What would the infusion rate be in ml per minute?

   a.) 66.6 ml / minute
   b.) 6.6 ml / minute
   c.) 0.6 ml / minute
   d.) none of the above

S. You have a 70% solution of Dextrose 1000 ml. How many Kg of Dextrose is in 400 ml of this solution?

   a.) 280 Kg
   b.) 28 Kg
   c.) 2.8 Kg
   d.) 0.28 Kg

T. You receive an order for Vancomycin (Vancocin®) 10 mg/Kg 500 ml to be infused over 90 minutes. The patient is five foot eleven inches tall and weighs 165 lb. What dose is needed for this patient?

a.) 750 mg
b.) 500 mg
c.) 250 mg
d.) 125 mg

U. The doctor orders Codeine gr $\frac{1}{4}$. How many milligrams is this equivalent to?

a.) 15 mg
b.) 30 mg
c.) 60 mg
d.) none of the above

V. You receive a prescription for Metronidazole (Flagyl®) 250 mg/5 ml po qid 240 ml. You find that you will have to compound this using 500 mg tablets. How many tablets will be needed to fill this order completely?

a.) 22 tablets
b.) 24 tablets
c.) 42 tablets
d.) 48 tablets

W. You are asked by the Pharmacist to add 45 mEq of Ca Gluconate in an IV bag of D5%W 1000 ml. You have a concentrated vial of Ca Gluconate 4.4 mEq/ml 50 ml. How many ml of this concentrated vial needs to be added to the IV bag?

a.) 1.2 ml
b.) 10.2 ml
c.) 0.12 ml
d.) 2.4 ml

ROUTES & FORMULATIONS

The way in which the body absorbs and distributes drugs varies with the route of administration.

Drugs are contained in products called **formulations**. There are many drug formulations and many different **routes** to administer them.

Routes are classified as enteral or parenteral.

Oral administration is called **enteral**. Enteral refers to anything involving the **alimentary** tract, i.e., from the mouth to the rectum. This tract is involved with digesting foods, absorbing nutrients, and eliminating unabsorbed wastes. There are three enteral routes: **oral, sublingual,** and **rectal**.

Any route other than oral, sublingual, and rectal is considered a parenteral administration route.

The term parenteral means next to, or beside the enteral. It refers to any sites that are outside of or beside the enteral or alimentary tract.

For each route, there are various formulations used to deliver the drug via that route.

Different dosage forms affect onset times, length of action, or concentrations of a drug in the body. Some drugs are formulated in more than one dosage form with each form producing different characteristics in these areas. A consideration for selecting a particular route or dosage form the type of effect desired. A **local effect** occurs when the drug activity is at the site of administration (e.g., eyes, ears, nose, skin). A **systemic effect** occurs when the drug is introduced into the circulatory system by any route of administration and carried to the site of activity.

Route	Dosage Form
Subcutaneous	Solutions
	Suspensions
	Emulsions
	Implants
Vaginal	Solutions
	Ointments
	Creams
	Aerosol foams
	Powders
	Suppositories
	Tablets
	Sponge
	IUDs

FORMULATIONS

Route	Dosage Form
Oral	Tablets
	Capsules
	Bulk Powders
	Solutions
	Suspensions
	Elixirs
	Syrups
Sublingual	Tablets
Rectal	Solutions
	Ointments
	Suppositories
Intraocular	Solutions
	Suspensions
	Ointments
	Inserts
	Contact lenses
Intranasal	Solutions
	Suspensions
	Sprays
	Aerosols
	Inhalers
	Powders
Inhalation	Aerosols
	Powders
Intravenous	Solutions
Intramuscular	Suspensions
Intradermal	Emulsions
Dermal	Solutions
	Tinctures
	Collodions
	Liniments
	Ointments
	Creams
	Gels
	Lotions
	Pastes
	Plasters
	Powders
	Aerosols
	Transdermal patches

ROUTES

Enteral Routes are in red.

Parenteral routes are in blue.

The term is followed by the organ(s) of absorption.

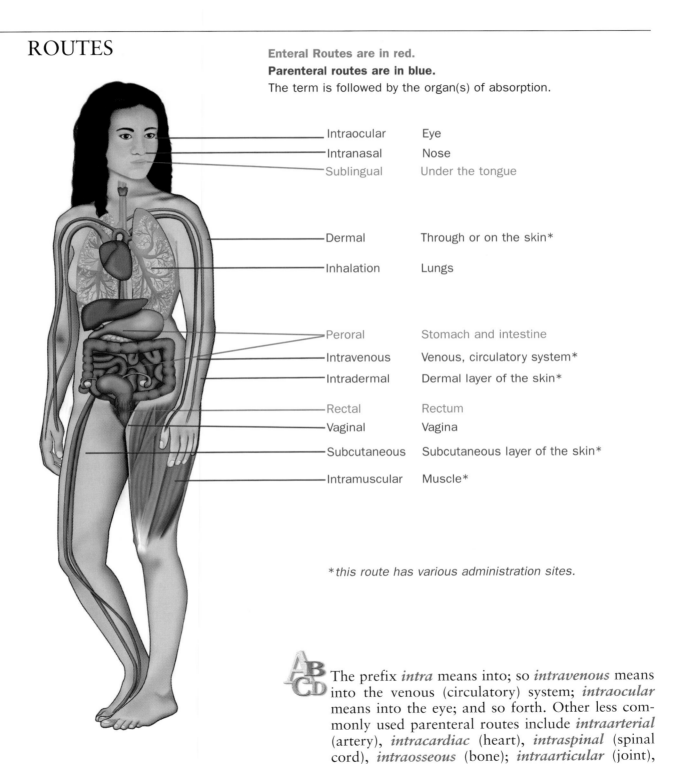

Intraocular	Eye
Intranasal	Nose
Sublingual	Under the tongue
Dermal	Through or on the skin*
Inhalation	Lungs
Peroral	Stomach and intestine
Intravenous	Venous, circulatory system*
Intradermal	Dermal layer of the skin*
Rectal	Rectum
Vaginal	Vagina
Subcutaneous	Subcutaneous layer of the skin*
Intramuscular	Muscle*

this route has various administration sites.

The prefix *intra* means into; so *intravenous* means into the venous (circulatory) system; *intraocular* means into the eye; and so forth. Other less commonly used parenteral routes include *intraarterial* (artery), *intracardiac* (heart), *intraspinal* (spinal cord), *intraosseous* (bone); *intraarticular* (joint), and *intrarespiratory* (lung).

ORAL FORMULATIONS

Oral administration is the most frequently used route of administration.

Oral dosage forms are easy to use, carry, and administer. The term used to specify oral administration is **peroral** or **PO** (per os). This indicates that the dosage form is to be swallowed and that absorption will occur primarily in the stomach and the intestine.

When formulations are orally administered, they enter the stomach, which is very acidic.

The stomach has a pH around 1-2. Certain drugs cannot be taken orally because they are **degraded** (chemically changed to a less effective form) or destroyed by stomach acid and intestinal enzymes. Additionally, the absorption of many drugs is affected by the presence of food in the stomach.

Drugs administered by liquid dosage forms generally reach the circulatory system faster than drugs formulated in solid dosage forms.

This is because the processes of **disintegration** and **dissolution** are not required. Oral liquids include solutions, suspensions, syrups, and elixirs. Solid oral dosage forms include tablets, capsules, and bulk powders.

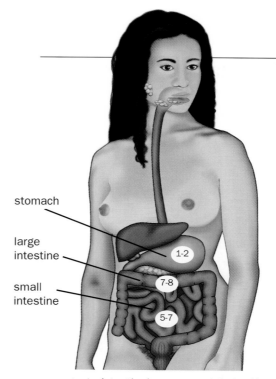

gastrointestinal organs and their pH

Gastrointestinal Action

The disintegration and dissolution of tablets, capsules, and powders generally begins in the stomach, but will continue to occur when the stomach empties into the intestine. **Controlled-release** or **extended-release** formulations are made so that dissolution occurs over a period of hours and provides a longer duration of effect compared to plain tablets. **Enteric** coated tablets serve a different function. They are used when the drug can be degraded by the stomach acid. The enteric coating will not let the tablet disintegrate until it reaches the higher pHs of the intestine.

pH the pH scale measures the *acidity* or the opposite *(alkalinity)* of a substance. 7 is the neutral midpoint of the scale, values below which represent increasing acidity, and above which represent increasing alkalinity.

Most oral dosage forms are intended for systemic effect, but not all For example, antacids have a local effect confined to the gastrointestinal tract.

Inactive Ingredients

Oral formulations contain various ingredients beside the active drug. These include binders, effervescent salts, lubricants, fillers, diluents, and disintegrants. They are added to help in the manufacture of the formulation and to help it disintegrate and dissolve when administered. A sample breakdown of ingredients is illustrated at right. Note, however, that each formulation is different.

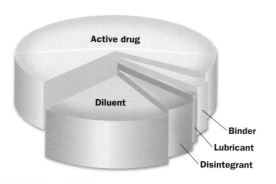

degradation the changing of a drug to a less effective or ineffective form.

adsorb attachment of one chemical to another.

SOLID FORMULATIONS

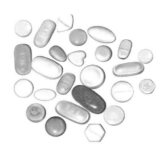

Tablets are hard formulations in which the drug and other ingredients are machine compressed under high pressure into a shape. Tablets vary in size, weight, hardness, thickness, and disintegration and dissolution characteristics depending upon their intended use. Most tablets are manufactured for peroral use, and many are coated to give an identifying color or logo on the formulation. **Sugar-coated** tablets are coated with a sweet glaze. **Film-coated** tablets are coated with a non-sweet coating. **Multiple compressed** tablets contain one drug in an inner layer and another drug (or the same drug) compressed at a lower pressure over it as an outer layer. They are used when a rapid release is desired for one drug (the outer layer) and a slower release is desired for the other drug (the inner layer). Other popular tablets are **chewable** and **effervescent.**

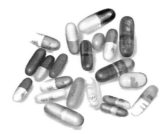

Capsules contain the drug and the other ingredients packaged in a gelatin shell. There are several capsule sizes. The capsule size used in any formulation is based on the amount of material to be placed inside the capsule. The gelatin shell dissolves in the stomach and releases the contents of the capsule. The freed contents must still undergo disintegration and dissolution before the drug is absorbed into the circulatory system. There are some capsule formulations that contain liquid instead of powders inside the gelatin shell; these are called soft capsules or soft-gel capsules. The active drug is already dissolved in the liquid.

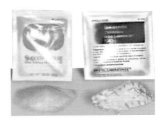

Bulk powders (e.g., Goody's BC powders) contain the active drug in a small powder paper or foil envelope. The patient empties the envelope into a glass of water or juice and drinks the contents. Most of the drug and ingredients dissolve in the water before the patient takes it.

LIQUID FORMULATIONS

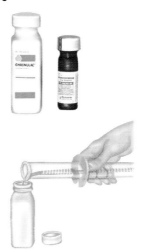

Solutions are made up of one or more solvents containing one or more dissolved substances. A solvent is a liquid which can dissolve another substance to form a solution. Solutions, elixirs, and syrups contain the drug and other ingredients already dissolved in the liquid. Elixirs are sweetened water and alcohol solutions that are generally less thick or viscous than water. Syrups are generally sugar-based solutions which are more viscous than water.

Suspensions are formulations where the drug cannot completely dissolve in the liquid. The drug particles are suspended in the liquid formulation. When suspensions are administered, the particles must dissolve before the drug is absorbed into the circulatory system. There are some suspensions that are intended for local activity: (e.g., activated charcoal, kaolin). These suspensions are orally administered to **adsorb** excessive intestinal fluid. In these suspensions, the particles will not dissolve.

SUBLINGUAL

The mouth is the route of administration for certain drugs where a rapid action is desired.

Formulations used in the mouth are generally fast dissolving uncoated tablets which contain highly water soluble drugs. These tablets are placed under the tongue (**sublingual** administration). When the drug is released from the tablet, it is quickly absorbed into the circulatory system since the membranes lining the mouth are very thin and there is a rich blood supply to the mouth.

Nitroglycerin is the best known example of a sublingual tablet formulation.

Nitroglycerin is sublingually administered since it is degraded in the stomach and intestine. Nitroglycerin is also available in a **translingual aerosol** that permits a patient to spray droplets of nitroglycerin under the tongue. There are also some steroid sex hormones that are sublingually administered.

Sublingual administration has certain limitations.

For various reasons (including the condition of the mouth, the patient, etc.), other routes of administration are considered more convenient for many drugs that would otherwise be candidates for sublingual administration. An additional consideration is that holding a drug in the mouth for almost any period of time is unpleasant since most drugs have a bitter taste.

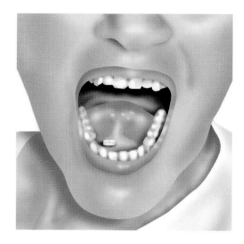

Using Sublingual Tablets

Sublingual tablets are highly water soluble, so patients should first take a sip of water to wet their mouth if it is dry.

The tablet is then placed far under the tongue and the mouth is closed and must remain closed until the tablet dissolves and is absorbed. No food or beverages can be taken until the drug is fully absorbed.

 water soluble the property of a substance being able to dissolve in water.

 Like many medical terms, *sub* is a Latin word meaning under; *trans* means across or over; and *lingua* means tongue.

RECTAL

Drugs are administered via the rectum either for a local effect or to bypass degradation caused by oral administration.

Local effects may include the soothing of inflamed hemorrhoidal tissues, promoting laxation, and enemas. Rectal administration for systemic activity is preferred when the drug is destroyed by stomach acid or intestinal enzymes, or if oral administration is unavailable (if the patient is vomiting, unconscious or incapable of swallowing oral formulations). Rectal administration is used to achieve a variety of systemic effects, including: asthma control, antinausea, antimotion sickness, and anti-infective.

The most common rectal administration forms are suppositories, solutions, and ointments.

Suppositories are semi-solid dosage forms that dissolve or melt when inserted into the rectum. Suppositories are manufactured in a variety of shapes and are used in other routes of administration such as vaginal or urethral. Most rectal solutions are used as enemas or cleansing solutions. Ointments are intended to be spread around the anal opening and are most often used to treat inflamed hemorrhoidal tissues.

Rectal dosage forms have certain significant disadvantages.

They are not preferred by most patients. They are inconvenient. Moreover, rectal absorption of most drugs is frequently erratic and unpredictable.

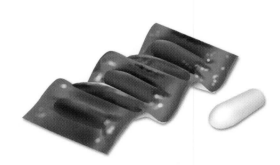

Suppositories

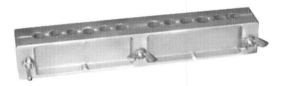

Mold used for making suppositories

Enemas

Enemas create an urge to defecate due to the injection of fluid into the rectum. A **cleansing** enema injects water or a cleansing solution. A **retention** enema injects an oil that is held in the rectum to soften the stool. Frequent use of enemas is discouraged as it can can have significant adverse effects.

 hemorrhoid painful swollen veins in the anal/rectal area, generally caused by strained bowel movements from hard stools.

PARENTERAL ROUTES

Parenteral routes of administration are used for a variety of reasons.

If an orally administered drug is poorly absorbed, or is degraded by stomach acid or intestinal enzymes, then a parenteral route may be indicated. Parenteral routes are also preferred when a rapid drug response is desired, as in an emergency situation. Parenteral routes of administration are also useful when a patient is uncooperative, unconscious, or otherwise unable to take a drug by an enteral route.

There are disadvantages of formulations given by parenteral routes.

One is cost. Most parenterals are more expensive than enteral route formulations. Another is that many parenterals require skilled personnel to administer them. A third disadvantage is that once a parenteral drug is administered, it is most difficult to remove the dose if there is an adverse or toxic reaction. Finally, parenteral administration has risks associated with invading the body with a needle (infection, thrombus, etc.).

Several parenteral routes require a needle and some type of propelling device (syringe, pump, gravity fed bag) to administer a drug.

These routes of administration are the **intravenous, intramuscular, intradermal,** and **subcutaneous.** These injectable routes have several characteristics in common. The formulations that can be used with injectables are limited to **solutions, suspensions,** and **emulsions.** Any other dosage formulation cannot pass through the syringe. These formulations must be **sterile** (bacteria-free) since they are placed in direct contact with the internal body fluids or tissues where infection can easily occur. The pH of the formulation must also be carefully maintained. This is commonly done by adding ingredients to the formulation as a **buffer** system. A fourth characteristic is that limited volumes of formulation can be injected. Too great an injection volume can cause pain and cell death (necrosis).

PARENTERALS

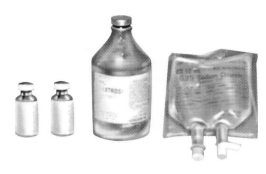

Which Parenteral?

Besides meaning any route other than oral, sublingual, and rectal, "parenteral" is commonly used to describe drugs administered through syringes. It is also used to describe the various bottles, vials, and bags used in preparing and delivering solutions for intravenous administration. It is possible to say that parenterals are prepared and parenterally administered at parenteral sites. As a result, extreme care must be taken when using the word parenteral so that the intended meaning is clear to all.

---

necrosis the death of cells.

sterile a sterile condition is one which is free of *all* microorganisms, both harmful and harmless.

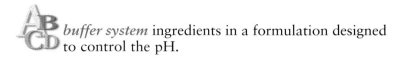

buffer system ingredients in a formulation designed to control the pH.

ROUTES

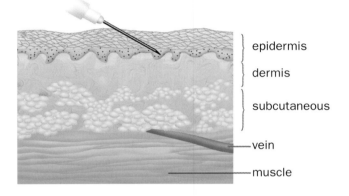

epidermis

dermis

subcutaneous

vein

muscle

Intradermal

Intradermal injections are administered into the top layer of the skin at a slight angle using short needles.

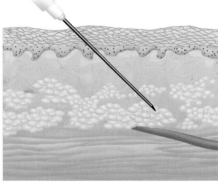

Subcutaneous

Subcutaneous injections are administered to the subcutaneous tissue of the skin using 3/8 inch to 1inch needles.

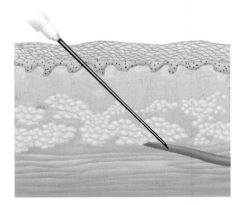

Intravenous

Intravenous injections are administered directly into veins.

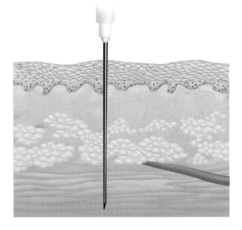

Intramuscular

Intramuscular injections are administered into muscle tissue using one to one-and-a-half inch needles.

INTRAVENOUS FORMULATIONS

Intravenous dosage forms are administered directly into a vein and therefore the blood supply.

Solutions are the most common formulation intravenously administered. Most solutions are **aqueous** (water based), but they may also have glycols, alcohols, or other non-aqueous solvents in them.

Injectable suspensions are difficult to formulate because they must possess syringeability and injectability.

Syringeability refers to the ease with which the suspension can be drawn from a container into a syringe. Injectability refers to the properties of the suspension while being injected, properties such as flow evenness, freedom from clogging, etc.

Emulsions are formulations that contain both aqueous and non-aqueous (oil) components.

Fat emulsions and total parenteral nutrition (TPN) emulsions are used to provide triglycerides, fatty acids, and calories for patients who cannot absorb them from the gastrointestinal tract.

Dry powder formulations are also manufactured for intravenous use, but they must be reconstituted with a suitable solvent to make a liquid formulation.

Some drugs are not stable in liquid form, and so these drugs are put into the powder form and reconstituted just prior to use. There are several solvents that might be used to reconstitute the dry powders. The appropriate solvent is indicated in the product information insert. The most common solvents are Sterile Water for Injection USP, Bacteriostatic Water for Injection USP, Sodium Chloride Injection USP, and Ringer's Injection USP.

COMPLICATIONS

There are a number of complications that can occur from intravenous administration. Some have already been mentioned: **sterility, excessive volumes, maintaining pH.** Additional complications are thrombosis, phlebitis, air emboli, and particulate material.

➡ **Thrombus** (blood clot) formation can result from many factors: extremes in solution pH, particulate material, irritant properties of the drug, needle or **catheter trauma,** and selection of too small a vein for the volume of solution injected.

➡ **Phlebitis,** or inflammation of the vein, can be caused by the same factors that cause thrombosis.

➡ **Air emboli** occur when air is introduced into the vein. The human body is generally not harmed by very small amounts of air injected into the venous system, but *air injected into the veins can be fatal,* and it is necessary to remove all air bubbles from formulation and administration sets before use.

➡ **Particulate material** can include small pieces of glass that chip from the formulation vial or rubber that comes from the rubber closure on injection vials. Although great care is taken to eliminate the presence of particulate material, a final filter in the administration line just before entering the venous system is an important precaution.

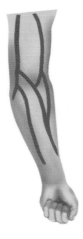

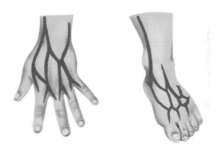

Intravenous Sites

Several sites on the body are used to intravenously administer drugs: the veins of the antecubital area (in front of the elbow), the back of the hand, and some of the larger veins in the foot. On some occasions, a vein must be exposed by a surgical cut.

aqueous water based.

solvent a liquid that dissolves another substance in it.

trauma an injury.

DEVICES

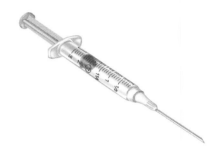

Syringes

Simple syringe and needle setups can be used to inject formulations over a short period of time (generally up to about 2 minutes). There are a variety of syringe sizes and needle sizes; syringe size is selected based on the volume of the formulation to inject. The needle size is generally based on the route of administration being used (IV, IM, SC, ID). Needle sizes of 16G to 20G are commonly used for intravenous injections. Some products come from the manufacturer already assembled and prefilled.

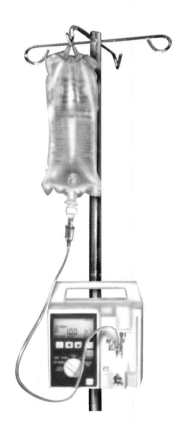

Infusion

Infusion is the gradual intravenous injection of a volume of fluid into a patient. The fluid consists of a primary fluid and whatever drug(s) are prescribed. The primary fluid is generally a large volume (500 ml to 1000 ml) bag or bottle of electrolyte solution such as D5W (dextrose 5% in water) or 1/2NS (one-half normal saline, 0.45% sodium chloride in water). It is intravenously infused at a rate of 2 ml to 3 ml per minute. The fluid bag has an administration set that includes an injection port between the bag and the needle. A simple syringe and needle may be used to inject a drug through the injection port into the primary fluid, or a second small plastic bag containing the drug can be piggybacked onto the primary fluid administration set.

Infusion Pumps

Administration devices that were dependent upon gravity have been shown to have a variable delivery rate. To ensure a constant delivery rate, controlled rate infusion pumps are used. Beginning in the late 1980s, patients were allowed to operate these pumps for occasional self-administration of analgesics. The term patient-controlled analgesia (PCA) was coined to describe this. PCA devices can provide either on-demand dosing or a constant infusion rate of drug as well as the on-demand feature.

INTRAMUSCULAR

Drugs are often given by the intramuscular route to patients unable to take them by oral administration.

This route is also used for drugs that are poorly absorbed from the gastrointestinal tract. It is generally considered less hazardous and easier to use than the intravenous route. However, patients generally experience more pain from intramuscular administration than intravenous administration.

Intramuscular (IM) injections are made into the muscle fibers that are under the subcutaneous layer of the skin.

Needles used for the injections are generally 1 inch to 1.5 inches long, and are generally 19 to 22 gauge in size. The principal sites of injection are the **gluteal** (buttocks), **deltoid** (upper arm), and **vastus lateralis** (thigh) muscles. When giving intramuscular injections into the gluteus maximus, one must be aware of the thickness of gluteal fat, particularly in female patients and an appropriate size needle must be used. Otherwise, the injection will not reach the muscle.

The site of injection should be as far as possible from major nerves and blood vessels to avoid nerve damage and accidental intravenous administration.

Injuries that can occur following intramuscular injection are abscesses, cysts, embolism, hematoma, skin sloughing, and scar formation. To avoid injury, when a series of injections are given, the injection site is changed or rotated. Generally only limited volumes can be given by intramuscular injection: 2 ml in the deltoid and thigh muscles, and up to 5 ml in the gluteus maximus.

Intramuscular injections generally result in lower but longer lasting blood concentrations than after intravenous administration.

Part of the reason is that intramuscular injections require an absorption step, which delays the time to peak concentrations. Also, when a formulation is injected, a **depot** forms inside the muscle tissue where the drug deposits. Absorption from this depot is dependent on many factors such as muscle exercise, particle size of the drug, and the salt form of the drug used in the formulation.

FORMULATIONS

Drugs for intramuscular injection are formulated as:

➡ solutions;
➡ suspensions;
➡ **colloids** in aqueous and oleaginous (oil-based) solvents;
➡ oil-in-water **emulsions;**
➡ water-in-oil emulsions.

Colloids and suspensions both contain insoluble particles in solution, but the particles in colloids are about 100 times smaller than those in suspensions.

Emulsions are mixtures of two liquids, generally oil and water, which do not dissolve into each other. One liquid is spread through the other by mixing or shaking and the use of a stabilizing substance called an **emulsifier**.

Different salt forms of the drug may also be used to take advantage of a slower dissolution rate or a lower solubility.

All these things can be varied to achieve the desired absorption rate. In general, aqueous solutions have a faster absorption rate than oleagineous solutions. Both of these have a faster absorption rate than colloids or suspensions.

INJECTION SITES

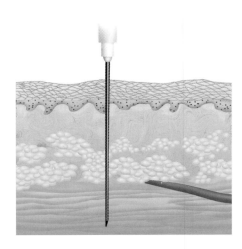

When administering intramuscular injections, it is necessary to adjust for any layers of body fat (especially in the gluteal area) and to use a size of needle that will penetrate to the muscle.

Z-Tract Injection

This is a technique used for medications that stain the skin (e.g., iron dextran injection) or irritate tissues (e.g., diazepam). The skin is pulled to one side prior to injection. Then the needle is inserted and the injection is performed. Once the needle is removed, the skin is released so that the injection points in the skin and muscle are no longer aligned. This keeps the drug from entering the subcutaneous tissue and staining or irritating the skin. A Z-track injection is generally 2 to 3 inches deep.

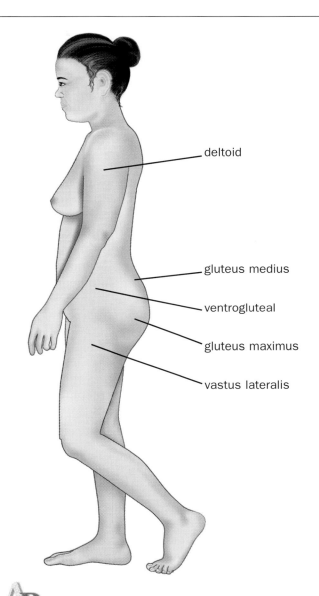

deltoid

gluteus medius

ventrogluteal

gluteus maximus

vastus lateralis

colloids particles up to a hundred times smaller than that those in suspensions that are, however, likewise suspended in a solution.

emulsions mixture of two liquids that do not dissolve into each other in which one liquid is spread through the other by mixing and use of a stabilizer.

℞ Intramuscular injections are generally more painful than intravenous.

SUBCUTANEOUS

The subcutaneous (SC, SQ) route is a versatile route of administration that can be used for both short term and very long term therapies. The injection of a drug or the **implantation** of a device beneath the surface of the skin is made in the loose tissues of the upper arm, the front of the thigh, and the lower portion of the abdomen. The upper back also can be used as a site of subcutaneous administration. The site of injection is usually rotated when injections are given frequently. The maximum amount of medication that can be subcutaneously injected is about 2 ml. Needles are generally 3/8 to 1 inch in length and 24 to 28 gauge.

Absorption of drugs from the subcutaneous tissue is influenced by the same factors that determine the rate of absorption from intramuscular sites.

However, there are fewer blood vessels in the subcutaneous tissue than in muscle, and absorption may be slower than with intramuscular administration. On the other hand, absorption after subcutaneous administration is generally more rapid and predictable than after oral administration. There are several ways to change the absorption rate. Using heat, or massaging the site have been found to increase absorption rates of many drugs. Also, there are various drugs which have been shown to increase absorption rate. By contrast, epinephrine decreases blood flow, which in turn decreases the absorption rate.

Many different solution and suspension formulations are given subcutaneously, but insulin is the most important drug routinely administered by this route.

Insulin comes in many different formulations each having a characteristic rate of absorption. The rate is controlled by the same factors used for intramuscular formulations: slowly soluble salt forms, suspensions versus solutions, differences in particle size, viscosity (thickness) of the injection form, etc.

In spite of the advantages of this route of administration, there are some precautions to observe.

Drugs which are irritating or in very **viscous** (thick) suspensions may produce serious adverse effects (including abscesses and necrosis) and be painful to the patient.

INJECTION SITES

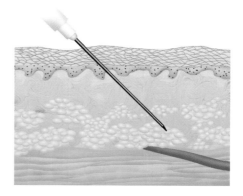

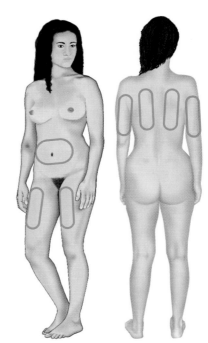

Subcutaneous injection sites are:

➡ lower abdomen;
➡ front of thigh;
➡ upper back;
➡ back of upper arm.

 viscosity the thickness of a liquid.

I ntradermal injections involve small volumes that are injected into the top layer of skin.

They are used for diagnostic reasons, desensitization, or immunization. Their effects are generally local rather than systemic.

An intradermal injection forms a *wheal,* or raised blister-like area, from which the drug will slowly be absorbed into the dermis.

The dermis is the layer of the skin just beneath the epidermis. It contains more blood vessels than the epidermis but fewer than most other injection sites. As a result, absorption is gradual.

The usual site for intradermal injections is the rear of the forearm.

Needles are generally 3/8 inches long and 23 to 26 gauge. For this route of administration, 0.1 ml of solution is the maximum volume that can be administered.

IMPLANTS

One of the most popular ways to achieve very long term drug release is to place the drug in a delivery system or device that is implanted into the body tissue. The subcutaneous tissue is the ideal tissue for implantation of such devices. Implantation generally requires a surgical procedure or a specialized injection device. The fact that the device will be in constant contact with the subcutaneous tissue requires that the device materials be **biocompatible,** i.e., not irritating, and won't promote infection or sterile abscess. An advantage of the subcutaneous tissue for the site of implantation is that the device can be easily removed if necessary.

There are many devices that are used in subcutaneous implantation. Norplant® are silicone rods that provide contraception for up to five years. Several pellet formulations (Oreton ®, Percorten ®) are also available, as well as a mini-pump (Alzet ®) which can deliver drug solutions for up to twenty-one days, as well as other devices.

Sometimes **ports** and **pumps** are placed in subcutaneous tissue and an attached delivery catheter is placed in a vein, cavity, artery, or CNS system. This allows for the injection of intravenous fluids, total parenteral nutrition (TPN) solutions, chemotherapy agents, or antibiotics.

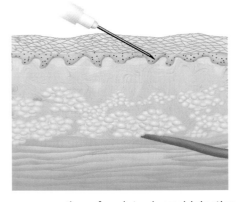

cross-section of an intradermal injection

 biocompatibility not irritating or infection or abscess causing to body tissue.

wheal a raised blister-like area on the skin, as caused by an intradermal injection.

OPHTHALMIC FORMULATIONS

Drugs are administered to the eye for local treatment of various eye conditions and for anesthesia.

Formulations that are used include aqueous solutions, aqueous suspensions, ointments, and implants. *Every ophthalmic product must be manufactured to be sterile in its final container.* Also, because of the sensitivity of the eye, various elements of the formulation, including pH and viscosity, must be carefully controlled.

A major problem of ophthalmic administration is the immediate loss of a dose by natural spillage from the eye.

The normal volume of tears in the eye is estimated to be 7 microliters, and if blinking occurs, the eye can hold up to 10 microliters without spillage. The normal commercial eyedropper dispenses 50 microliters of solution. As a result, *more than half of a dose will be expelled from the eye by overflow.* The ideal volume of drug solution to administer would be 5 to 10 microliters. However, microliter dosing eye droppers are not generally available to patients.

Other problems include lacrimal (tear) drainage and too rapid absorption by the eyelid lining.

Tears wash the eyeball as they flow from the **lacrimal gland** across the eye and drain into the **lacrimal canalicula** (tear ducts). In man, the rate of tear production is approximately 2 microliters per minute, and so the entire tear volume in the eye turns over every 2 to 3 minutes. This rapid washing and turnover accounts for loss of an ophthalmic dose in a relatively short period of time. It can also cause systemic absorption because the drug drains into the lacrimal sac and is then emptied into the gastrointestinal tract. A similar and frequently occurring problem is caused by absorption of the drug into the **conjunctiva** (eyelid lining). The drug is then rapidly carried away from the eye by the circulatory system.

OPHTHALMIC ADMINISTRATION

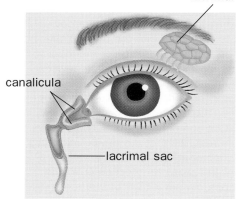

anatomy of the eye

Administration Considerations

➡ The eye is highly sensitive, requiring careful formulation for sterility, pH, viscosity, etc. to avoid irritation.

➡ The eye only holds a very small volume of liquid (7-10 microliters), so most eyedropper doses are lost through overflow.

➡ Systemic absorption can occur from drainage through the tear ducts or absorption through the eyelid.

 Ophthalmic administration is used to deliver a drug on the eye, into the eye, or onto the conjunctiva. Drug penetration into the eye (**transcorneal transport**) is not considered an effective process as it is estimated that only one-tenth of a dose penetrates into the eye.

A B C D *ophthalmic* related to the eye.

lacrimal gland the gland that produces tears for the eye.

lacrimal canalicula the tear ducts.

conjunctiva the eyelid lining.

transcorneal transport drug transfer into the eye.

Most ophthalmic solutions and suspensions are dispensed in eye dropper bottles.

Because of the problems of this route, patients must be shown how to properly instill the drops in their eyes, and every effort should be made to emphasize the need for instilling only one drop, not two or three.

To maintain longer contact between the drug and the surrounding tissue, suspensions, ointments, and inserts have been developed.

Ophthalmic suspensions are aqueous, with the particle size kept to a minimum to prevent irritation of the eye. Ointments tend to keep the drug in contact with the eye longer than suspensions. Most ophthalmic ointment bases are a mixture of mineral oil and white petrolatum and have a melting point close to body temperature. But ointments tend to blur patient vision as they remain viscous and are not removed easily by the tear fluid. Therefore, ointments are generally used at night as additional therapy to eye drops used during the day.

There are three types of devices commonly used to deliver ophthalmic dosages: hydrogel (soft) contact lenses, non-erodible inserts, and soluble inserts.

Hydrogel contact lenses are placed in a solution containing a drug such as an antibiotic, and the lenses absorb some of the drug solution. The lenses are then placed in the eye and the drug will release from the lenses over a period of time. **Ocusert®** is a non-erodible ocular insert designed to deliver pilocarpine at a controlled rate for up to 7 days. The insert is placed between the eyeball and the lower eyelid. With the Ocusert, patients use a fraction of the amount of pilocarpine they would with drop therapy. The biggest disadvantage of the insert is its tendency to float on the eyeball, particularly in the morning after waking. Soluble ophthalmic drug inserts are dried solutions that have been fashioned into a film or rod. These solid inserts are placed between the eyeball and the lower eyelid, and as they absorb tears, they slowly erode away. **Lacrisert®** is a soluble insert used in the treatment of moderate to severe **dry eye syndrome.**

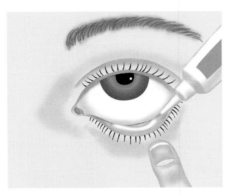

using an eye dropper

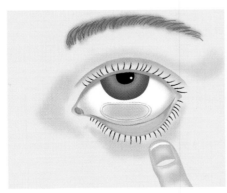

using an ointment

Ocusert

R Ophthalmic ointment tubes are typically small, holding approximately 3.5 g of ointment and fitted with narrow gauge tips which permit the extrusion of narrow bands of ointment.

INTRANASAL FORMULATIONS

The adult nasal cavity has a capacity of about 20 ml, a very large surface area for absorption, and a very rich blood supply.

The formulations used for intranasal administration are primarily used for their decongestant activity on the **nasal mucosa**, the cellular lining of the nose. The drugs that are typically used are decongestants, antihistamines, and corticosteroids.

The intranasal absorption of some drugs produces blood concentrations similar to when the drug is intravenously administered.

Because of this, intranasal administration is being investigated as a possible route of administration for insulin in the treatment of diabetes mellitus and for glucagon in the treatment of hypoglycemia. Intranasal administration also serves as a possible alternate route for drugs that are seriously degraded or poorly absorbed by oral administration.

Intranasal formulations include solutions, suspensions, sprays, aerosols, and inhalers.

Each product is formulated so it will not irritate the mucosa. Generally solutions or suspensions are administered by drops or as a fine mist from a nasal spray or aerosol container. Nasal sprays are preferred to drops because drops are more likely to drain into the back of the mouth and throat and be swallowed. The plastic spray bottle which is gently squeezed is used to issue a spray. A nasal inhaler is a tube which is inserted into the nostril opening. The tube contains a material that is saturated with the drug. As the patient inhales, the drug is vaporized and pulled into the nasal cavity.

DEVICES

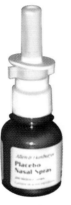

nasal spray

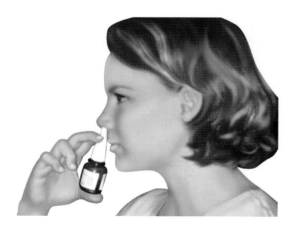

using a nasal spray

 nasal mucosa the cellular lining of the nose.

nasal cavity the cavity behind the nose and above the roof of the mouth that filters air and moves mucous and inhaled contaminants outward and away from the lungs.

nasal inhaler a device which contains a drug that is vaporized by inhalation.

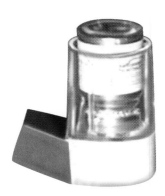

nasal aerosol

Atomizer

Atomizers are devices which breaks a liquid up into a spray. One type of atomizer uses a squeeze bulb to blow air across a liquid solution causing the liquid to vaporize. As the liquid vaporizes, the air stream created by the bulb also carries the spray out of the device and into the nose.

Insufflator

In instances where a powder is to be intranasally administered, an insufflator is used. Squeezing the rubber bulb causes a turbulence within the powder reservoir forcing some of the powder into the air stream and out of the device.

There are three ways a dosage can be lost following nasal administration.

The nasal lining contains enzymes which can metabolize and degrade some drugs. In addition, normal mucous flow, which protects the lungs by moving mucus and inhaled contaminants away from the lungs and out the nostril, will carry dosage with it as well. Finally, nasal administration often causes amounts of the drug to be swallowed. In some cases, enough drug will be swallowed to be equal to an oral dose. This may lead to a systemic effect from the drug even though it is intranasally administered.

Intranasal dosage forms should not be used for prolonged periods.

This may lead to chronic swelling (**edema**) of the nasal mucosa which aggravates the symptoms the dosage forms were intended to relieve. As a result, intranasal administration should be for short periods of time (no longer than 3 to 5 days). Patients should be advised not to exceed the recommended dosage and frequency of use.

Ways Intranasal Dosage Is Lost

✔ enzymes in the mucosa metabolize certain drugs.

✔ normal mucous flow removes dosage.

✔ amounts of the drug are swallowed.

 Because it can lead to irritation and swelling, intranasal administration is generally kept to limited volumes for short periods of time.

INHALATION FORMULATIONS

Inhalation dosage forms are intended to deliver drugs to the pulmonary system (lungs).

The lungs have a large surface area for absorption and a rich blood supply. This route avoids the problems of degradation and poor absorption found with the oral route. However, there is enough inconsistency in the absorption of drugs from the lungs that this route is not considered an alternative to intravenous administration.

Gaseous or volatile anesthetics are the most important drugs administered via this route.

Other drugs administered affect lung function, act as bronchodilators (bronchial tube decongestants), or treat allergic symptoms. Examples of drugs administered by this route are adrenocorticoid steroids (beclomethasone), bronchodilators (epinephrine, isoproterenol, metaproterenol, albuterol), and antiallergics (cromolyn).

Most of the inhalation dosage forms are aerosols that depend on the power of compressed or liquefied gas to expel the drug from the container.

Aerosols are easy to use, and have no danger of contamination. However, they are not very effective in delivering a drug to the respiratory tract. This is not due to poor aerosol design, but to the physical barriers of the airway and lungs that any inhalation dosage form must overcome to be effective.

Particle size is the critical factor with these dosage forms.

Large particles (about 20 microns) hit in the back of the mouth and throat and are eventually swallowed rather than inhaled. Particles from 1 to 10 microns reach the bronchioles. Smaller particles (0.6 micron) penetrate to the alveolar sacs of the lungs where absorption is rapid, but retention is limited since a large fraction of the dose is exhaled. The particles that reach the alveolar sacs and remain there are responsible for providing systemic effects. Breathing patterns and the depth of breathing also play important roles in the delivery of inhaled aerosols into the lung.

ABSORPTION

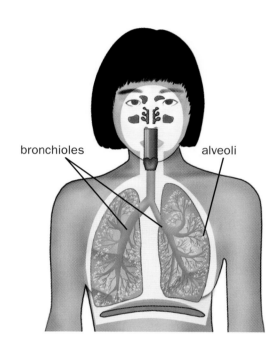

bronchioles

alveoli

For an inhalation dosage form to reach the alveoli of the lungs it has to pass through a series of twists, turns, and increasingly smaller passageways as it travels from the mouth to the lungs. When the drug reaches the alveoli, it will be absorbed directly into the circulatory system. Because of the difficult route, varying amounts of inhalation dosages are swallowed and wind up in the gastrointestinal system.

inspiration breathing in.

alveolar sacs (alveoli) the small sacs of specialized tissue that transfer oxygen out of inspired air into the blood and carbon dioxide out of the blood and into the air for expiration.

DEVICES

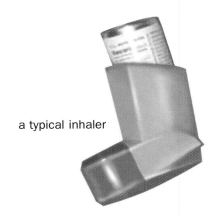

a typical inhaler

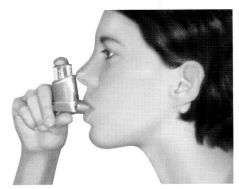

using an inhaler

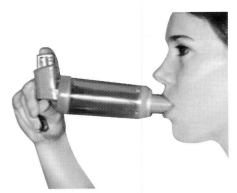

using an inhaler with spacer

Metered Dose Inhalers

Aerosols to administer powerful drugs use special metering valves that deliver a fixed dose when the aerosol is activated. These are called "metered dose inhalers." The amount of drug released with each activation is regulated by an valve that has a fixed capacity or dimensions.

Adapters and Spacers

Coordination is required on the part of the patient between breathing in (**inspiration**) and activation of the aerosol. Extender devices or spacers have been developed to assist patients who cannot coordinate these two processes. The spacer goes between the aerosol's mouthpiece and the patient's mouth. The spacer allows the patient to separate activation of the aerosol from inhalation by 3 to 5 seconds.

Powder Inhalers

Some drugs are administered in powder form using a special inhalation device such as a **Rotahaler.** The device automatically releases the drug when the user inhales.The powdered drug is supplied in hard gelatin capsules that are placed in the inhaler. The patient squeezes the inhaler to pierce the capsule and release the powder. When the patient inhales from the device, the powder is mixed with the inspired air by a small propeller and is then delivered to the lungs with the inspired air.

Some patients may not be able to use inhaled powders and humid conditions may also make inhaling powder difficult.

DERMAL FORMULATIONS

The skin is the largest and heaviest organ in the body and accounts for about 17% of a person's weight.

It forms a barrier that protects the underlying organ systems from trauma, temperature, humidity, harmful penetrations, moisture, radiation, and microorganisms. Dosage forms that are applied to the skin are called **dermal** or **percutaneous** forms.

Most dermal dosage forms are used for local (topical) effects on or within the skin.

Formulations are used as protectants, lubricants, emollients, or drying agents, or for the specific effect of the drug present. Examples of treatments using dermal formulations include minor skin infections, itching, burns, diaper rash, insect stings and bites, athlete's foot, corns, calluses, warts, dandruff, acne, psoriasis, and eczema.

Dermal administration has a number of advantages.

It provides an ease of administration not found in other routes, and usage by patients is generally good. It can also provide continuous drug administration. In addition, dermal formulations can be easily removed if necessary. The major disadvantage of this route of administration is that the amount of drug that can be absorbed will be limited to about 2 mg/day. This is often a significant limitation if the route is being considered for systemic therapy.

Basic rules of dermal absorption:

➥ More drug is absorbed when the formulation is applied to a larger surface area.
➥ Formulations or dressings that increase the hydration of the skin generally improve absorption.
➥ The greater the amount of rubbing in (inunction) of the formulation, the greater the absorption.
➥ The longer the formulation remains in contact with the skin, the greater will be the absorption.

---

percutaneous the absorption of drugs through the skin, often for a systemic effect.

topical applied for local effect, usually to the skin.

hydrates absorbs water.

THE SKIN

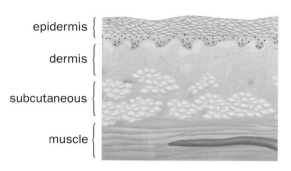

epidermis
dermis
subcutaneous
muscle

The skin is composed of three layers of tissue:
➥ epidermis;
➥ dermis;
➥ subcutaneous tissue.

The skin is generally 3- 5 millimeters thick, though it is thicker in the palms and soles of the feet and thinner in the eyelids and genitals. Within the skin are several other elements: hair follicles, sebaceous glands, sweat glands, and nails.

The outer layer of skin is called the **stratum corneum**. In normal skin, the cells of this layer are continually replaced by new cells from underneath. As new cells develop, they displace the outer cells that have died. The turnover time from cell development to shedding of the dead cells (**sloughing**) is about 21 days.

The skin's outer layer is a barrier to drug penetration. It is about 10 micrometers thick, but can swell to approximately three times that by absorbing as much as five times its weight in water. When the stratum corneum absorbs water (**hydrates**), it becomes easier for drugs to penetrate. For that reason, certain dressings are designed to do this. Also, some skin conditions such as eczema and psoriasis can hydrate the stratum corneum and increase the absorption of some drugs.

FORMULATIONS

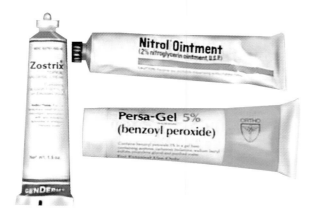

Ointments, Creams, Gels, and Lotions

Ointments, creams, gels, and lotions are the most popular dermal formulations. Physically, they appear to be very similar in consistency and texture, but there are differences. **Ointments** have drugs that have been incorporated into a base. There are several different types of bases ranging from petrolatum to polyethylene glycols. **Creams** are semisolid emulsions, and are less viscous and lighter in texture than ointments. Creams have an added feature in that they "vanish" or disappear with rubbing. **Gels** are dispersions of solid drugs in a jelly-like liquid vehicle. **Lotions** are suspensions of solid drugs in an aqueous vehicle.

Solutions, Tinctures, Collodions, and Liniments

Dermal **solutions** and **tinctures** are generally used as anti-infective agents. *Solutions are aqueous and tinctures are alcoholic.* Both are generally dispensed in small volumes, and should be packaged in containers that make them convenient to use. Dropper bottles (glass bottles with an applicator tip) are most often used. Examples of solutions and tinctures are Coal Tar Solution, Hydrogen Peroxide, Povidone-Iodine, Iodine Tincture, and Compound Benzoin Tincture.

Collodions are liquid preparations of pyroxylin dissolved in a solvent mixture of alcohol and ether. Pyroxylin looks like raw cotton and is slowly but completely soluble in the solvent mixture. When applied to the skin, the solvent rapidly evaporates, leaving a protective film on the skin that contains a thin layer of the drug. **Liniments** are alcoholic or oleaginous solutions generally applied by rubbing.

Pastes, Powders, Plasters

Pastes are generally used for their protective action and for their ability to absorb discharges from skin lesions. Pastes contain more solid material than ointments, and are stiffer and less penetrating. Medicinal **powders** are a mixture of drug and an inert (inactive) base such as talcum or corn starch. Powders have different dusting and covering capability. **Plasters** are solid or semisolid adhesive masses that are spread on a suitable backing material. They provide prolonged contact at the site of application. Some of the common backing materials used are paper, cotton, felt, linen, muslin, silk, and moleskin. The backing is cut into different shapes appropriate to cover the body surface area.

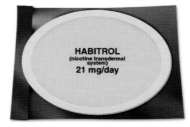

Transdermal Patches, Tapes, and Gauzes.

Transdermal systems (patches, tapes, and gauzes) *deliver drugs through the skin for a systemic effect.* The systems can be divided into two kinds: those that control the rate of drug delivery to the skin, and those that allow the skin to control the rate of absorption. The first type is for powerful drugs that must have their absorption rate controlled by a device. The second type is for less powerful drugs. The largest problems with transdermal patches are skin sensitivity experienced by some patients, and technical difficulties associated with the adhesiveness of the systems to different skin types and under various conditions.

Aerosols

Percutaneous aerosols are generally used to apply anesthetic and antibiotic dosages for local effect.

VAGINAL FORMULATIONS

Vaginal administration has many of the same characteristics found with other parenteral routes of administration.

It avoids the degradation that occurs with oral administration; doses can be retrieved if necessary; and it has the potential of long term drug absorption. However, vaginal administration leads to variable absorption since the vagina is a physiologically and anatomically dynamic organ with pH and absorption characteristics changing over time. Another disadvantage of this route is that administration of a formulation during menstruation could predispose the patient to **Toxic Shock Syndrome.** There is also a tendency of some dosage forms to be expelled after insertion into the vagina.

Formulations for this route of administration are: solutions, powders for solutions, ointments, creams, aerosol foams, suppositories, tablets, contraceptive sponges and IUDs.

Powders are used to prepare solutions for vaginal douches used to cleanse the vagina. The powders are supplied either as bulk or unit packages and are dissolved in a prescribed amount of water prior to use. Most douche powders are used for their hygienic effects, but a few contain antibiotics.

Vaginal administration gives the opportunity for long term administration.

This potential has been explored in the area of contraception protection using **intrauterine devices (IUDs).** The first IUD was developed in 1970 and was effective for 21 days. The vaginal ring was worn until the onset of menstruation, removed during menstruation, and then reinserted for another 21 days. Several IUDs have been marketed since that time, including the Progestasert.

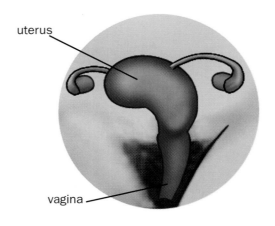

uterus

vagina

The Vagina

The vagina is a cylinder-like organ that leads from the cervix and uterus to an external opening. It is used for intercourse, the release of menstrual fluids, and as the lower portion of the birth canal.

Toxic Shock Syndrome (TSS)

Toxic shock syndrome is a rare and potentially fatal disease that results from a severe bacterial infection of the blood. In women, it can be caused when bacteria natural to the vagina move into the bloodstream. Though primarily associated with the use of super-absorbency tampons, it has also been associated with various vaginal dosage forms. Its symptoms include a high fever, nausea, skin rash, faintness and muscle ache. It is treated with antibiotics and other medicines.

Suppositories

Vaginal suppositories are employed as contraceptives, feminine hygiene antiseptics, bacterial antibiotics, or to restore the vaginal mucosa. Vaginal suppositories are inserted high in the vaginal tract with the aid of a special applicator. The suppositories are usually globe, egg, or cone-shaped and weigh about 5 grams.

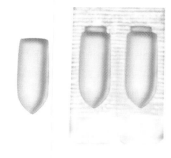

Suppositories are made from a variety of bases. Cocoa butter is a popular oleaginous base, but is difficult to formulate as a suppository. Glycerinated gelatin (glycerin and gelatin) is excellent for prolonged local effects since it softens slowly. However, **polyethylene glycols** (polyols or **PEGs**) are the most popular of all bases. They dissolve when inserted into a body cavity, so the base does not need to be formulated to melt at body temperature. This allows convenient storage without refrigeration. They also do not melt in the fingers while being inserted, nor do they leak from the vaginal opening.

Ointments, creams, and aerosol foams

Vaginal ointments, creams, and aerosol foams typically contain antibiotics, estrogenic hormonal substances, and contraceptive agents.

Creams and foams are placed into a special applicator tube, and the tube is then inserted high in the vaginal tract. The applicator plunger is depressed and the formulation is deposited.

IUD

The progestasert IUD (intrauterine device) releases an average of 60 micrograms of progesterone per day for a period of one year. This IUD is replaced annually to maintain contraception.

Tablets

Vaginal tablets, also called inserts, have the same activity and are inserted in the same manner as vaginal suppositories. Patients should be instructed to dip the tablet into water before insertion. Also, because tablets are generally used at bedtime and can be messy if the formulation is an oleaginous base, it should be recommended to patients that they wear a sanitary napkin to protect nightwear and bed linens. These same instructions should be given to patients receiving vaginal suppositories.

Contraceptive Sponge

A unique formulation for vaginal administration is the contraceptive sponge. Though it was voluntarily removed from the U.S. market by the manufacturer, it is marketed elsewhere and may be marketed in the U.S. again. The sponge is made of polyurethane and contains a spermicidal agent. Contraception occurs by the action of the drug and the physical blockage of the cervix by the sponge. The sponge is designed to provide contraceptive protection for a 24 hour period. Before its removal from the market, the sponge was found to have occasional removal problems after use and a few cases of toxic shock were associated with it.

 contraceptive device or formulation designed to prevent pregnancy.

IUD an intrauterine contraceptive device that is placed in the uterus for a prolonged period of time.

REVIEW

KEY CONCEPTS

- ✔ The way in which the body absorbs and distributes drugs varies with the route of administration.

- ✔ A local effect occurs when the drug activity is at the site of administration (e.g., eyes, ears, nose, skin). A systemic effect occurs when the drug is introduced into the circulatory system.

- ✔ Enteral refers to anything involving the tract from the mouth to the rectum. There are three enteral routes: oral, sublingual, and rectal. Oral administration is the most frequently used.

- ✔ The stomach has a pH around 1-2. Certain drugs cannot be taken orally because they are degraded or destroyed by stomach acid and intestinal enzymes.

- ✔ Drugs administered by liquid dosage forms generally reach the circulatory system faster than drugs formulated in solid dosage forms.

- ✔ Oral formulations contain various ingredients beside the active drug. These inactive ingredients include binders, effervescent salts, lubricants, fillers, diluents, and disintegrants.

- ✔ Formulations used in the mouth are generally fast dissolving uncoated tablets which contain highly water soluble drugs.

- ✔ The most common rectal administration forms are suppositories, solutions, and ointments.

- ✔ Any route other than oral, sublingual, and rectal is considered a parenteral administration route. These routes are often preferred when oral administration causes drug degradation or when a rapid drug response is desired, as in an emergency situation.

- ✔ The parenteral routes requiring a needle are intravenous, intramuscular, intradermal, and subcutaneous. These solutions must be sterile (bacteria-free), have an appropriate pH, and be limited in volume.

- ✔ Intravenous dosage forms are administered directly into a vein (and the blood supply).

- ✔ Most solutions are aqueous (water based), but they may also have glycols, alcohols, or other non-aqueous solvents in them.

- ✔ Fat emulsions and TPN emulsions are used to provide triglycerides, fatty acids, and calories for patients who cannot absorb them from the gastrointestinal tract.

- ✔ Infusion is the gradual intravenous injection of a volume of fluid into a patient.

- ✔ Intramuscular injections generally result in lower but longer lasting blood concentrations than after intravenous administration.

- ✔ The subcutaneous (SC, SQ) route can be used for both short term and very long term therapies. Insulin is the most important drug routinely administered by this route.

- ✔ Intradermal injections involve small volumes that are injected into the top layer of skin.

- ✔ Every ophthalmic product must be manufactured to be sterile in its final container.

- ✔ Inhalation dosage forms are intended to deliver drugs to the pulmonary system (lungs).

- ✔ Most dermal dosage forms are used for local (topical) effects on or within the skin.

- ✔ A potential side effect of vaginal administration is Toxic Shock Syndrome.

SELF TEST

MATCH THE TERMS.   *answers can be checked in the glossary*

aqueous
buffer system
degradation
emulsions
hydrates
local effect
nasal inhaler
nasal mucosa
ophthalmic
percutaneous
solvent
sterile
sublingual
systemic effect
topical
trauma
viscosity
water soluble

a condition which is free of all microorganisms.
a device which contains a drug that is vaporized by inhalation.
a liquid that dissolves another substance in it.
absorbs water.
an injury.
applied for local effect, usually to the skin.
ingredients in a formulation designed to control the pH.
mixture of two liquids that do not dissolve into each other.
the absorption of drugs through the skin, often for a systemic effect.
related to the eye.
the cellular lining of the nose.
the changing of a drug to a less effective or ineffective form.
the property of a substance being able to dissolve in water.
the thickness of a liquid.
under the tongue
water based.
when a drug is introduced into the circulatory system.
when drug activity is at the site of administration.

CHOOSE THE BEST ANSWER.   *answers are in the back of the book*

1. Which of the pH values listed below indicates a substance may be alkaline?
   a. pH 1-2
   b. pH 3-4
   c. pH 5-6
   d. pH 7-8

2. Which of the following routes is least likely to give a systemic effect?
   a. oral (po)
   b. sublingual (sl)
   c. rectal (pr)
   d. intradermal (id)

3. Which pathway would the use of a metered dose inhaler (MDI) follow?
   a. mouth, trachea, alveoli, bronchioles
   b. mouth, bronchioles, trachea, alveoli
   c. mouth, trachea, bronchioles, alveoli
   d. none of the above

4. The Norplant® device is made of cylindrical silicone rods that slowly release progesterone to provide contraception for up to 5 years. The method of implantation for these rods is:
   a. intradermal
   b. subcutaneous
   c. intramuscular
   d. intrathecal

PARENTERALS

In parenteral therapy, there are special requirements for how formulations are packaged and how they are administered.

In Chapter 7, *Routes and Formulations*, the methods by which parenteral formulations are administered were reviewed. This chapter will review how these formulations are prepared and packaged.

Parenterals are packaged as two types of products: *large volume parenteral* (LVP) solutions and *small volume parenteral* (SVP) solutions.

LVP solutions are typically bags or bottles containing larger volumes of intravenous solutions. Common uses of LVP solutions without additives include: correction of electrolyte and fluid balance disturbances, nutrition, and vehicles for administering other drugs.

SVP solutions are generally contained in ampules or vials.

Their contents are withdrawn by syringe and either added to an LVP container or injected directly into the patient. SVP solutions are administered directly into the patient by several routes and for reasons that include inability to take oral medications, degradation of some drugs by the gastrointestinal tract, and when rapid and/or continuous action is required (see Chapter 7, *Routes and Formulations*).

CHARACTERISTICS

Because intravenous products are administered directly into the bloodstream, there are a number of special considerations and precautions that must be taken.

✔ **Solutions for injection must be sterile, that is, free from bacteria and other microorganisms.**

Techniques that maintain sterile conditions and prevent contamination must be followed. These are called **aseptic techniques.**

✔ **Solutions must be free of all visible particulate material.**

Examples of such contaminants are glass, rubber cores from vials, cloth or cotton fibers, metal, and plastic. Undissolved particles of an active drug may be present in intravenous suspensions, but no contaminants should be present.

Inspections

Parenteral solutions should always be visually inspected before use. Formulated or admixed solutions should be inspected after compounding. Visual inspection can show two of the six characteristics of parenteral solutions: particulate material, and stability (if lack of stability is indicated by precipitation or crystallization in the solution). Inspection is generally performed against a brightly lit white background.

Visual inspection cannot reveal anything about the sterility, pH, osmolality, presence of pyrogens, or chemical degradation of the drug. Special equipment and skilled personnel are needed to determine these factors. Since sterilty cannot be determined visually, good aseptic technique must be used when dealing with parenteral solutions.

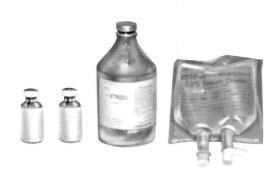

✔ **All parental solutions must be pyrogen-free.**

Intravenous solutions can cause **pyretic** (fever) reactions if they contain pyrogens. Pyrogens are chemicals that are produced by microorganisms. They are soluble in water and are not removed by sterilizing or filtering the solution.

✔ **The solution must be stable for its intended use.**

Most admixtures are prepared hours in advance of when they are to be administered. So the stability of a particular drug in a particular intravenous solution must be factored into the admixture preparation. This information is generally available in a number of reference sources.

✔ **The pH of intravenous solution should not vary significantly from physiological pH, about 7.4.**

Sometimes, other factors may be more important, such as when acidic or alkaline solutions are needed to increase drug solubility or used as a therapeutic treatment themselves.

✔ **Intravenous solutions should be formulated to have an osmolarity similar to that of blood.**

Osmolarity is the characteristic of a solution determined by the number of dissolved particles in it (see page 156). It is measured in terms of **osmoles** (Osmol) or **milliosmoles** (mOsmol) per liter.

Blood has an osmolarity of approximately 300 mOsmol per liter. Both 0.9% sodium chloride solution and 5% dextrose solution have a similar osmolarity. When a solution has an osmolarity equivalent to that of another, it is called **isotonic.**

Intravenous solutions that have greater osmolarity than blood are called **hypertonic** to it, and those with lower osmolarity, **hypotonic.** Both may cause damage to red blood cells, pain, and tissue irritation. However, it is at times necessary to administer such solutions. In these cases, the solutions are usually given slowly and/or through large, free flowing veins to minimize the reactions.

 aseptic techniques techniques that maintain sterile condition.

pyrogens chemicals produced by microorganisms that can cause *pyretic* (fever) reactions in patients.

osmolarity a characteristic of a solution determined by the number of dissolved particles in it.

isotonic when a solution has an osmolarity equivalent to that of another.

hypertonic when a solution has a greater osmolarity than that of another.

hypotonic when a solution has a lesser osmolarity than that of another.

LVP SOLUTIONS

Large volume parenteral (LVP) solutions are intravenous solutions packaged in containers holding 100 ml or more.

There are three types of containers: glass bottle with an air vent tube, glass bottle without an air vent tube, and plastic bags. Plastic bags are available in different sizes. The most common sizes are 50, 100, 250, 500, and 1,000 ml. The top of the bag has a flap with a hole it to hang the bag on an administration pole. At the other end of the bag are two ports of about the same length. One is the administration set port, and the other is the medication port. Graduation marks to indicate the volume of solution in the bag are on its front. They are marked at 25 ml to 100 ml intervals depending on the overall size of the bag.

The administration set port has a plastic cover on it to maintain the sterility of the bag.

The cover is easily removed. Solution will not drip out of the bag through this port because of a plastic diaphragm inside the port. When the spike of the administration set is inserted into the port, the diaphragm is punctured, and the solution will flow out of the bag into the administration set. This inner diaphragm cannot be resealed once punctured.

The medication port is covered by a protective rubber tip.

Drugs are added to the LVP solution through this port using a needle and syringe. There is an inner plastic diaphragm about one half inch inside the port, just like the administration set port. This inner diaphragm is also not self-sealing when punctured by a needle, but the protective rubber tip prevents solutions from leaking from the bag once the diaphragm is punctured. The plastic bag system is not vented to outside air. It collapses as the solution is administered, so a vacuum is not created inside.

Piggybacks

Medications are often administered with piggybacks, which are small volumes of fluid (usually 50-100 ml) infused into the administration set of an LVP solution. Piggybacks are typically infused over a period of thirty to sixty minutes. Some medications are also administered directly into a **volume control chamber**, which is a container in the administration line that holds measured amounts of solution from the IV bag.

ADMINISTRATION

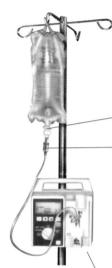

Administration Set

The basic method to administer a LVP solution is to use an administration set. The set contains a spiked plastic device to pierce a **port** on the IV container.

This connects to a **sight** or **drip chamber** that may be used to set the **flow rate**, the rate ordered by the physician at which the solution is to be administered to the patient (generally measured in ml/hour). A clamp pinching the tubing also regulates flow. The line then leads to a rubber injection port to which a needle may be attached or to an **infusion pump** which will control the flow rate.

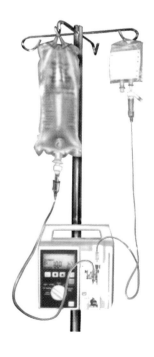

DEVICES

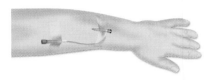

Heparin Lock

In some instances, a patient may not have a primary LVP solution, yet must receive piggyback medications. This is done through a heparin lock, which is a short piece of tubing attached to a needle or intravenous catheter. When the tubing is not being used for the piggyback, heparin is used to fill the tubing. This drug prevents blood from clotting in the tube.

Other Devices

Infusion pumps, syringe pumps, and **ambulatory pumps** are devices used to administer LVP solutions and control flow rates.

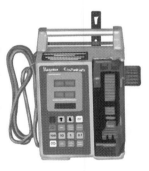

Administration sets are threaded through infusion pumps, and the pumps control the gravity flow. Syringe pumps expel solutions from a syringe into an administration set such as a heparin lock. An ambulatory pump is about the size of a hand. It allows patients to have some freedom of movement compared to being restricted to an infusion pump attached to an administration pole. Infusion pumps have made the infusion process much more accurate and easier to administer and have been a major factor in the growth of home infusion.

Plastic bags have advantages not found with glass bottles.

They do not break. They weigh less. They take up less storage space, and they take up much less disposal space. As a result, glass LVP solution bottles are rarely used.

Some drugs and solutions may not be used with plastic because they interact with it.

In these cases, glass IV bottles are used. They are packaged with a vacuum, sealed by a solid rubber closure, and the closure is held in place by an aluminum band. Graduation marks are along the sides of the bottle and are usually spaced every 20 ml to 50 ml. The solution bottle is hung on an administration pole in an inverted position using the aluminum or plastic band on the bottom of the bottle.

Solutions flow from the containers to the patient through the administration set.

For solutions to flow out of a glass container, air must be able to enter the container to relieve the vacuum as the solution leaves. Some bottles have air tubes built into the rubber closure for this. Some bottles do not, and then an administration set with a filtered airway in the spike must be used.

Common LVP Solutions

Many different intravenous solutions are commercially available. However, four solutions are commonly used either as LVP solutions or as the primary part of an admixture solution. The solutions are:

- ➡ **sodium chloride solution,**
- ➡ **dextrose solution,**
- ➡ **Ringer's solution,**
- ➡ **Lactated Ringer's solution.**

Various combinations of different strengths of sodium chloride and dextrose solutions are also available, e.g., 5% dextrose and 0.45% sodium chloride, or 5% dextrose and 0.2% sodium chloride.

ABCD *flow rate* the rate (in ml/hour or ml/minute) at which the solution is administered to the patient.

heparin lock an injection device which uses heparin to keep blood from clotting in the device.

piggybacks small volume solution added to an LVP.

infusion the slow continuous introduction of a solution into the blood stream.

SVP SOLUTIONS

Small volume parenteral (SVP) solutions are usually 100 ml or less and are primarily used as vehicles for delivering medications. When a drug is added to a parenteral solution, the drug is referred to as the additive, and the final mixture is referred to as the **admixture**.

The phrase "small volume parenterals" can also refer to formulations packaged for parenteral administration: ampules, vials, and prefilled syringes.

Liquid drugs are supplied in prefilled syringes, heat-sealed ampules, or in glass vials sealed with a rubber closure. Powdered drugs are supplied in vials and must be reconstituted (dissolved in a suitable solvent) before being added to the intravenous solution.

Ampules are sealed glass containers with a neck that must be snapped off.

Most ampules are weakened around the base of the neck for easy breaking. These will have a colored band around the base of the neck. Some ampules, however, must first be scored and weakened with a file or the top may shatter. It is useful to wrap a gauze pad around the top of the ampule when opening. This will provide some protection to the fingers if the ampule shatters and will also reduce the possibility of glass splinters becoming airborne. A 5 micron (μm) **filter needle** should be used when withdrawing the contents of an ampule, since glass particles may have fallen inside when the top was snapped off. The filter needle should be removed and replaced with the regular needle before injecting the drug into any solution.

ADDING SVPs TO LVPs

Generally the LVP solution is used as a continuous infusion because of its large volume and slow infusion rates. SVP solutions can be introduced into the on-going LVP infusion by injecting the SVP into the rubber injection port or the volume control chamber of the administration set. However, most often the medication is introduced into the LVP solution, or into a minibag and used as a piggyback.

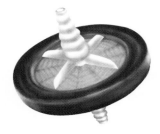

Filters

A filter similar to the one above is often placed between the syringe and needle before the medication is introduced into the bottle or bag. Double ended filtered needles are also used to transfer solutions from a vial directly into a bottle or bag. This eliminates the need of using a syringe.

 admixture the resulting solution when a drug is added to a parenteral solution.

lyophilized freeze-dried.

diluent a liquid that dilutes a substance or solution.

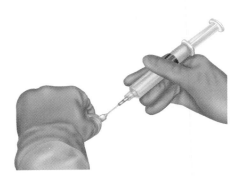

Using a Needle and Syringe to Add a Drug to an LVP:

1. Remove the protective covering from the LVP package.

2. Assemble the needle and syringe.

3. If the drug in the SVP is in powder form, reconstitute it with the recommended diluent.

4. Swab the SVP with an alcohol swab and draw the necessary volume of drug solution.

5. Swab the medication port of the LVP with an alcohol swab.

6. Insert the needle into the medication port and through the inner diaphragm. The medication port should be fully extended to minimize the chance of going through the side of the port.

7. Inject the SVP solution

8. Remove the needle.

9. Shake and inspect the admixture.

Drugs and other additives to intravenous solutions are packaged in vials.

They are available either in liquid form or as **lyophilized** (freeze dried) powders. Powders must be reconstituted with a suitable solution (**diluent**) before use. Vials are made of glass or plastic and have a rubber stopper through which a needle is inserted to withdraw or add to the contents. Before withdrawing solution from a vial, an equal volume of air is usually drawn up in the syringe and injected into the vial. Some medications are packaged under pressure or can produce gas (and pressure) upon reconstitution. In such cases, air is not injected into the vial before withdrawing the solution.

Vials may be prepared for single-dose or multidose use.

Single-dose vials do not contain preservatives and should be discarded after one use. Multidose vials contain a preservative to inhibit bacterial contamination once the vial has been used. Also, the rubber closure will reseal on a multidose vial. These vials can be used for a number of doses of variable volume.

There are two varieties of prefilled syringes.

One type, a cartridge type package, is a single syringe and needle unit which is to be placed in a special holder before use. Once the syringe and needle unit is used, they are discarded but the holder can be used again with a new unit. Another type of prefilled syringe consists of a glass tube closed at both ends with rubber stoppers. The prefilled tube is placed into a specially designed syringe that has a needle attached to it. After using this type of prefilled syringe, all of the pieces are discarded.

Ready to mix systems

Ready-to-mix systems consist of a specially designed minibag with an adapter for attaching a drug vial. The admixing takes place just prior to administration. The major advantages of ready-to-mix systems include a significant reduction in waste and lower potential for medication error because the drug vial remains attached to the minibag and can be rechecked is necessary. However, the systems do cost more, and there is the potential that the system will not be properly activated so that the patient receives only the diluent or a partial dose.

SYRINGES

The basic parts of a syringe are the barrel, plunger, and tip.

The barrel is a tube that is open at one end and tapers into a hollow tip at the other end. The plunger is a piston-type rod with a slightly cone-shaped stopper that passes inside the barrel of the syringe. The tip of the syringe provides the point of attachment for a needle. The volume of solution inside a syringe is indicated by graduation lines on the barrel. Graduation lines may be in milliliters or fractions of a milliliter, depending on the capacity of the syringe. The larger the capacity, the larger the interval between graduation lines. Special purpose syringes, such as **insulin syringes**, have graduation lines in both milliliters and insulin units to reflect their intended use.

There are several common types of syringe tips.

Slip-lok tips allow the needle to be held on the syringe by friction. The needle is reasonably secure, but it may slip off if not properly attached or if considerable pressure is used. **Luer-lock** tips have a collar with grooves that lock the needle in place. **Eccentric** tips, which are off-center, are used when the needle must be parallel to the plane of injection such as in an intradermal injection.

Syringes come in sizes ranging from 1 to 60 ml.

As a rule, the syringe size is the next size larger than the volume to be measured. For example, a 3 ml syringe should be selected to measure 2.3 ml, or a 5 ml syringe to measure 3.8 ml. In this way, the graduation marks on the syringe will be in the smallest possible amounts for the volume measured. Syringes should not be filled to capacity because the plunger can be easily dislodged.

SYRINGES

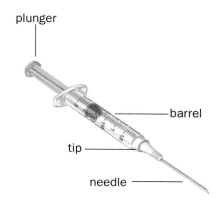

A syringe with graduation marks

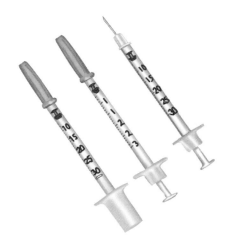

Insulin syringes, with and without needle and barrel caps.

Measuring Volume

The volume of solution in a syringe is measured to the edge of the plunger's stopper while the syringe is held upright and all the air has been removed from the syringe.

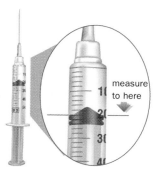

measure to here

Disposable needles should always be used when preparing admixtures as they are presterilized and individually wrapped to maintain sterility.

NEEDLES

Components

A needle has three parts: the **hub**, the **shaft**, and the **bevel**. The hub is at one end of the needle and is the part that attaches to the syringe. It is designed for quick and easy attachment and removal. The shaft is the long, slender stem of the needle that is beveled at one end to form a point called the "bevel." The hollow bore of the needle shaft is known as the **lumen**.

Sizes

Needle sizes are indicated by length and **gauge**. The length of a needle is measured in inches from where the shaft meets the hub to the tip of the bevel. Needle lengths range from 3/8 inch to three and a half inches. Some special use needles are even longer. The gauge of a needle, used to designate the size of the lumen, ranges from 27 (the smallest) to 13 (the largest). *In other words, the higher the gauge number, the smaller is the lumen.*

Needle sizes are chosen based on both the viscosity of the parenteral solution and the type of rubber closure on the container. Needles with a relatively small lumens can be used for most solutions. However, some viscous solutions require large lumens. One problem with this, however, is that large needles are more likely to damage the rubber closures of solution containers, causing particles to fall into the container and contaminate the solution. This is called **"coring."** As a result, small gauge needles are used if the rubber closure can be easily cored.

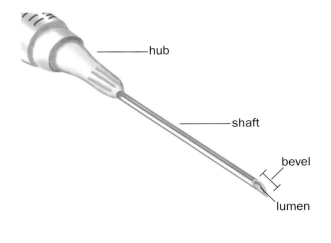

hub
shaft
bevel
lumen

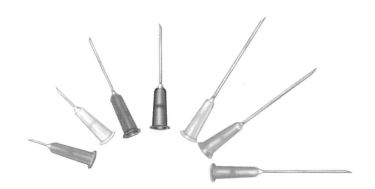

different size needles

bevel an angled surface, as with the tip of a needle.

gauge a measurement—with needles, the higher the gauge, the thinner the lumen.

lumen the hollow center of a needle.

coring when a needle damages the rubber closure of a parenteral container, causing fragments of the closure to fall into the container and contaminate its contents.

FILTERS

Filters are often used to remove contaminating particles from solutions.

They can be attached at the end of a syringe or can be part of the needle. They are divided into two basic groups: **depth filters** and **membrane filters**. Depth filters work by passing the solution through twisting channels that trap particles. A membrane filter looks like paper and consists of many small pores of a uniform size that trap particles larger than the pores. Filters have a wide range of pore sizes. Common ones are 0.22, 0.45, 1, 5, or 10 μm (microns).

Membrane filters are intended to filter a solution only as it is expelled from a syringe.

1. A regular needle is attached to the syringe.

2. The solution is pulled into the syringe.

3. Air bubbles are removed from the syringe.

4. The needle is removed from the syringe.

5. A membrane filter is then attached to the syringe.

6. Another needle is placed on the end of the filter.

7. Air is eliminated from the filter chamber by holding the syringe in a vertical position so that the needle is pointing upward. The air in the filter chamber is then expelled by slowly pushing in the plunger. Air must be expelled before the filter becomes wet; otherwise, the air will not pass through the filter. Do not pull back on the plunger when the membrane filter is being used because the filter may rupture.

8. Once air has been expelled, pressure should be slowly and continuously applied to push the solution through the filter.

MEMBRANE FILTERS

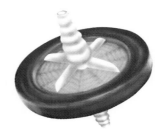

a membrane filter

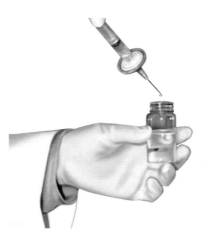

a membrane filter attached to a syringe

DEPTH FILTERS

The depth filter is rigid enough so the solution may be filtered either as it is pulled into or expelled from the syringe, but not both ways in the same procedure. If the drug solution is to be filtered as the solution is pulled into the syringe, the following steps are used:

1. The filter needle is attached to the syringe.

2. The solution is pulled into the syringe.

3. The filter needle is removed.

4. A new needle is attached to the syringe.

5. The solution is expelled from the syringe.

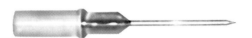

The depth filter is inside the clear hub of this filter needle.

FINAL FILTERS

A filter that filters a solution immediately before it enters the patient's vein is called a **final filter**. Some administration sets contain final filters as components. Some filters are designed to be attached to administration sets and serve as final filters.

membrane filter a filter that attaches to a syringe and filters solution through a membrane as the solution is expelled from the syringe.

depth filter a filter placed inside a needle hub that can filter solutions being drawn in or expelled, but not both.

final filter a filter that filters solution immediately before it enters a patient's vein.

LAMINAR FLOW HOODS

Microorganisms invisible to the eye are present in natural air and on most surfaces, even those that appear clean. Unless aseptic technique is used to prepare parenteral solutions, contamination can easily occur from the environment in which the product is being prepared or from the person preparing it.

The best way to reduce the environmental risk is to use a laminar flow hood which establishes and maintains an ultraclean work area.

Room air is drawn into a horizontal hood and passed through a prefilter to remove relatively large contaminants such as dust and lint. The air is then channeled through a high efficiency particulate air (HEPA) filter that removes particles larger than 0.3 μm (microns). The purified air then flows over the work surface in parallel lines at a uniform velocity (i.e., laminar flow). The constant flow of air from the hood prevents room air from entering the work area and removes contaminants introduced into the work area by material or personnel.

The surfaces of the hood's work area are clean, not sterile.

Therefore, it is necessary to use techniques which maintain the sterilty of all sterile items. These are called **aseptic techniques.** They apply to the technician, the laminar flow hood, and all substances and materials involved in the procedure.

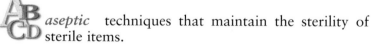

aseptic techniques that maintain the sterility of sterile items.

laminar flow continuous movement at a stable rate in one direction.

HEPA filter a high efficiency particulate air filter.

Types of Laminar Flow Hoods

There are two models of laminar flow hoods: the console model and the bench model. The console model sits on the floor and the work area ranges in width from 3 to 8 feet. The bench (counter top) model is also available in several different sizes. In this model, room air enters at the top of the unit and is channeled downward through the HEPA filter and out horizontally across the work surface.

SAFE PRACTICES

Positioning of material and working inside a hood aseptically requires training, practice, and attention to details.

- ✔ **Never sneeze, cough, talk directly into a hood.**
- ✔ **Close doors or windows.** Breezes can disrupt the air flow sufficiently to contaminate the work area.
- ✔ **Perform all work at least 6 inches inside the hood** to derive the benefits of the laminar air flow. Laminar flow air begins to mix with outside air near the edge of the hood.
- ✔ **Maintain a direct, open path between the filter and the area inside the hood.**
- ✔ **Place nonsterile objects, such as solution containers or your hands, downstream from sterile ones.** Particles blown off these objects can contaminate anything downstream from them.
- ✔ **Do not put large objects at the back of the work area next to the filter.** They will disrupt air flow.

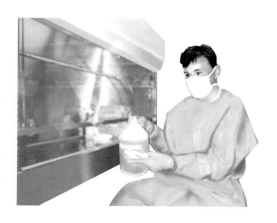

AIR FLOW

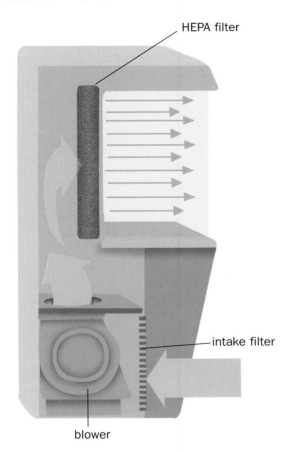

HEPA filter

intake filter

blower

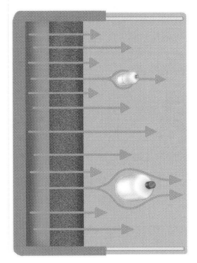

view from above

The illustration at left shows how the laminar air flow hood draws in air through its filters and channels it outward in parallel lines.

The illustration above shows how air is channeled around objects on the work surface. Note that there is a "dead" area behind the large container.

BIOLOGICAL SAFETY HOODS

Biological safety hoods protect both personnel and the environment from contamination. It is used in the preparation of hazardous drugs. A biological safety cabinet functions by passing air through a HEPA filter and directing it down toward the work area. As the air approaches the work surface, it is pulled through vents at the front, back, and sides of the hood. A major portion of the air is recirculated back into the cabinet and a minor portion passes through a secondary HEPA filter and is exhausted into the room.

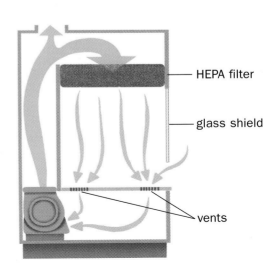

HEPA filter

glass shield

vents

ASEPTIC TECHNIQUE

Personnel involved with admixing parenteral solutions must use good aseptic technique.

Aseptic techniques are the sum total of methods and manipulations required to minimize the contamination of sterile products. Contamination can be from microorganisms and/or particulate material. Working in a laminar flow hood does not, by itself, guarantee aseptic technique. The guidelines on these pages must also be followed, along with any facility and manufacturer guidelines that apply.

Turn On Flow Hood

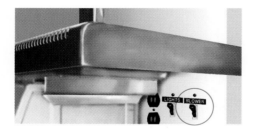

✔ Turn the laminar flow hood on and let it operate for at least 30 minutes before use in order to produce a particle free environment. Maintain a designated "clean" area around the hood.

Cleaning Flow Hood

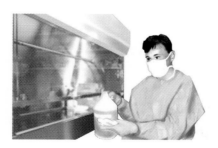

✔ Clean the inside of the hood with a suitable disinfectant such as 70% isopropyl alcoho. Cleaning is started with long side-to-side motions on the back surface of the hood working from top to bottom.

✔ Then the sides of the hood are cleaned using back-to-front motions again working from the top to the bottom of each side.

✔ Then the surface of the hood is cleaned using back-to-front motions.

Clothing and Barriers

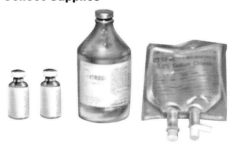

✔ Wear clean lint-free garments or **barrier** clothing, including gowns, hair covers, and a mask.

✔ Wear **sterile gloves.**

✔ Follow facility or manufacturer guidelines for putting on and removing barrier clothing. Unless barriers are put on properly, they can easily become contaminated.

Collect Supplies

✔ Assemble all necessary supplies checking each for expiration dates and particulate material.

✔ Plastic solution containers should be squeezed to check for leaks.

✔ Use only presterilized needles, syringes, and filters. Check the protective covering of each to verify they are intact.

Wash hands

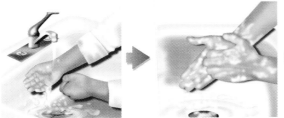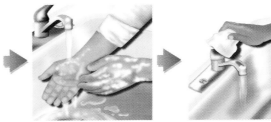

✔ Remove all jewelry and scrub hands and arms to the elbows with a suitable antibacterial agent.

✔ Stand far enough away from the sink so clothing does not come in contact with it.

✔ Turn on water. Wet hands and forearms thoroughly. Keep hands pointed downward.

✔ Scrub hands vigorously with an antibacterial soap.

✔ Work soap under fingernails by rubbing them against the palm of the other hand.

✔ Interlace the fingers and scrub the spaces between the fingers.

✔ Wash wrists and arms up to the elbows.

✔ Thoroughly rinse the soap from hands and arms.

✔ Dry hands and forearms thoroughly using a nonshedding paper towel.

✔ Use a dry paper towel to turn off the water faucet.

✔ After hands are washed, avoid touching clothes, face, hair, or any other potentially contaminated object in the area.

Position Supplies for Use

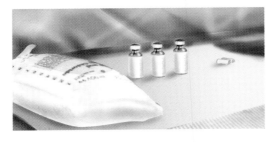

✔ Place supplies on a sterile cloth with smaller supplies closer to the HEPA filter and larger supplies further away from the filter.

✔ Space supplies to maximize laminar flow.

Sterilize Puncture Surfaces

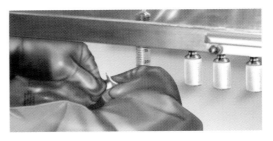

✔ Swab all surfaces that require entry (puncture) with an alcohol wipe. Avoid excess alcohol or lint that might be carried into the solution.

 Sterile supplies often have instructions for use as well as expiration dates. Always follow such instructions along with any facility or manufacturer instructions.

WORKING WITH VIALS

There are two types of parenteral vials that are used in making admixtures.

One contains the drug in solution. The other contains a powder that must be dissolved in a diluent to make a solution. In either case, a needle will be used to penetrate the rubber closure on the vial. To prevent coring and other problems, the techniques on these pages should be followed whenever you are transferring medications from vials.

CORING

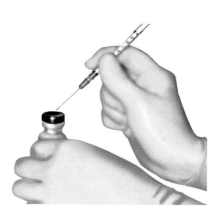

To prevent coring, follow these steps:

✔ Place the vial on a flat surface and position the needle point on the surface of the rubber closure so that the bevel is facing upward and the needle is at about a 45 to 60 degree angle to the closure surface.

✔ Put downward pressure on the needle while gradually bringing the needle up to an upright position. Just before penetration is complete, the needle should be at a vertical (90 degree) angle.

✔ Before the needle is withdrawn from the vial, the drug solution in the needle and the tip of the syringe should be cleared by drawing additional air into the syringe.

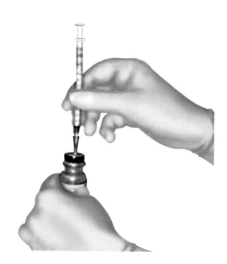

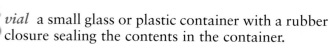 *vial* a small glass or plastic container with a rubber closure sealing the contents in the container.

coring when a needle damages the rubber closure of a parenteral container, causing fragments of the closure to fall into the container and contaminate its contents.

Preparing admixtures for a specific prescription is referred to as *extemporaneous compounding.* Extemporaneous means not prepared in advance.

VIAL WITH SOLUTION

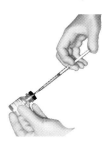 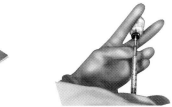 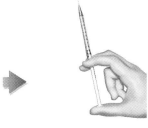

✔ Draw into the syringe a volume of air equal to the volume of drug to be withdrawn. This will offset the pressure in the vial and help in withdrawing the solution.

✔ Penetrate the vial without coring and inject the air.

✔ Turn the vial upside down. Using one hand to hold the vial and the barrel of the syringe, pull back on the plunger with the other hand to fill the syringe. Fill the syringe with a slight excess.

✔ Withdraw the needle from the vial. With the needle end up, tap the syringe to allow air bubbles to come to the top of the syringe. Press the plunger to remove air and excess solution.

✔ Transfer the solution into the intravenous bag or bottle, minimizing coring.

VIAL WITH POWDER

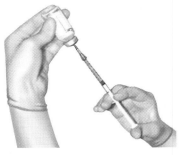 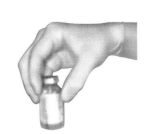 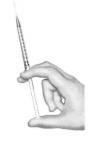

✔ Determine the correct volume of diluent and withdraw it from its vial following the steps outlined above.

✔ Inject the diluent into the medication vial.

✔ Once the diluent is added, a little air should be withdrawn to create a slight negative pressure in the vial. This lowers the chance that aerosol droplets will be sprayed when the needle is withdrawn.

✔ Unless shaking is not recommended, shake the vial until the drug is dissolved.

✔ Reinsert the needle and remove the proper volume of drug solution. Do not inject air before withdrawing the drug solution at this point because the vial is already pressurized.

✔ Remove all air bubbles from the syringe, and transfer the reconstituted solution to the final container.

WORKING WITH AMPULES

Ampules are always broken open at the neck.

Ampules have a colored stripe around the neck if they are prescored to indicate the neck has been weakened by the manufacturer to facilitate opening. Some ampules are not prescored by the manufacturer, and the neck must first be weakened (scored) with a fine file.

TO OPEN AN AMPULE

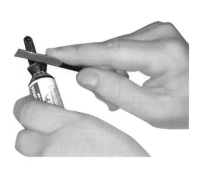 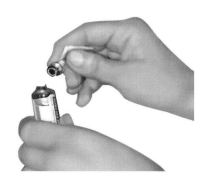

✔ If the ampule is not pre-scored, use a fine file to lightly score the neck at its narrowest point. Do not file all the way through the glass.

✔ Hold the ampule upright and tap the top to settle the solution in the ampule.

✔ Swab the neck of the ampule with an alcohol swab.

✔ Wrap a gauze pad around the neck of the ampule. Grasp the ampule on each side of the neck with the thumb and index finger of each hand.

✔ Quickly snap the ampule moving your hands outward and away. If the ampule does not snap easily, rotate it slightly and try again.

✔ Inspect the opened ampule for glass particles that may have fallen inside.

Note: Hands may be clean but are never sterile. Once they touch a sterile surface, it is no longer sterile. The outside surface of the above ampule would no longer be sterile. In situations where all surfaces must be sterile, hands would be gloved.

ampules sealed glass containers with an elongated neck that must be snapped off.
sharps needles, jagged glass or metal objects, or any items that might puncture or cut the skin.

TRANSFERRING SOLUTION

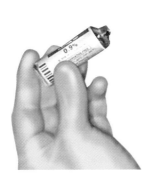

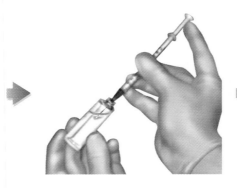

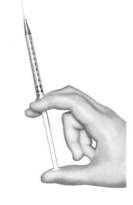

✔ Hold the ampule at about a 20-degree angle.
✔ Insert the needle into the ampule. Avoid touching the opening of the ampule with the needle point.

✔ Position the needle in the solution. Place its beveled edge against the side of the ampule to avoid pulling glass particles into the syringe.
✔ Withdraw solution but keep needle submerged to avoid withdrawing air into the syringe.

✔ Withdraw needle from ampule and remove all air bubbles from the syringe.
✔ Transfer the solution to the final container using a filter needle or membrane filter.

DISPOSAL

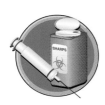

Discarded gloves, needles, syringes, ampules, vials, and prefilled syringes used in preparing parenterals pose a source of contamination and must be disposed of properly. In many health care facilities and other locations, such containers often have a label with **"Sharps"** on it, indicating objects that might puncture or cut the skin of anyone who handles them.

✔ Always separate sharps from other refuse for disposal.
✔ Receptacles that are easy to identify and are leakproof, punctureproof, and sealable should be used exclusively for this type of hazardous waste.
✔ Needles should not be clipped or recapped in order to prevent aerosolization or accidental needle sticks.
✔ Excess solutions should be returned to their original vial, an empty vial, or some other suitable, closed container.

UNITS OF MEASUREMENT

There are different ways to express the amount of drug in a parenteral solution.

Each method of expressing the concentration is related to a particular property of the solution. The common concentrations and their units are listed on these pages.

MOLARITY

Molarity is an expression of the number of moles of a drug in a volume of solution. A mole is the number of grams equal to the **molecular weight** of the drug. The molecular weight is the sum of the atomic weights of all the atoms that make up the molecule. Potassium chloride (KCl) has a molecular weight of 74.6. So, one mole of potassium chloride is 74.6 grams.

Parenteral concentrations are generally expressed as **mole/liter** (written as mol/L, or M). A 1M solution of potassium chloride contains 74.6 grams of the drug in 1000 ml (1 liter) of solution.

Some molarity concentrations are expressed as millimoles per liter. A millimole is one-thousandth of a mole.

Salt Forms

Drugs come in different salt forms for a variety of reasons, and the salt form and **"waters of hydration"** must be factored into determining the molecular weight of a drug. For example, chloride comes as the sodium salt, the potassium salt, and the calcium salt.

Waters of hydration are water molecules that can attach to drug molecules. For example, calcium chloride ($CaCl_2$) exists in three different forms, **anhydrous** (no waters), **dihydrate** (2 associated waters), and **hexahydrate** (six waters of hydration). *The dihydrate form is the one used in making parenteral solutions.*

OSMOLES

Another expression for concentration is the osmole (Osmol). An osmole is equal to the molecular weight of the drug divided by the number of **ions** formed when a drug dissolves in solutions.

$$osmole = \frac{molecular\ weight}{ions}$$

For example, potassium chloride forms two ions when it dissolves in solutions. Therefore, 1 Osmol of potassium chloride would be its molecular weight (74.6 grams) divided by two: 37.3 grams. Anhydrous calcium chloride forms three ions when it dissolves in solution: one calcium ion and two chloride ions. 1 Osmol would be its molecular weight (111.0 grams) divided by three: 37.0 grams.

Most Osmol solutions are expressed as Osmol/liter (written as Osmol/L). Some concentrations are expressed as mOsmol/L. A milliosmole is one-thousandth of an osmole.

molecular weight the sum of the atomic weights of one molecule.

ion molecular particles that carry electric charges.

anhydrous without water molecules.

waters of hydration water molecules that attach to drug molecules.

equivalent weight a drug's molecular weight divided by its valence, a common measure of electrolytes.

valence the number of positive or negative charges on an ion.

EQUIVALENTS

Another expression of concentration is the **equivalent (Eq)**. It is used to describe concentrations of electrolytes such as potassium chloride, sodium chloride, sodium acetate, etc.

When an electrolyte dissolves in solution, it divides into **ions,** particles which carry electric charges that can be positive or negative. The number of positive *or* negative charges (but not both added together) is called the **valence** of the ions. It indicates the ions' ability to combine with other atoms or molecules.

An equivalent weight is equal to the molecular weight of the drug divided by the valence of the ions that form when the drug is dissolved.

$$\text{equivalent} = \frac{\text{molecular weight}}{\text{valence}}$$

As with molar solutions, equivalent solutions are expressed as **Eq/liter** (written as Eq/L). Equivalent concentrations are also expressed as milliequivalents (mEq) per liter. A milliequivalent is one-thousandth of an equivalent weight.

EXAMPLE

Potassium chloride (KCl) splits into one potassium ion (K^+) and one chloride ion (Cl^-).

➥ **KCl's valence is 1** since there is either one positive charge on the potassium ion or one negative charge on the chloride ion.
➥ **The equivalent weight of KCL is 74.6 grams divided by one: 74.6 grams.**

EXAMPLE

Anhydrous calcium chloride ($CaCl_2$, 110.0 grams) splits into one calcium ion having two positive charges (++) and two chloride ions, each having one negative charge (-).

➥ **Its valence is 2.**
➥ **The equivalent weight of $CaCl_2$ is 111.0 grams divided by two: 55.5 grams.**

PERCENTAGE WEIGHT PER VOLUME

Percentage concentrations refer to the drug's weight per 100 ml if the drug is a solid, or the drug's volume per 100 ml if the drug is a liquid.

$$\text{solid: \%} = \frac{\text{weight (gm)}}{\text{100ml}}$$

$$\text{liquid: \%} = \frac{\text{volume (ml)}}{\text{100ml}}$$

For example, a 5% dextrose solution contains 5 grams of dextrose (a solid) in 100 ml of solution. A 5% acetic acid solution (common household vinegar) contains 5 ml of acetic acid (a liquid) per 100 ml of solution.

Percentage concentrations are applied to other formulations besides parenteral solutions. A 10% zinc oxide ointment would have 10 grams of zinc oxide (a solid) in 100 grams of ointment.

INTERNATIONAL UNITS

Because the potency and purity of drugs from biological sources vary depending on the source, they are measured by **units of activity** rather than by weight. Units may be abbreviated as IU, or U, and are expressed for example as 2,000 U, 1,000,000 U, etc. Drugs commonly measured in international units include penicillin, insulin, heparin, and some vitamins.

SPECIAL SOLUTIONS

PARENTERAL NUTRITION SOLUTIONS

Parenteral nutrition solutions are complex admixtures used to provide nutritional support to patients who are unable to take in adequate nutrients through their digestive tract. These admixtures are composed of dextrose, fat, protein, electrolytes, vitamins, and trace elements. They are hypertonic solutions. Base parenteral nutrition solutions are available in 2,000 and 3,000 ml sizes. The base solution consists of:

➡ an amino acid solution (a source of protein);
➡ a dextrose solution (a source of carbohydrate calories).

These solutions, sometimes referred to as **macronutrients,** make up most of the volume of a parenteral nutrition solution. Several electrolytes, trace elements, and multiple vitamins (together referred to as **micronutrients**) may be added to the base solution to meet individual patient requirements. Common electrolyte additives include sodium chloride (or acetate), potassium chloride (or acetate), calcium gluconate, magnesium sulfate, and sodium (or potassium) phosphate. Multiple vitamin preparations containing both water-soluble and fat-soluble vitamins are usually added on a daily basis. A trace element product containing zinc, copper, manganese, selenium, and chromium may be added.

Intravenous fat (lipid) emulsion is required as a source of essential fatty acids. It is also used as a concentrated source of calories. Fat provides nine calories per gram, compared to 3.4 calories per gram provided by dextrose. Intravenous fat emulsion may be admixed into the parenteral nutrition solution with amino acids and dextrose, or piggybacked into the administration line. When intravenous fat emulsion is admixed with the base solution, the resulting solution is referred to as a **total nutrient admixture (TNA)**, or **total parenteral nutrition (TPN) admixture**.

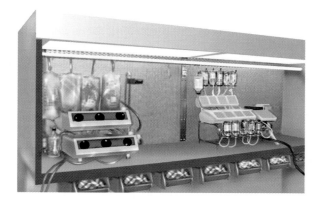

TPN preparation system

Administration

TPN solutions are generally (though not always) administered via the subclavian vein under the collar bone over 8 to 24 hours. Slow administration using this vein minimizes the adverse effects that may occur with such a hypertonic solution. The subclavian vein is large and close to the heart, so the solution is diluted rapidly by the large volume of blood in the heart.

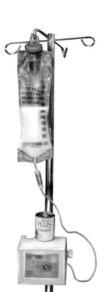

To assure their accurate delivery, nutrition solutions are almost always administered with an intravenous infusion pump. Parenteral nutrition solutions are commonly administered through an in-line filter in the administration set positioned as close to the patient as possible. However, intravenous fat emulsions, either alone or as part of a TPN solution, can be administered through an in-line filter only if it has a pore size of 1.2 micron or larger. An alternative is to piggyback the intravenous fat emulsion into the primary line below the in-line filter.

macronutrients amino acids and dextrose in the base parenteral nutrition solution.

micronutrients electrolytes, vitamins, and trace elements added to a base parenteral nutrition solution.

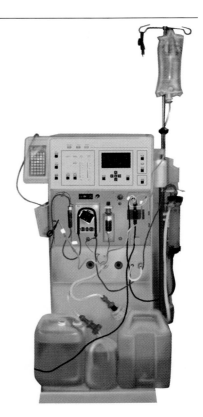

DIALYSIS SOLUTIONS

Dialysis refers to the passage of small particles through membranes. This is caused by **osmosis,** the action in which a drug in a solution of a higher concentration will move through a **permeable** membrane (one that can be penetrated) to a solution of a lower concentration.

Like irrigation solutions, dialysis solutions are not administered into the venous system and are supplied in containers larger than 1000 ml capacity. **Peritoneal dialysis solutions** are used by patients who do not have functioning kidneys. The solution is administered directly into the **peritoneal cavity (**the cavity between the abdominal lining and the internal organs) to remove toxic substances, excess body waste, and serum electrolytes through osmosis. *These solutions are hypertonic to blood so the water will not move into the circulatory system.*

Peritoneal solutions are administered several times a day. The solution is permitted to flow into the abdominal cavity, and then remains in the cavity for 30 to 90 minutes. It is then drained by a siphon into discharge bottles. This procedure is repeated many times a day and may use up to 50 liters of solution.

IRRIGATION SOLUTIONS

Irrigation solutions are not administered directly into the venous system but are subject to the same stringent controls as intravenous fluids. They are packaged in containers that are larger than 1000 ml capacity and are designed to empty rapidly. **Surgical irrigating solutions** (splash solutions) are used to:

➡ bathe and moisten body tissues,
➡ moisten dressings,
➡ wash instruments.

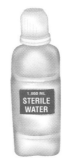

They are typically Sodium Chloride for Irrigation or Sterile Water for Irrigation. **Urologic solutions** are used during operations to:

➡ maintain tissue integrity,
➡ remove blood to maintain a clear field of vision.

Sterile Water for Irrigation, 1.5% glycine, and 3% sorbital solutions are commonly used because they are **non-hemolytic (**do not damage blood cells).

 osmosis the action in which drug in a higher concentration solution passes through a permeable membrane to a lower concentration solution.

dialysis movement of particles in a solution through permeable membranes.

REVIEW

KEY CONCEPTS

✔ Parenterals are packaged as two types of products: large volume parenteral (LVP) solutions and small volume parenteral (SVP) solutions.

✔ LVP solutions are typically bags or bottles containing larger volumes of intravenous solutions. SVP solutions are generally contained in ampules or vials.

✔ Solutions for injection must be sterile, free of all visible particulate material, pyrogen-free, stable for their intended use, have a pH around 7.4, and in most (but not all) cases isotonic.

✔ The flow rate is the rate at which the solution is administered to the patient.

✔ Piggybacks are small volumes of fluid (usually 50-100 ml) infused into the administration set of an LVP solution.

✔ Infusion pumps, syringe pumps, and ambulatory pumps are devices used to administer LVP solutions and control flow rates.

✔ When a drug is added to a parenteral solution, the drug is referred to as the additive, and the final mixture is referred to as the admixture.

✔ The volume of solution in a syringe is measured to the edge of the plunger's stopper while the syringe is held upright and all air has been removed from the syringe.

✔ Syringes come in sizes ranging from 1 to 60 ml. As a rule, a syringe size is used that is one size larger than the volume to be measured.

✔ Needle sizes are indicated by length and gauge. The higher the gauge number, the smaller is the lumen (the hollow bore of the needle shaft). Large needles may be needed with highly viscous solutions but are more likely to cause coring.

✔ Syringe filters are often used to remove contaminating particles from solutions.

✔ A laminar flow hood establishes and maintains an ultraclean work area for the preparation of IV admixtures.

✔ Aseptic techniques maintain the sterilty of all sterile items and are used in preparing IV admixtures.

✔ Biological safety hoods are used in the preparation of hazardous drugs and protect both personnel and the environment from contamination.

✔ Percentage concentrations refer to the drug's weight per 100 ml if the drug is a solid, or the drug's volume per 100 ml if the drug is a liquid.

✔ Equivalent (Eq) or milliequivalent (mEq/l) are used to describe concentrations of electrolytes in solution.

✔ Parenteral nutrition solutions are complex admixtures composed of dextrose, fat, protein, electrolytes, vitamins, and trace elements. They are hypertonic solutions. Most of the volume of TPN solutions is made up of macronutrients: amino acid solution (a source of protein) and a dextrose solution (a source of carbohydrate calories).

✔ Peritoneal dialysis solutions are used by patients who do not have functioning kidneys to remove toxic substances, excess body waste, and serum electrolytes through osmosis.

SELF TEST

MATCH THE TERMS.   *answers can be checked in the glossary*

admixture

aseptic techniques

bevel

dialysis

diluent

gauge

HEPA filter

hypertonic

hypotonic

ion

isotonic

osmolarity

pyrogens

a characteristic of a solution determined by the number of dissolved particles in it.

when a solution has a lesser osmolarity than that of another.

a high efficiency particulate air filter.

a liquid that dilutes a substance or solution.

a needle measurement–the higher the gauge, the thinner the lumen.

when a solution has an osmolarity equivalent to that of another.

an angled surface, as with the tip of a needle.

chemicals produced by microorganisms that can cause fever reactions in patients.

molecular particles that carry electric charges.

movement of particles in a solution through permeable membranes.

techniques that maintain sterile condition.

the resulting solution when a drug is added to a parenteral solution.

when a solution has a greater osmolarity than that of another.

CHOOSE THE BEST ANSWER.   *answers are in the back of the book*

1. An intravenous solution that is formulated to have an osmolarity equivalent to that of blood is
   a. isotonic to it.
   b. hypotonic to it.
   c. hypertonic to it.
   d. none of the above

2. You are to use 2.4 ml of diluent to reconstitute a vial of medication. What size of syringe should be used?
   a. 20 ml
   b. 10 ml
   c. 5 ml
   d. 3 ml

3. When using the laminar flow hood, a technician should work inside the hood at least
   a. two inches
   b. four inches
   c. six inches
   d. eight inches

4. Of the following needles, which size of needle is most likely to cause coring?*
   a. 13 G
   b. 16 G
   c. 20 G
   d. 23 G

COMPOUNDING

Extemporaneous compounding is the on-demand preparation of a drug product according to a physician's prescription, formula, or recipe.

As we mentioned in the preceding chapter, extemporaneous means "not prepared in advance." Such compounding is done to meet the special needs of particular patients. It requires specialized knowledge of the physical and chemical properties of drugs and their vehicles. It also requires proper training and skill. This chapter will focus on the terminology, equipment, and basic principles of extemporaneous compounding.

There are various types of compounding.

It can mean the preparation of suspensions, dermatologicals, and suppositories; the conversion of one dose or dosage form into another; the preparation of select dosage forms from bulk chemicals; the preparation of intravenous admixtures, parenteral nutrition solutions, and pediatric dosage forms from adult dosage forms; the preparation of radioactive isotopes; or the preparation of cassettes, syringes, and other devices with drugs for administration in the home setting.

The demand for pharmaceutical compounding has grown substantially.

Reasons for this include the growth of home health care, the unavailability of certain drug products, orphan drugs, veterinary compounding, and biotechnology-derived drug products. Newly evolving dosage forms and therapies also suggest that compounding will become more common in pharmacy practice.

Technicians, under pharmacist supervision, are increasingly involved in compounding.

Specific responsibilities will vary from environment to environment. Therefore, it is necessary to know and understand the specific responsibilities and requirements that apply to your job.

SPECIAL NEEDS

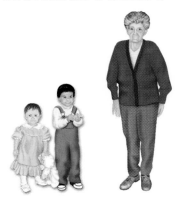

Compounding is done for many special reasons, including for:

- ➡ Pediatric patients requiring diluted adult strengths of drugs.

- ➡ Patients needing an oral solution or suspension of a product that is only available in another form.

- ➡ Patients with sensitivity to dyes, preservatives, or flavoring agents found in commercial formulations.

- ➡ Dermatological formulations with fortified (strengthened) or diluted concentrations of commercially available products.

- ➡ Specialized dosages for therapeutic drug monitoring.

- ➡ Care for hospice patients in pain management.

- ➡ Compounding for animals.

Accuracy and Stability In Compounding

Different units of the same manufactured product must essentially have the same content and characteristics, and they are tested to confirm this. However, there is no such testing or proof for extemporaneously compounded products. As a result, compounding accuracy and the stability of the compounded product are issues. The USP defines **stability** of drug forms as the chemical and physical integrity of the dosage unit, and when appropriate, the ability of the unit to maintain protection against microbiological contamination.

The supervising pharmacist must determine that a product can be accurately compounded and *will be stable for its expected use. Accuracy is then essential* in all weighings, measurements, and other activities in the compounding process.

SECTION 503A

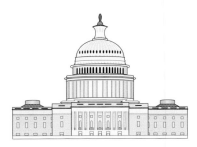

This law gives the following definitions of compounding and manufacturing:

Compounding is defined as "the preparation, mixing, assembling, packaging, or labeling of a drug or device (i) as the result of a practitioner's prescription drug order or initiative based on the practitioner-patient-pharmacist relationship in the course of professional practice, or (ii) for the purpose of, or as an incident to, research, teaching, or chemical analysis and not for sale or dispensing. Compounding also includes the preparation of drugs or devices in anticipation of prescription drug orders based on routine, regularly observed prescribing patterns."

Manufacturing is defined as "the production, preparation, propagation, conversion, or processing of a drug or device, either directly or indirectly, by extraction from substances of natural origin or independently by means of chemical or biological synthesis, and includes any packaging or repackaging of the substance(s) or labeling or relabeling of its container, and the promotion and marketing of such drugs or devices. Manufacturing also includes the preparation and promotion of commercially available products from bulk compounds for resale by pharmacies, practitioners, or other persons."

In 1997, a major piece of federal legislation was passed that preserves the right of pharmacists to compound.

The legislation was titled the **FDA Modernization Act of 1997**, and became effective November 21, 1998. The legislation added to the Food, Drug and Cosmetic Act a provision (Section 503A) which clearly establishes that compounding by pharmacists is legal. Previously, the FDA considered compounding a form of manufacturing and subject to the same **Good Manufacturing Practices (GMP)** that applied to the large pharmaceutical manufacturers. Meeting these regulations would have effectively eliminated compounding from pharmacy.

The new law guarantees the continued availability of compounded drug products as a part of individual patient treatment.

It preserved the pharmacist-patient-practitioner (triad) relationship as the basis for the practice of compounding. It also seeks to prevent manufacturing under the pretense of compounding.

Effects of the Law

✔ preserved the pharmacist-patient-practitioner relationship as the basis for the practice of compounding;

✔ allowed for **anticipatory** (in advance of expected need) **compounding;**

✔ set criteria for the drug substances used in compounding;

✔ described a foundation for addressing interstate distribution of compounded drugs;

✔ limited advertising and promotion to compounding services.

extemporaneous compounding the on-demand preparation of a drug product according to a physician's prescription, formula, or recipe.
stability the chemical and physical integrity of the dosage unit, and when appropriate, its ability to withstand microbiological contamination.
anticipatory compounding compounding in advance of expected need.

EQUIPMENT

Each individual compounded prescription can be viewed as a four step process: measure, mix, mold, and package.

Not all steps are needed in every compounded prescription, but they indicate the type of equipment necessary for compounding.

To Measure

Balance, weights, weighing containers, volumetric glassware (graduates, pipets, flasks), syringes, buret.

To Mix

Beakers, Erlenmeyer flasks, spatulas, funnels, sieves, mortar and pestle.

To Mold

Hot plates, suppository molds, capsule shells, ointment slabs.

To Package

Prescription bottles, capsule vials, suppository boxes, ointment jars.

Degree of Error

Class A balances can weigh as little as 120 mg of material with a 5% error. 5% is generally considered an acceptable error in most pharmaceutical processes.

Small Quantities

When a prescription calls for a ingredient weighing less than 120 mg, a precise amount of the drug is mixed with an inert (inactive) powder, so that a fraction of the resulting mix weighing at least 120 mg will contain the amount of drug needed. This fraction of the mixed powders is called an **aliquot**.

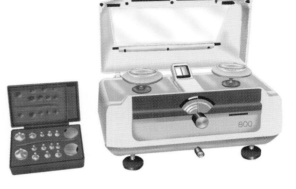

Balance

A balance is used to determine the weight of a powder, dosage form, liquid, etc. Most pharmacies have a **Class A** prescription balance. The Class A balance is a 2 pan torsion type balance which uses both internal and external weights. The balance has a **rider** which adds the internal weights to the right hand pan. The rider is always calibrated in the metric system (grams), though some riders also have calibration marks in the apothecary system (grains).

Sensitivity

Class A balances have a sensitivity requirement of up to **6 mg.** The sensitivity of a balance is the amount of weight that will move the balance pointer one division mark.

Capacity

Class A balances have a minimum weighable quantity of 120 mg and most have a maximum weighable quantity of 60 grams, though some will weigh up to 120 grams.

Weights

A proper set of metric weights is essential for prescription compounding. These are usually brass cylindrical weights ranging from 1 gram to 50 gram and fractional weights of 10 mg to 500 mg. Weights should be stored in their box. They must be handled with forceps (not with fingers!) to prevent soiling and erosion of the weights.

calibrate to set, mark, or check the graduations of a measuring device.

aliquot a portion of a mixture.

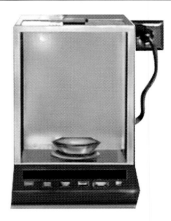

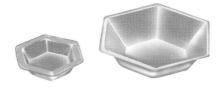

Electronic or Analytical balance

A way to weigh smaller quantities than 120 mg with acceptable accuracy is to use either an electronic or analytical balance. Electronic balances come in a variety of sizes and shapes. Most are top-loading balances and have sensitivities around 1 mg. Analytical balances may be found in some pharmacies, but are generally found in research laboratories. They have extremely high sensitivities and are designed to weigh milligram and microgram quantities of materials.

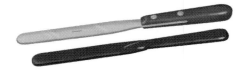

Spatulas

Spatulas are used to transfer solid ingredients. They are also used as the mixing instruments in semisolid dosage forms such as ointments and creams. Spatulas are available in a variety of sizes and are made of stainless steel, hard rubber, or plastic. Stainless steel spatulas can be corroded with certain materials such as iodine and in these cases, the rubber or plastic spatulas should be used. Always check that spatulas are clean before use.

Weighing Papers or Weighing Boats

Weighing papers or weighing boats should always be placed on the balance pans before any weighing is done. These protect the pans from damage and also provide a convenient way to transfer the weighed material from the balance to another vessel. Weighing papers are made of nonabsorbable glassine paper and weighing boats are made of polystyrene. When using weighing papers, the paper should be diagonally creased from each corner and then flattened and placed on the pans. This ensures a collection trough in the paper. New weighing papers or weighing boats should be used with each new drug to prevent contamination.

Mortar and Pestle

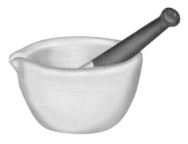

The mortar and pestle is made of three types of materials: glass, wedgewood; and porcelain. Wedgewood and porcelain mortars are earthenware, relatively course in texture, and are used to grind crystals and large particles into fine powders. The process of grinding powders to reduce the particle size is call trituration. Glass mortars and pestles are preferable for mixing liquids and semi solid dosage forms.

VOLUMETRIC EQUIPMENT

In compounding, liquid drugs, solvents, or additives are measured in volumetric glassware or plasticware.

Volumetric means "measures volume." Common volumetric vessels are **pipets, cylindrical** and **conical graduates, burets, syringes,** and **volumetric flasks.** The volume capacity is etched on the vessel, and some devices will have graduation marks.

Volumetric vessels are either TD or TC, "to deliver" or "to contain."

Volumetric pipets, burets, and syringes are TD vessels. Volumetric flasks and cylindrical and conical graduates are TC vessels, although in practice they are also used as TD vessels.

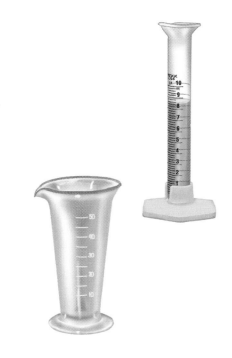

Graduates

Graduates, both cylindrical and cone shaped, are used for measuring and transferring liquids. Cylindrical graduates are the preferred device because they are more accurate. Graduates are available in sizes ranging from 5 ml to 4000 ml. When selecting a graduate, always choose the smallest graduate capable of containing the volume to be measured. Avoid measurements of volumes that are below 20 percent of the capacity of the graduate because the accuracy is unacceptable. For example a 100 ml graduate cannot accurately measure volumes below 20 ml. When measuring small volumes, such as 20 ml and less, it is often preferable to use a syringe or pipet.

Volumetric Flasks

Volumetric flasks have slender necks and wide bulb-like bases. Volumetric flasks are single volume glassware and come in sizes ranging from 5 ml to 4000 ml. There is a calibration mark etched on the neck of the flask, that when filled to that mark, the flask contains the volume marked on it.

Volumetric flasks are hard to use if dissolving solids in liquid because of the narrowness of the neck. If solids are to be dissolved, partially fill the flask with liquid to affect dissolution, and then fill the flask with more liquid to the calibration mark.

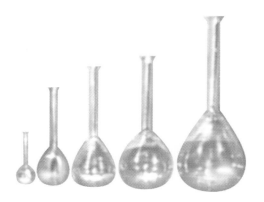

volumetric measures volume.

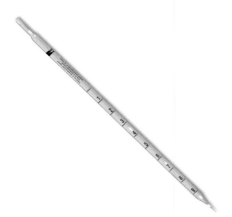

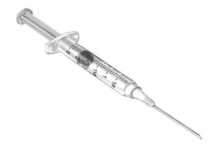

Pipets

Pipets are thin glass tubes recommended for the delivery of all volumes less than 5 ml and required for delivering volumes less than 1 ml (in the absence of an appropriate syringe). A rubber pipet bulb is used to draw liquid into the pipet. There are two basic types of pipets:

➡ The single volume or transfer pipet is the most accurate and simplest to use, but is limited to the measurement of a single fixed volume. They are normally used for the accurate transfer of 1.0, 2.0, 5.0, 10.0, and 25.0 ml of liquid.

➡ The calibrated volumetric pipet is graduated from a point near the tip to the capacity of the pipet. It can deliver multiple volumes of liquid with good volumetric precision.

Syringes

Syringes come in sizes from 0.5 ml to 60 ml and in a variety of materials and styles. For most compounding tasks involving small volumes, a disposable hypodermic syringe made of plastic is used. Syringes have graduation marks on the barrel for measuring partial volumes. As when selecting a graduate, choose the smallest syringe capable of containing the volume to be measured.

 Erlenmeyer flasks (right), beakers, and prescription bottles, regardless of markings, are *not volumetric glassware*, but are simply 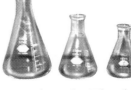 containers for storing and mixing liquids. The designated volume is only the *approximate* capacity of the vessel.

USING A BALANCE

In order to obtain an accurate weight of components on the prescription balance, appropriate techniques must be used. The following steps should always be taken to insure accuracy.

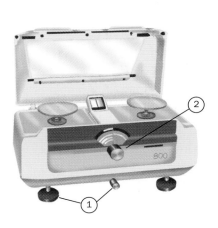

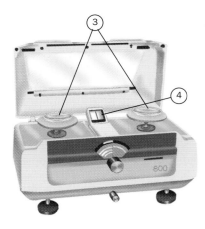

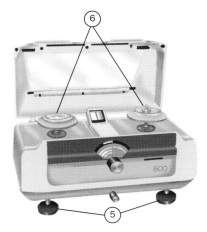

1. Arrest the balance by turning the arrest knob. Level the balance front to back by turning the leveling screw feet all the way into the balance and then moving them the same direction until the 4 sides of the balance are equidistant from the benchtop. For balances with leveling bubbles, move the leveling screw feet until the bubble is in the middle of the tube.

2. Set the internal weights to zero. This is done by turning the calibrated dial to zero.

3. Use weighing boats or glassine weighing papers. If using weighing papers, fold diagonally. Then gently flatten and place one on each weighing pan.

4. Unlock the balance by releasing the arrest knob and note the rest point of the pointer on the index. If the pointer does not rest at the center of the index, then it will be necessary to level the balance from left to right.

5. Level the balance left to right by adjusting the leveling screw feet. To shift the pointer left, grasp both the screw feet between thumbs and forefingers and rotate so that thumbs move inward. To shift the pointer to the right, rotate both screw feet so that forefingers move toward the back of the balance. Continue adjusting the screw feet slowly until the pointer rests at the center of the index.

6. Arrest the balance and place the required weights in the boats on the right pan. Place the material to be weighed in the boats on the left pan.

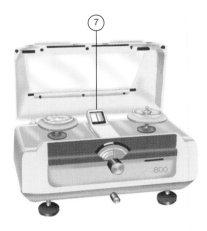

7. Release the balance and note the shift of the pointer on the index. If the pointer shifts left, too much of the drug is on the pan and a portion should be removed. If it shifts right, there is too little drug and more should be added.

8. Once you are satisfied that you have made an accurate measurement, double check to make sure that you have weighed the correct substance (check the label) and that you have used the correct weights (internal and external).

Basic Guidelines

There are some general rules about using a balance that help to maintain the balance in top condition.

✔ Always cover both pans with weighing papers or use weighing boats. These protect the pans from abrasions, eliminate the need for repeated washing, and reduce loss of drug to porous surfaces.

✔ A clean paper or boat should be used for each new ingredient to prevent contamination of components.

✔ The balance must be readjusted after a new weighing paper or boat has been placed on each pan. Weighing papers taken from the same box can vary in weight by as much as 65 mg. If the new zero point is not established, an error of as much as 65 mg can be made. On 200 mg of material, this is more than 30%. Weighing boats also vary in weight.

✔ Always arrest the balance before adding or removing weight from either pan. Although the balance is noted for its durability, repeated jarring of the balance will ultimately damage the working mechanism of the balance and reduce its accuracy.

✔ Always clean the balance, close the lid, and arrest the pans before storing the balance between uses.

✔ Always use the balance on a level surface and in a draft-free area.

ABCD *arrest knob* the knob on a balance that prevents any movement of the balance.

LIQUID MEASUREMENT

Selecting a Liquid Measuring Device

✔ *Always use the smallest device (graduate, pipet, syringe) that will accommodate the desired volume of liquid.* This will minimize the potential for errors of measurement associated with misreading the scale.

✔ Use a graduated pipet or syringe to measure/deliver volumes less than 1 ml.

✔ Remember that oily and viscous liquids will be difficult to remove from graduates and pipets, and at best require long drainage time. Consider using a syringe instead, or measuring by weight rather than volume.

✔ Never use prescription bottles, non-volumetric flasks, beakers, or household teaspoons as measurement devices.

✔ Liquids have a **meniscus** when they are poured into containers. The surface of the liquid curves downward toward the center. If the container is very narrow, the meniscus can be quite large. When reading a volume of a liquid against a graduation mark, *hold the graduate so the meniscus is at eye level and read the mark at the bottom of the meniscus.* Viewing the level from above will create the incorrect impression that there is more volume in the graduate.

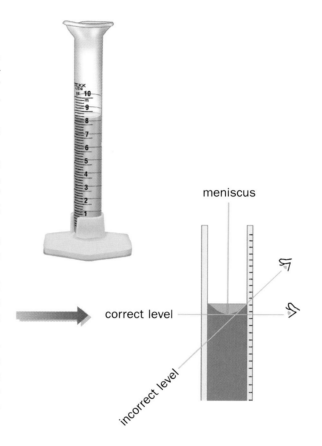

meniscus

correct level

incorrect level

Droppers

Medicine droppers can be used to deliver small doses of liquid medication. But the medicine dropper must first be calibrated because the drop size will vary from dropper to dropper and from liquid to liquid. Personal factors can also contribute to the inaccuracy of droppers. Two individuals dispensing the same liquid from identical droppers may produce drops of different sizes because of variations in the pressure, speed of dropping, and the angle at which the dropper is held.

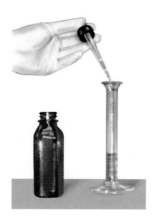

To calibrate a medicine dropper, slowly drop the final drug formulation into a small cylindrical graduate (10 ml), and count the number of drops needed to add several milliliters (ml) to the graduate. Calculate the average number of drops per ml. Some commercially produced medications are packaged with a marked dropper which as has already been calibrated for that preparation.

Graduates

Cylindrical graduates are more accurate than conical graduates. The following steps will help to maximize accuracy when using either a cylindrical or conical graduate.

1. Either place the graduate on a flat surface that will allow you to view it at eye level or hold the graduate by the base with the left hand (for a right handed person) and elevated so that the desired mark is at eye level.

2. Hold the solution container with the right hand and pour the liquid to be measured into the center of the graduate. This will avoid the error resulting from liquid adhering to the wall of the graduate (especially viscous liquids).

3. As the surface of the liquid approaches the desired mark, decrease the flow rate or use a dropper or pipet to bring the level to final volume. The final volume should be determined by aligning the bottom of the meniscus with the desired graduation mark.

4. Transfer the liquid from the graduate to the appropriate vessel or container, allowing about 15 seconds for aqueous and hydro-alcoholic liquids to drain. Approximately 60 seconds (or more) will be required for more viscous liquids such as syrups, glycerin, propylene glycol, and mineral oil.

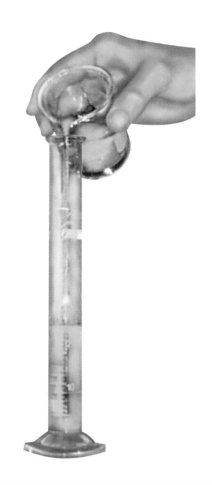

Special Precautions When Using Graduates

✔ While graduates are volumetric devices, they are not mixing devices. They should not be used as the container to dissolve solids in liquids. A solution should be prepared in a beaker or flask, and then returned to the graduate for final volume adjustments.

✔ Do not assume that the final volume of a prescription will be the sum of the individual volumes of ingredients. This is particularly important with the admixture of aqueous and nonaqueous solutions such as alcohol and water. When these solutions are mixed, the total volume is less than the sum of the two volumes.

 meniscus the curved surface of a column of liquid.

LIQUID MEASUREMENT (cont'd)

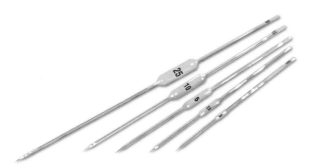

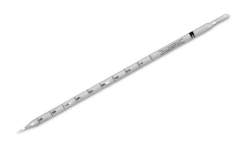

Single Volume Pipets

Single volume pipets have only one graduation mark, and that is the indicated volume of the pipet (e.g., 5 ml, 10 ml, etc.). As a result, the pipet is filled, and then emptied. There is no partial filling done with a single volume pipet. The steps in using a single volume pipet are:

1. Using a rubber bulb for suction, draw the liquid into the pipet until it is above the graduation mark.

2. Remove the pipet from the solution.

3. Wipe the end of the pipet with a tissue or Kimwipe.

4. While holding the pipet in a vertical position, release the pressure inside the bulb and allow the liquid to flow into a waste beaker until the bottom of the meniscus coincides with the graduation mark. Droplets which remain suspended from the tip of the pipet can be removed by touching the pipet to the inside of the waste beaker.

5. Allow the pipet to drain for 30 seconds (or up to 5 minutes for viscous liquids) while touching the tip of the pipet to the inner side of the receiving vessel.

Calibrated Volumetric Pipets

The calibrated volumetric pipet is filled and emptied the same way as with a single volume pipet. However, it has multiple graduation marks that allow partial volumes to be transferred by noting the meniscus level before and after delivery. For example, you can deliver 1.50 ml of a liquid by filling the pipet to 8.50 ml and then allowing it to drain until the meniscus reaches 7.00 ml. A second delivery could be made by allowing the meniscus to reach 5.50 ml. The final graduation of the pipet is usually some distance above the pipet tip so that delivery is performed from graduation to graduation and not from graduation to tip as with the single volume pipet.

From a practical standpoint, *the calibrated pipet is the preferred pipet for compounding.* Just about any prescription requiring small volumes can be compounded with just three basic sizes of pipets: a 1 ml pipet subdivided in 1/100 ml graduations, a 2 ml pipet subdivided in 1/10 ml graduations, and a 5 ml pipet subdivided in 1/10 ml graduations.

Syringes

Syringes come in a variety of sizes ranging from 0.5 ml (calibrated in 0.01 ml graduations) to 60 ml (calibrated in 2 ml graduations). Syringes may be used to deliver a wide range of liquid volumes with a high degree of accuracy. Measurements made with syringes are more accurate and precise than those made with cylindrical graduates. They are especially useful for measuring and delivering viscous liquids. Besides being easy to use, plastic disposable syringes are unbreakable and economical. Like graduates and pipets, select a syringe that equals or barely exceeds the volume to be measured.

Liquids are pulled into the syringe by pulling back on the plunger. The tip of the syringe must be fully submerged in the liquid to prevent drawing air into the syringe. Generally, an excess of solution is drawn into the syringe so that any air bubbles may be expelled by holding the syringe tip up, tapping the syringe until the air bubbles rise into the hub, and depressing the plunger to expel the air. This ensures that the hub will be completely filled with solution and the volume of delivery will be accurate.

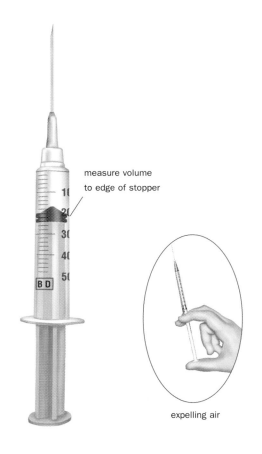

measure volume to edge of stopper

expelling air

Oral Syringes

Oral syringes are available for accurately dispensing a dose of liquid medication to the patient. They are especially useful when administering non-standard doses. Oral syringes have tips that are larger than hubs on standard syringes so needles can't be placed on these syringes. After the dose is drawn into the syringe, a syringe cap is placed on the tip to prevent leakage and prevent contamination.

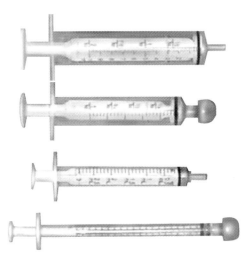

MIXING SOLIDS AND SEMI-SOLIDS

Mixing Powders

When mixing two powders of unequal size, a technique called **geometric dilution** is used. The smaller amount of powder is diluted in steps by additions of the larger amount of powder. If the two powders are just mixed together without this technique, a **homogenous** (fully and evenly combined) mixture will not result.

To correctly mix the powders, the smaller amount of powder is first **triturated** with an approximate equal portion of the large amount of powder in a mortar. Trituration is the fine grinding of a powder. This first triturate is then mixed with an approximate equal portion of the large amount of powder, and these are again triturated in the mortar. This dilution process is continued until all of the two powders have been mixed in the mortar.

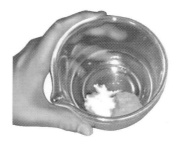

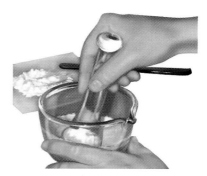

Aliquots

When a prescription calls for less than 120 mg. of an ingredient, a weighable amount of the drug is first triturated with an inert powder, so that a weighable aliquot (portion) of the triturate will contain the amount of drug needed. A simple proportion equation is used to determine the amount of drug and inert powder to be triturated, and the resulting aliquot needed.

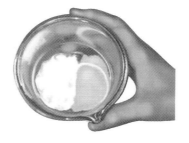

Ointment Slabs

Some ointments and creams are prepared on ointment slabs which are porcelain or ground glass plates, often square or rectangular, that provide a hard nonabsorbable surface for mixing compounds. Spatulas are used to mix the drug into the ointment using the technique of geometric dilution. Many times drugs are **levigated** prior to being incorporated into an ointment to reduce the grittiness of the final formulation.

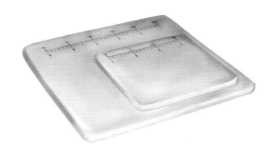

trituration the fine grinding of a powder.
levigation triturating a powdered drug with a solvent in which it is insoluble to reduce its particle size.
geometric dilution a technique for mixing two powders of unequal size.

Levigation

Levigation is a technique used to reduce the particle size of a powdered drug by triturating it with a solvent in which the drug is insoluble. This is generally done before the drug is incorporated into a formulation such as a suspension, an ointment, a suppository base, etc. For example, hydrocortisone (used in ointments) is levigated with glycerin before being incorporated into an ointment base. This reduces the size of the hydrocortisone particles so the resulting ointment will be smooth, not gritty. Levigation can be done in a mortar or on an ointment slab.

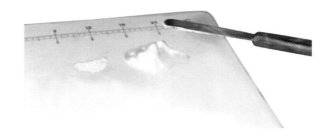

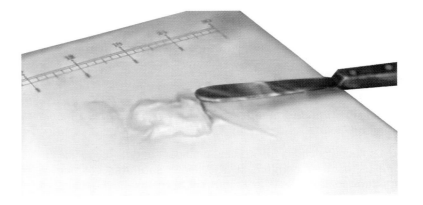

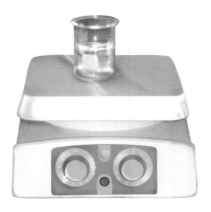

Hot Plates

Sometimes solids are mixed by melting them together in a beaker on a hotplate. The hotplate needs to be a special low temperature (25°C to 120°C) hotplate, and not a standard laboratory type hotplate; those hotplates heat at 125°C to 150°C at their lowest setting. If a low temperature hotplate is not available, a water bath or steam bath will suffice. Most solids and semi-solids used in pharmaceutical compounding will completely melt by 70°C. The melt is removed from the hotplate and allowed to cool to room temperature with constant stirring using a stirring rod, spatula, or magnetic stirring bar. Forced cooling in cold water, ice water, or ice will change the consistency and texture of the final product.

COMPOUNDING PRINCIPLES FOR SELECT FORMS

Solutions

Solutions are probably the most common compounded products. Solutions are clear liquids (but not necessarily colorless liquids) in which the drug is completely dissolved. The simplest compounded solution is the addition of a drug in liquid form to a liquid vehicle. This involves the careful measurement of the drug using graduates or syringes, and then diluting the drug to the final volume. The resulting mixture should be gently shaken to ensure adequate mixing. Water is the most common solvent for pharmaceutical solutions, but ethanol, glycerin, propylene glycol, or a variety of syrups may be used, depending on the product requirements.

When solids are to be dissolved in solution, they must be carefully weighed, using a prescription balance. Most solids dissolve easily in a solvent. However, some may need to be triturated first to reduce the particle size and increase the dissolution rate. Others require that the solvent be heated (but not overheated, since some drugs decompose at higher temperatures). Some drugs require vigorous shaking, stirring, or **sonication** (the application of sound waves using sonic mixing equipment).

The solubility of the drug must be known before attempting to dissolve it in a solution. If a drug is not soluble in a vehicle, then no amount of mixing will help.

When a solution contains the maximum amount of drug it can accommodate at room temperature, it is called a **saturated solution.** A **supersaturated** solution is one that contains a larger amount of solute than the solvent can normally accommodate at room temperature. These types of solutions are made by preparing a saturated solution at a higher temperature than room temperature, filtering out excess drug, and then reducing the temperature back to room temperature. Saturated and supersaturated solutions are physically unstable and tend to precipitate the excess solute under refrigeration or when other drugs are added to the solution.

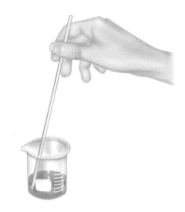

Most solutions require gentle shaking or stirring for adequate mixing.

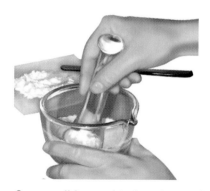

Some solids need to be triturated before mixing in a solution.

 sonication exposure to high frequency sound waves.

saturated solution a solution containing the maximum amount of drug it can contain at room temperature.

supersaturated solution a solution containing a larger amount of drug than it normally contains at room temperature.

Syrups

A syrup is a concentrated or nearly saturated solution of sucrose in water. Syrups containing flavoring agents are known as flavoring syrups (e.g. Cherry Syrup, Acacia Syrup, etc.); medicinal syrups are those which contain drugs (e.g. Guaifenesin Syrup).

Syrup USP (sometimes referred to as Simple Syrup) contains 850 grams of sucrose and 450 ml of water in each liter of syrup. Although very concentrated, the solution is not saturated. Since 1 gram of sucrose dissolves in 0.5 ml water, only 425 ml of water would be required to dissolve the 850 grams of sucrose. This slight additional water makes the syrup more stable over a range of temperatures and allows refrigeration without crystallization.

When a reduction in calories or sucrose properties is desired, syrups can be prepared from sugars other than sucrose (e.g., glucose, fructose), non-sugar polyols (e.g., sorbitol, glycerin, propylene glycol, mannitol), or other non-nutritive artificial sweeteners (e.g., aspartame, saccharin). Non-nutritive sweeteners do not produce the same viscosity as with sugars and polyols, so viscosity enhancers such as methylcellulose are added. Polyols, though less sweet than sucrose, produce good viscosity and have some preservative and solvent qualities. A 70% sorbitol solution is a commercially available syrup vehicle.

Syrups are primarily made by two methods, with or without heat. Using heat is a faster method, but it cannot be used with heat sensitive ingredients. When using heat, the temperature must be carefully controlled to avoid overheating sucrose and making the syrup darker in color and more likely to ferment. When making syrups without heat, stirring or shaking generally provides the energy to produce the solution. In this case, a vessel that is about twice as large as the final volume of the product is needed to provide room for adequate mixing.

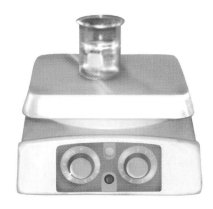

Supersaturated solutions require heating.

Elixirs

Elixirs are hydroalcoholic solutions. That is, they contain alcohol and water. The alcohol serves as the solvent for the drug. The amount of alcohol used will vary with the amount of drug to be dissolved. Because of the alcohol content, elixirs will be inappropriate for certain patients.

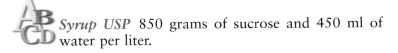

Syrup USP 850 grams of sucrose and 450 ml of water per liter.

Suspensions

The term suspension refers to a "two-phase" system consisting of a finely divided solid dispersed in a liquid. The smallest particle size that can be suspended is approximately 0.1 micrometer. The primary concern in formulating suspensions is that they tend to settle over time, so the dose is unevenly dispersed in the liquid. A well formulated suspension remains dispersed or settles very slowly, and can be redispersed easily with shaking. The settling properties of a suspension are controlled by (1) the addition of **flocculating agents** to enhance particle "dispersability" and (2) the addition of **thickening agents** to reduce the settling (sedimentation rate) of the suspension.

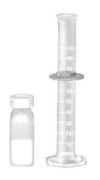

➡ Flocculating agents are electrolytes which carry an electrical charge. The flocculating agent imparts the electrical charge upon the suspended particle; since all of the particles will have the same charge, there is a slight repulsion between the particles as they settle. What results are clusters of particles or floccules which are loosely associated with each other and may be easily redispersed by shaking.

➡ Suspending or thickening agents are added to suspensions to thicken the suspending medium, thereby reducing the sedimentation rate of the floccules. Typical suspending agents carboxymethylcellulose, methylcellulose, bentonite, and tragacanth.

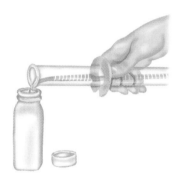

Most solid drugs are levigated in a mortar to reduce the particle size as much as possible before adding it to the vehicle. Common levigating agents are alcohol or glycerin. A portion of the vehicle is added to the mortar, and mixed until a uniform mixture results. This mixture is then put into the final container or a volumetric measuring device as necessary. The mortar and pestle is rinsed with portions of the remaining vehicle, and each rinsing is added to the final container or volumetric measuring device until the final volume is reached. Suspensions should be dispensed in containers that contain enough air space for adequate shaking. The bottle should contain the auxiliary label "Shake well."

mixing

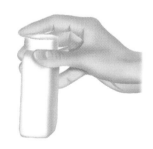

shaking

flocculating agent electrolytes used in the preparation of suspensions.

suspending agent a thickening agent used in the preparation of suspensions.

Ointments and Creams

Ointments and creams are used for many different purposes, e.g., as protectants, antiseptics, emollients, antipruritics, kerotolytics, and astringents. Ointments are simple mixtures of a drug(s) in an ointment base. A cream is a semi-solid emulsion. A particular ointment base is chosen for its fundamental properties, or for its potential to serve as a drug delivery vehicle.

If the base is to be a drug delivery vehicle, the primary consideration will be its ability to release drug. The release of a drug from the base is dependent on the type of base into which the drug is incorporated, as well as the solubility of the drug in the base material. Oleaginous (oil based) bases generally release substances slowly and unpredictably, since water cannot penetrate them well enough to dissolve the drug and allow for diffusion. Water **miscible** or aqueous bases tend to release drugs more rapidly.

Ointments are generally compounded on an ointment slab. In the simple case of combining two ointments or creams, each component is carefully weighed and placed on an ointment slab. The ointments are combined by geometric dilution using two spatulas to mix the ointments. One spatula will be used to continually remove ointment from the other spatula. Using the spatula, transfer the mixture into an ointment jar just big enough for the final volume. When filling the ointment jar, use the spatula to bleed out air pockets. Wipe any excess material from the outside of the jar, including the cap screw threads.

Drugs in powder or crystal form, such as salicylic acid, precipitated sulfur, or hydrocortisone, need to be triturated or levigated in a mortar and pestle before incorporating them into an ointment base. This will prevent a gritty texture in the final product. Another technique to reduce particle size is to dissolve the drug (if soluble) in a very small amount of solvent, and then let the solvent evaporate.

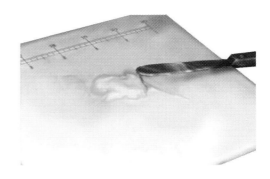

Ointments are generally compounded on an ointment slab.

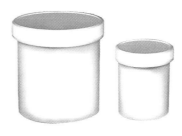

Ointment jars.

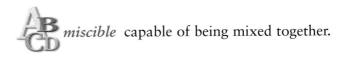

miscible capable of being mixed together.

COMPOUNDING PRINCIPLES FOR SELECT FORMS (cont'd)

Emulsions

An emulsion is an unstable system consisting of at least two **immiscible** liquids, one of which is dispersed in the form of small droplets throughout the other, and a stabilizing agent. The dispersed liquid is known as the **internal or discontinuous phase,** whereas the liquid serving as the **dispersion medium** is known as the **external or continuous phase.**

Oil-in-Water (o/w)

When oils, petroleum hydrocarbons, and/or waxes are the dispersed phase, and water or an aqueous solution is the continuous phase, the system is called an oil-in-water (o/w) emulsion. An o/w emulsion is generally formed if the aqueous phase makes up greater than 45% of the total weight, and a **hydrophilic emulsifier** is used.

Water-in-Oil (w/o)

When water or aqueous solutions are dispersed in an oleaginous (oil based) medium, the system is known as a water-in-oil (w/o) emulsion. W/O emulsions are generally formed if the aqueous phase constitutes less than 45% of the total weight and an **lipophilic emulsifier** is used.

Emulsifiers

Emulsions will separate into two distinct phases or layers over time. Some separation can be overcome with shaking. However, some separation results in emulsions that "break" and these cannot be redispersed. Emulsions are stabilized by adding an emulsifier or emulsifying agents. Emulsifiers provide a protective barrier around the dispersed droplets. Some commonly used emulsifying agents include: tragacanth, sodium lauryl sulfate, sodium dioctyl sulfosuccinate, and polymers known as the Spans and Tweens.

There are various methods used to make emulsions. Each requires that energy be put into the system in the form of either shaking, heat, or the action of a mortar and pestle.

emulsion elements before mixing

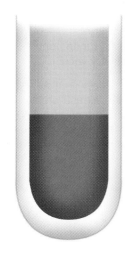

a close-up after mixing

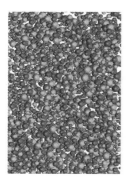

ABCD *immiscible* cannot be mixed.
emulsifier a stabilizing agent in emulsions.
water-in-oil an emulsion in which water is dispersed through an oil base.
oil-in-water an emulsion in which oil is dispersed through a water base.
hydrophilic emulsifier a stabilizing agent for water based dispersion mediums.
lipophilic emulsifier a stabilizing agent for oil based dispersion mediums.

Methods

The **Continental method** is one method for preparing emulsions. In this method, the **initial or primary emulsion** is formed from oil, water, and a "gum" type emulsifier which is usually acacia. The primary emulsion is formed from 4 parts oil, 2 parts water, and 1 part emulsifier. The 4 parts oil and 1 part emulsifier represent their total amounts for the final emulsion. In a dry Wedgewood or porcelain mortar, the 1 part gum is triturated with the 4 parts oil until the powder is thoroughly levigated. Then the 2 parts water are added, and the mixture is vigorously and continually triturated until the primary emulsion is formed (usually 3-4 minutes). It appears as creamy white and produces a "cracking" sound as it is triturated. Additional ingredients are incorporated after the primary emulsion is formed, and the product is then brought to the final volume with the external phase vehicle.

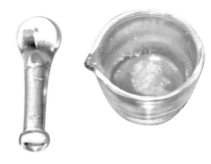

gum and water in preparation for the Wet Gum method

In the **Wet Gum method,** the primary emulsion is formed by triturating the 1 part gum with 2 parts water to form a **mucilage,** and then slowly adding the 4 parts oil. After all the oil is added, the mixture is triturated for several minutes to form the primary emulsion. Then other ingredients may be added as in the continental method.

Some emulsions will have a consistency of a lotion or a cream (a semi-solid formulation). The method of choice in making these types of emulsions is the **beaker method.** The ingredients of the formulation are divided into water soluble and oil soluble components. All oil soluble components are dissolved in the oily phase in one beaker and all water soluble components are dissolved in the water phase in a separate beaker. Both phases are then heated to approximately 70°C using a low temperature hotplate or steam bath. The two beakers are removed from the heat, and the internal phase is slowly added to the external phase with continual stirring. The product is allowed to cool to room temperature but is constantly stirred with a stirring rod, spatula or magnetic stirring bar.

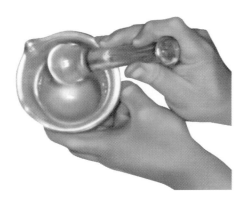

forming the mucilage

 primary emulsion the initial emulsion formed in a preparation to which ingredients are added to create the final volume.

mucilage a wet, slimy preparation formed as an initial step in a wet emulsion preparation method.

COMPOUNDING PRINCIPLES FOR SELECT FORMS (cont'd)

Suppositories

There are three classes of suppository bases based on their composition and physical properties:

➡ **Oleaginous** bases

➡ **Water soluble** or **miscible** bases

➡ **Hydrophilic** bases

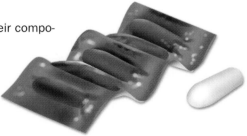

Oleaginous

A well-known oleaginous base is cocoa butter (theobroma oil USP). At room temperature, cocoa butter is a solid, but at body temperature, it melts to a bland, nonirritating oil. Cocoa butter is no longer the base of choice because preparing suppositories with it is difficult, and the suppositories require refrigeration. Synthetic triglycerides can be used that do not have the formulation difficulties of cocoa butter, but they are more expensive. There are also newer bases composed of mixtures of fatty acids that do not have the formulation problems or the expense.

Water Soluble or Miscible

Water soluble or miscible bases contain glycerinated gelatin or polyethylene glycol (PEG) polymers. Glycerinated gelatin is a useful suppository base, particularly for vaginal suppositories. Glycerinated gelatin suppositories are gelatinous solids that tend to dissolve or disperse slowly to provide prolonged release of active ingredients. **Polyethylene glycol (PEGs)** polymers are chemically stable, non-irritating, miscible with water and mucous secretions, and can be formulated by molding or compression in a wide range of hardnesses and melting points. Like glycerinated gelatin, they do not melt at body temperature, but dissolve slowly to provide a prolonged release of drugs.

Polyethylene glycols are available in various molecular weight ranges. Those of 200, 400, or 600 molecular weight are liquids. Those with molecular weights over 1000 are solids. Certain PEGs may be used individually as suppository bases but, more commonly, formulas call for compounds of two or more molecular weights mixed in various proportions to give a desired hardness or dissolution time. Since PEGs suppositories dissolve in body fluids and need not be formulated to melt at body temperature, they can be formulated with much higher melting points and can be safely stored at room temperature.

Hydrophilic

Hydrophilic bases are mixtures of oleaginous and water miscible bases. They generally contain a small percentage of cholesterol or lanolin to assist water absorption.

Molding

Suppositories are usually prepared by **compression molding** or **fusion molding.** Compression molding is a method of preparing suppositories by mixing the suppository base and the drug ingredients and forcing the mixture into a special compression mold. The method requires that the capacity of the molds first be determined by compressing a small amount of the base into the dies and weighing the finished suppositories. When active ingredients are added, it is necessary to leave out a portion of the suppository base, based on the amount of the active ingredients.

Fusion molding is a method in which the drug is dispersed or dissolved in a melted suppository base. The fusion method can be used with all types of suppositories and must be used with most of them. In this method, the suppository base is melted on a low temperature hotplate, and the drug (if soluble) is dissolved in the melted base. If the drug is not soluble, it is pushed through a sieve into the melted base. The sieve reduces the drug to a very fine powder. The mixture is then removed from the heat, and poured into a suppository mold, overfilling each cavity. The mixture is allowed to congeal (harden).

a suppository mold

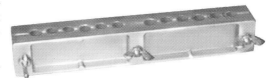

Suppository molds

There are two types of suppository molds: metal (aluminum or steel) molds or plastic molds. The metal molds come in a variety of cavity sizes, from six to one hundred. The two halves of the mold are held together with screws. When the suppository mixture has congealed, the excess mass can be removed with a hot spatula or knife scraped flat across the top surface of the mold. The screws on the mold are unscrewed, and the mold is separated. Never open a mold by prying it apart with a knife or spatula. This will damage the matching mold faces which have been accurately machined to give a tight seal. The suppositories are removed from the mold, generally wrapped in foil paper, and put in a suppository box.

Plastic suppository molds come in long strips and can be torn into any number of cavities. When the suppository has hardened in the cavity, the plastic mold is heat sealed, torn into individual suppository cavities, and put in a suppository box.

a suppository box

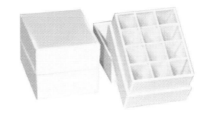

 compression molding a method of making suppositories in which the ingredients are compressed in a mold.

fusion molding a suppository preparation method in which the active ingredients are dispersed in a melted suppository base.

COMPOUNDING PRINCIPLES FOR SELECT FORMS (cont'd)

Capsules

Hard gelatin capsules consist of a body and a cap which fits firmly over the body of the capsule. For human use, eight sizes of capsules are available. The capacity of each size varies according to the bulk density of the drug packaged inside the capsule. To aid in the selection of the appropriate size, a table, with the capacity of five common drugs for that particular size capsule, is printed on the box of the empty capsules. As a guide, the relative sizes and fill capacities of capsules are:

Size	Volume (ml)
000	1.37
00	.95
0	.68
1	.5
2	.37
3	.3
4	.2
5	.13

In general, the smallest capsule capable of containing the final volume is used since patients often have difficulty swallowing large capsules.

When filling a small number of capsules, the **"punch"** method is used. The ingredients are triturated to the same particle size and then mixed by geometric dilution. Since some powder will be lost in the punching process, calculate for the preparation of at least one extra capsule. The powder is placed on a powder paper or an ointment slab and smoothed with a spatula to a height approximately half the length of the capsule body. The body of the capsule is held vertically and the open end is repeatedly pushed or "punched" into the powder until the capsule is filled. The cap is then replaced to close the capsule. Each filled capsule is weighed using an empty capsule as a counterweight. Powder is added or removed until the correct weight has been placed in the capsule.

Capsule filling machines are available which allow the filling of 100 capsules at a time. The machines come with a capsule loader which correctly aligns all of the capsules in the machine base. The powder is poured onto the base plate and special spreaders and combs are used to fill the individual capsules. All of the caps are simultaneously returned to the capsule bodies, and the batch is complete. When using a capsule filling machine, it takes practice to ensure that each capsule has the same amount of drug. There is a tendency to overfill the capsules in the center, and underfill the capsules around the ends.

The Punch method

Other Compounding Tips:

➥ It is a good practice to remove the exact number of empty capsules needed from the capsule box before compounding begins. This will avoid preparing the wrong number of capsules and will prevent the contamination of other empty capsules with drug particles that cling to hands.

➥ The simplest method to keep a capsule free of moisture during compounding is to use the body of one capsule as a holder for other capsule bodies during the filling operation. This avoids the capsules coming into contact with the fingers. Another way of protecting the capsules is to wear **finger cots** or rubber gloves.

➥ To remove traces of drug from the outside of the filled capsules, roll them between the folds of clean towel or shake in a towel that has been gathered into the form of a bag.

➥ Liquids that do not dissolve gelatin, e.g., alcohol and fixed oils, may be dispensed in capsules. By calibrated dropper or pipet, the correct volume of liquid is delivered into the empty capsule body. To ensure proper sealing, none of the liquid should touch the edge of the capsule and the size of the capsule should be chosen so that the liquid does not completely fill the body. The capsule is sealed by moistening the lower portion of the inside of the cap with warm water using a camel's hair brush. The moistened cap is placed on the body and given a half turn. The capsules should be placed on a paper and inspected for leakage.

➥ Capsules will absorb moisture and soften in high humidity. In a dry atmosphere they become brittle and crack. To protect capsules from the extremes of humidity, dispense them in plastic or glass vials, and store in a cool, dry place. A piece of cotton may be added to keep the capsules from rattling.

 punch method a method for filling capsules by repeatedly pushing or "punching" the capsule into an amount of drug powder.

finger cots protective coverings for fingers.

REVIEW

KEY CONCEPTS

✔ Extemporaneous compounding is the on-demand preparation of a drug product according to a physician's prescription, formula, or recipe.

✔ Class A balances can weigh as little as 120 mg of material with a 5% error.

✔ Electronic or analytical balances are used to weigh quantities smaller than 120 mg.

✔ Weighing papers or weighing boats should always be placed on the balance pans before any weighing is done.

✔ Liquid drugs, solvents, or additives are measured in volumetric glassware or plasticware.

✔ For small volumes, a disposable hypodermic syringe made of plastic is used.

✔ Erlenmeyer flasks (right), beakers, and prescription bottles, regardless of markings, are not volumetric glassware.

✔ Always use the smallest device (graduate, pipet, syringe) that will accommodate the desired volume of liquid.

✔ When reading a volume of a liquid against a graduation mark, hold the graduate so the meniscus is at eye level and read the mark at the bottom of the meniscus.

✔ Medicine droppers can be used to deliver small liquid doses but must first be calibrated.

✔ When aqueous and nonaqueous solutions such as alcohol and water are mixed, the total volume may be less than the sum of the two volumes.

✔ Measurements made with syringes are more accurate and precise than those made with cylindrical graduates.

✔ Trituration is the fine grinding of a powder. Levigation is the trituration of a powdered drug with a solvent in which the drug is insoluble to reduce the particle size of the drug.

✔ Water is the most common solvent for pharmaceutical solutions, but ethanol, glycerin, propylene glycol, or a variety of syrups may be used.

✔ A saturated solution is a one that contains the maximum amount of drug it can accommodate at room temperature.

✔ A supersaturated solution is one that contains a larger amount of solute than it can normally accommodate at room temperature. Supersaturated solutions require heating.

✔ Suspensions are a "two-phase" compound consisting of a finely divided solid dispersed in a liquid.

✔ An emulsion is an unstable system consisting of at least two immiscible (unmixable) liquids, one that is dispersed as small droplets throughout the other, and a stabilizing agent.

✔ There are three classes of suppository bases based on their composition and physical properties: oleaginous bases, water soluble or miscible bases, and hydrophilic bases.

✔ Compression molding is a method of preparing suppositories by mixing the suppository base and the drug ingredients and forcing the mixture into a special compression mold.

✔ When preparing capsules, the smallest capsule capable of containing the final volume is used since patients often have difficulty swallowing large capsules.

SELF TEST

MATCH THE TERMS.

answers can be checked in the glossary

arrest knob

flocculating agent

geometric dilution

hydrophilic emulsifier

levigation

lipophilic emulsifier

meniscus

punch method

stability

suspending agent

Syrup USP

trituration

the chemical and physical integrity of the dosage unit and its ability to withstand contamination.

the knob on a balance that prevents any movement of the balance.

the curved surface of a column of liquid.

the fine grinding of a powder.

triturating a powdered drug with a solvent in which it is insoluble to reduce its particle size.

a technique for mixing two powders of unequal size.

850 grams of sucrose and 450 ml of water per liter.

electrolytes used in the preparation of suspensions.

a thickening agent used in the preparation of suspensions.

a stabilizing agent for water based dispersion mediums.

a stabilizing agent for oil based dispersion mediums.

a method for filling capsules.

CHOOSE THE BEST ANSWER.

answers are in the back of the book

1. When using a Class A Torsion balance
   a. the weight goes on the left pan and the powder goes on the right pan
   b. the weight goes on the right pan and the powder goes on the left pan
   c. no need to place weights, as the weight can be adjusted internally
   d. Class A Torsion balances only have one pan to weigh powders

2. The term triturate refers to
   a. the use of a levigating agent to reduce particle size
   b. the grinding of large particles into fine powders
   c. the method of mixing two powders of unequal size
   d. adding a tri-hydrate to reduce particle size

3. Of the following capsules, which one would hold the most volume?
   a. size 5
   b. size 3
   c. size 1
   d. size 0

4. Which of the following would be used in a suppository for the prolonged release of active ingredients?
   a. oleaginous
   b. miscible
   c. hydrophilic
   d. hydroalchoholic

HOW DRUGS WORK

Drugs produce their individual effects on the body as either desired effects or undesired effects.

Once they are in the blood, drugs are circulated throughout the body. The properties of both the drug and the body influence where the drug will go, and what concentration it will have at each place. The place where a drug causes an effect to occur is called the **site of action**. Some of the effects caused by the drug are desired effects, and some are undesired. *The objective of drug therapy is to deliver the right drug, in the right concentration, to the right site of action at the right time to produce the desired effect.*

When a drug produces an effect, it is interacting on a molecular level with cell material or structure.

The cell material directly involved in the action of the drug is called its **receptor**. The receptor is often described as a lock into which the drug molecule fits as a key, and only those drugs able to bind chemically to the receptors in a particular site of action can produce effects in that site. This is why specific cells only respond to certain drugs, even though their receptors are exposed to any drug molecules that are present in the body. This is also why drugs are **selective** in their action, that is, they only act on specific targeted receptors and the tissues they affect.

Receptors are located on the surfaces of cell membranes and inside cells.

There are many different types of receptors, having many different roles in the body's processes. Most receptors can be found throughout the body, though some occur in only a few places. Receptor activation is responsible for most of the pharmacological responses in the body.

---

 biopharmaceutics the study of the factors associated with drug products and physiological processes, and the resulting systemic concentrations of the drugs.

site of action the location where an administered drug produces an effect.

receptor the cellular material at the site of action which interacts with the drug.

selective (action) the characteristic of a drug that makes its action specific to certain receptors and the tissues they affect.

DRUG ACTION AT THE SITE OF ACTION

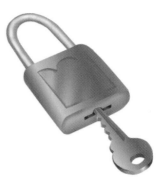

Like a lock and key, only certain drugs are able to interact with certain receptors.

Types of Action

When drugs interact with the site of action, they can:

➡ act through physical action, as with the protective effects of ointments upon topical application;

➡ react chemically, as with antacids that reduced excess gastric acidity;

➡ modify the metabolic activity of pathogens, as with antibiotics;

➡ change the osmolarity of plasma and draw water out of tissues and into the blood.

➡ incorporate into cellular material to interfere with normal cell function.

➡ join with other chemicals to form a complex that is more easily excreted.

➡ modify the biochemical or metabolic process of the body's cells or enzyme systems.

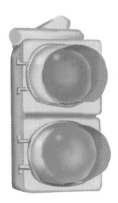

antagonists
block action

_____

agonists activate
receptors

Other Drug Actions

➥ Some drugs work by changing the ability of ions to move into or out of cells. For example, sodium or calcium ion channels can open and allow movement of the ions into nerve cells, stimulating them. With potassium channels, the opposite can happen. The channels can open and allow the movement of potassium ions out of nerve cells, obstructing their function.

➥ Some drugs modify the creation, release, or control of nerve cell hormones that regulate different physiological processes.

When drug molecules bind with a receptor, they can cause a reaction that stimulates or inhibits cell functions.

The pharmacological effects of this are called **agonism** or **antagonism**. **Agonists** are drugs that activate receptors and produce a response that may either accelerate or slow normal cell processes, depending on the type of receptor involved. For example, epinephrine-like drugs act on the heart to increase the heart rate, and acetylcholine-like drugs act on the heart to slow the heart rate. Both are agonists. **Antagonists** are drugs that bind to receptors but do not activate them. They block the receptors' action by preventing other drugs or substances from interacting with them.

The number of receptors available to interact with a drug will directly influence the effect.

A minimum number of receptors have to be occupied by drug molecules to produce the desired effect. If there are too few drug molecules to occupy the necessary number of receptors, there will be little or no effect. In this case, increasing the dosage will increase the effect. On the other hand, once all receptors are occupied, increasing the dosage will not increase the effect.

Receptors can be changed by drug use.

For example, extended stimulation of cells with an agonist can reduce the number or sensitivity of the receptors, and the effect of the drug is reduced. Extended inhibition of cell functions with an antagonist can increase the number or sensitivity of receptors. If the antagonist is stopped abruptly, the cells can have an extreme reaction to an agonist. To avoid such withdrawal symptoms, some drugs must be gradually discontinued.

_____

 agonist drugs that activate receptors to accelerate or slow normal cell function.

antagonist drugs that bind with receptors but do not activate them. They block receptor action by preventing other drugs or substances from activating them.

CONCENTRATION & EFFECT

It is difficult to measure the amount of a drug at the site of action and therefore to predict an effect based upon it.

One problem is that many factors influence a drug's movement from the site of administration to the site of action (metabolism, excretion, membrane permeability, etc.). It can also be physically impossible to measure the site of action either because of its unknown location or small size.

One way to monitor the amount of a drug in the body and its effect at the site of action is to construct a dose-response curve.

A specific dose of a drug is given to one subject and the effect or response is measured. When a series of such doses is given to a number of people, the results show that some people respond to low doses but others require larger doses for a response to be produced. This is due to human variability: different people have different characteristics that affect how a drug product behaves in them. Some differences are due to the product itself, but most come from how the drug is transported from the site of administration to the site of action, and how it interacts with the receptor.

Another way to monitor a drug's concentration in the body and its related effect is to determine its concentration in the body's fluids.

Of the body's fluids, blood is generally used because of its rapid and intensive interaction between the site of administration and the site of action. As a result, knowing a drug's concentration in the blood can be directly related to its effect and this is the most common way to analyze the potential effect of a drug.

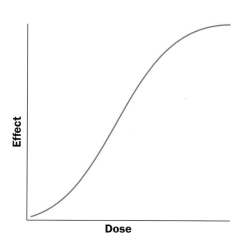

A typical dose-response curve shows that responses increase as the doses are increased.

Blood Concentration-Time Profiles

Blood concentration-time profiles have these applications:

➥ Manufacturers use their data to evaluate their drug products

➥ Pharmacy professionals use them to visualize the consequences of incorrectly compounding a formulation or of using the wrong route of administration.

➥ Researchers and clinicians use them to measure human variability in drug formulation performance (e.g., influence of age, gender, nationality, or disease).

➥ Physicians and pharmacists use them to monitor the drug therapy of patients.

ABCD *minimum effective concentration (MEC)* the blood concentration needed of a drug to produce a response.

onset of action the time MEC is reached and the response occurs.

therapeutic window a drug's blood concentration range between its minimum effective concentration and minimum toxic concentration.

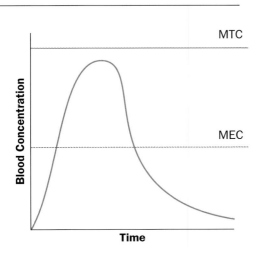

An advantage of using blood concentrations as a measure of "drug amount in the body" is that blood can be repeatedly sampled. When sampling covers several hours or more, a blood concentration-time profile can be developed. Plasma or serum concentrations can be used instead of blood concentrations, and the same profiles will also result.

For most drugs, changes in the blood concentration-time profile reflect changes in concentration at the site of action and therefore changes in effect.

There are exceptions to this. The concentration of some drugs in the site of action produces an action hours or days later. Other drugs show no relationship between blood concentrations and concentrations in the site of action. Still others don't depend on blood concentrations at all to produce an effect.

A Sample Profile

The illustration above shows a typical blood concentration–time curve for a drug given orally. The blood concentration begins at zero at the time the drug is administered (before it has been absorbed into the blood). With time, the drug leaves the formulation and enters the blood, causing concentrations to rise. To produce an effect, they must achieve a **minimum effective concentration (MEC).** This is when there is enough drug at the site of action to produce a response. The time this occurs is called the **onset of action.** With most drugs, when blood concentrations increase, so does the intensity of the effect, since *blood concentrations reflect the site of action concentrations that produce the response.*

Some drugs have an upper blood concentration limit beyond which there are undesired or toxic effects. This limit is called the **minimum toxic concentration (MTC).** The range between the minimum effective concentration and the minimum toxic concentration is called the **therapeutic window.** *When concentrations are in this range, most patients receive the maximum benefit from their drug therapy with a minimum of risk.*

The last part of the curve shows the blood concentrations declining as absorption is complete. The time between the onset of action and the time when the minimum effective concentration is reached by the declining blood concentrations is called the **duration of action.** The duration of action is the time the drug should produce the desired effect.

ADME PROCESSES & DIFFUSION

Blood concentrations are the result of four simultaneously acting processes: absorption, distribution, metabolism, and excretion.

These four processes are referred to as the **ADME** processes, but may also be called **disposition**. Metabolism and excretion combined are called **elimination**.

The transfer of drug into the blood from an administered drug product is called absorption.

When a drug product is first administered, absorption is the primary process. Distribution, metabolism, and excretion will also occur, but the amount of drug available for them is much less than the amount of drug available for absorption. So these processes have little effect. As more of the drug is absorbed into the blood, it is available to undergo the other processes and their roles increase.

A drug's distribution will be affected by physiological functions and its own properties.

Though blood may deliver the drug to body tissue, if the drug cannot penetrate the tissue's membranes, it will not interact with the receptors inside. The opposite situation can also occur. A drug may be able to enter a tissue, but if there is not enough blood flow to the tissue, little of the drug will enter. Distribution is also influenced by drug binding to proteins in the blood or in tissues.

The ADME processes are all illustrated by blood concentration–time curves.

Concentrations rise during absorption, but as absorption nears completion, metabolism and elimination become the primary processes, and they cause the blood concentration to decline.

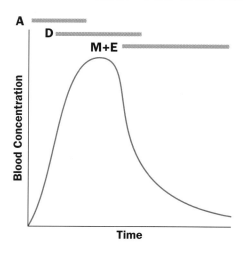

In the first part of a blood concentration–time curve, absorption is the primary process and concentrations rise. As absorption nears completion, metabolism and excretion become the primary processes, with distribution occurring throughout.

 disposition a term sometimes used to refer to all of the ADME processes together.

passive diffusion the movement of drugs from an area of higher concentration to lower concentration.

active transport the movement of drug molecules across membranes by active means, rather than passive diffusion.

hydrophobic water repelling; cannot associate with water.

hydrophilic capable of associating with or absorbing water.

lipoidal fat like substance.

 Even though the ADME processes occur simultaneously, they are studied separately to understand the critical factors responsible for each process.

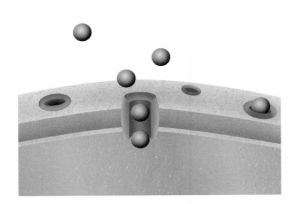

A diagram showing drug molecules penetrating a a cell membrane

Ionization and Unionization

Because they are weak organic acids and bases, most drugs will dissociate (come apart) and associate (attach to other chemicals) 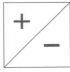 in solutions. When acids dissociate, they become ionized. When bases dissociate, they become unionized.

Unionized drugs penetrate biological membranes more easily than ionized drugs for these reasons:

➡ unionized drugs are more lipid soluble.

➡ charges on biological membranes bind or repel ionized drug.

➡ ionized drugs associate with water molecules, creating larger particles with reduced penetrating capability.

Besides the four ADME processes, a critical factor of drug concentration and effect is how drugs move through biological membranes.

Before an effective concentration of a drug can reach its site of action, it must overcome many barriers, most which are biological membranes.

Biological membranes are complex structures composed of lipids (fats) and proteins.

They are generally classified in three types: those made up of *several layers of cells*, such as the skin; those made up of *a single layer of cells*, as in the intestinal lining; and those of *less than one cell* in thickness, as in the membrane of a single cell.

Most drugs penetrate biological membranes by *passive diffusion*.

Drugs in the body's fluids will generally move from an area of higher concentration to an area of lower concentration until the concentrations in each area are balanced, or in a state of equilibrium. This process is called passive diffusion. It is the most common way a drug penetrates biological membranes and is a primary factor in the distribution process. This movement from higher to lower concentration causes most orally administered drugs to move from the intestine to the blood and from the blood to the site of action.

Drug concentration is not the only factor influencing diffusion.

Membranes are **lipoidal** (fat-like), and drugs that are more lipid (fat) soluble will penetrate them better than those that are not. These drugs are called **hydrophobic**. They hate or repel water and are attracted to fats. **Hydrophilic** drugs (drugs attracted to water) can also penetrate membranes, however. It is thought that they move through water-filled passages called **aqueous pores** which allow water (and any drug contained in it) into cells.

In addition to passive diffusion, some drugs may be carried across membranes by *specialized transport mechanisms*.

This type of **active transport** (as opposed to passive) is thought to explain how certain substances that do not penetrate membranes by passive diffusion nevertheless succeed in entering a cell.

ABSORPTION

O nce a drug is released from its dosage formulation, the process that transfers it into the blood is called *absorption*.

Absorption occurs to some extent with any route of administration. For example, even a drug in an intravenous suspension or emulsion must first be released from the dosage form to be absorbed into the blood. However, since most drugs are given orally, this page and the next several will look at the ADME processes from the perspective of oral administration.

One of the primary factors affecting oral drug absorption is the *gastric emptying time*.

This is the time a drug will stay in the stomach before it is emptied into the small intestine. Since stomach acid can degrade many drugs and since most absorption occurs in the intestine, gastric emptying time can significantly affect a drug's action. If a drug remains in the stomach too long, it can be degraded or destroyed, and its effect decreased. Gastric emptying time can be affected by a various conditions, including the amount and type of food in the stomach, the presence of other drugs, the person's body position, and their emotional condition. Some factors increase the gastric emptying time, but most slow it.

Once a drug leaves the stomach, its rate of movement through the intestines directly affects its absorption.

Slower than normal intestinal movement can lead to increased drug absorption because the drug is in contact with the intestinal membrane longer. Faster than normal intestinal movement can produce the opposite result since the drug moves through the intestinal tract too rapidly to be fully absorbed.

Bile salts and enzymes from the intestinal tract also affect absorption.

Bile salts improve the absorption of hydrophobic and certain other drugs. Enzymes added to the intestinal tract's contents from pancreatic secretions destroy certain drugs and consequently decrease their absorption. Enzymes are also present in the intestinal wall and destroy drugs that pass from the gut into the blood, decreasing their absorption.

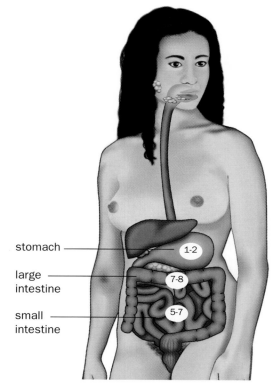

stomach

large intestine

small intestine

gastrointestinal organs and their pH

Most drugs are given orally and absorbed into the blood from the small intestine. The small intestine's large surface area makes absorption easier. However, there are many conditions in the stomach that can affect absorption positively or negatively before the drug even reaches the small intestine. Once in the intestines, there are many additional factors that can affect a drug's absorption.

 gastric emptying time the time a drug will stay in the stomach before it is emptied into the small intestine.

DISTRIBUTION

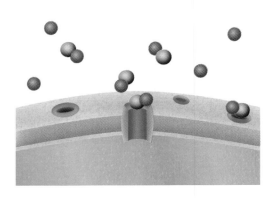

Protein Binding

Many drugs bind to proteins in blood plasma to form a complex that is too large to penetrate cell openings. So the drug remains inactive.

Protein binding can be considered a type of drug storage within the body. Some drugs bind extensively to proteins in fat and muscle, and are gradually released as the blood concentration of the drug falls. These drugs remain in the body a long time, and therefore have a long duration of action.

Selective Action

Though drugs are widely distributed throughout the body once they reach the bloodstream, they can have action that is selective to certain tissues or organs. This is due both to the specific nature of receptor action as well as to various factors that can affect the distribution of the drug. This is why drugs can be targeted to specific therapeutic effects.

Since most receptors can be found in multiple areas throughout the body, most drugs have multiple effects. This is why a drug may be used for different therapies. It is also one reason they have side effects. For example, terbutaline is used for bronchodilation. It will also delay labor in pregnant women.

Distribution involves the movement of a drug within the body once the drug has reached the blood.

Blood carries the drug throughout the body and to its sites of action, as well as to the organs responsible for the metabolism and excretion of the drug.

The blood flow rates to certain organs have a significant effect on distribution.

Drugs are rapidly distributed to organs having high blood flow rates such as the heart, liver, and kidneys. Distribution to areas such as muscle, fat, and skin is usually slower because they have lower blood flow rates.

The permeability of tissue membranes to a drug is also important.

Most tissue membranes are easily penetrated by most drugs. Small drug molecules (those having a low molecular weight) and drugs that are hydrophobic will generally diffuse through tissue membranes with ease. Some tissue membranes have specialized transport mechanisms that assist penetration. A few tissue membranes are highly selective in allowing drug penetration. The blood-brain barrier, for example, limits drug access to the brain and the cerebral spinal fluid.

Protein binding can also affect distribution.

Many drugs will "bind" to proteins in blood plasma, forming a complex. The large size of such complexes prevents the bound drug from entering its sites of action, metabolism, and excretion—making it inactive. Only free or "unbound" drug can move through tissue membranes. Another drug with a stronger binding characteristic can displace a less well bound drug, making it pharmacologically active again and increasing its effect.

 complex when molecules of different chemicals attach to each other, as in protein binding.

protein binding the attachment of a drug molecule to a plasma or tissue protein, effectively making the drug inactive, but also keeping it within the body.

METABOLISM

Drug metabolism refers to the body's process of transforming drugs.

The transformed drug is called a **metabolite**. Most metabolites are inactive and are excreted. However, the metabolites of some drugs are active, and they will produce effects on the individual until they are further metabolized or excreted.

The primary site of drug metabolism in the body is the liver.

Enzymes are complex proteins that cause chemical reactions in other substances. The enzymes produced by the liver interact with drugs and transform them into metabolites.

In response to the chronic administration of certain drugs, the liver will increase its enzyme production.

This is called **enzyme induction,** and it results in greater metabolism of a drug. As a result, larger doses of the drug must be administered to produce the same therapeutic effects. Some drugs decrease or delay enzyme activity, a process called **enzyme inhibition.** In this case, smaller doses of the drug will be needed to avoid toxicity from drug accumulation.

The liver may secrete drugs or their metabolites into bile that is stored in the gall bladder.

The gall bladder empties the bile (and any drugs or metabolites in it) into the intestine in response to food entering the intestinal tract. This is called **enterohepatic cycling.** Any drugs or metabolites contained in the bile may be reabsorbed or simply eliminated with the feces.

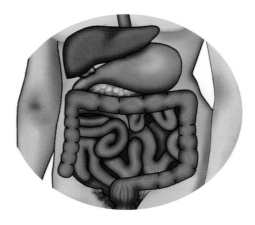

First Pass Metabolism

With oral administration, once a drug is absorbed from the enteral tract, it is immediately delivered to the liver. It will then be transferred into the general systemic circulation.

Before it reaches the circulatory system, however, the drug can be substantially degraded or destroyed by the liver's enzymes. This is called "first-pass metabolism" and is an important factor with orally administered drugs. Because of it, certain drugs must be administered by other routes. Any route other than oral either partially or completely bypasses first-pass metabolism.

---

metabolite the substance resulting from the body's transformation of an administered drug.

enzyme a complex protein that causes chemical reactions in other substances

enzyme induction the increase in enzyme activity that results in greater metabolism of drugs.

enzyme inhibition the decrease in enzyme activity that results in reduced metabolism of drugs.

first pass metabolism the substantial degradation of a drug caused by enzyme metabolism in the liver before the drug reaches the systemic circulation.

enterohepatic cycling the transfer of drugs and their metabolites from the liver to the bile in the gall bladder and then into the intestine.

EXCRETION

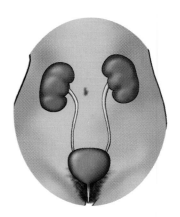

Factors Affecting Urinary Excretion

➡ If the kidney's process of filtration becomes impaired, excretion will be reduced and drugs will accumulate in the blood. In such cases, the dosage of drugs must be decreased or the dosage interval lengthened.

➡ Some drugs affect the excretion of others. In such cases, the affected drug will accumulate in the blood, and the dosage of the affected drug must be decreased or the dosage interval lengthened.

➡ The pH of the urine can affect the reabsorption of some drugs. A high pH can increase excretion of weak acids such as salicylates and phenobarbital. The opposite effect can occur with a low (acidic) pH.

Most drugs and their metabolites are excreted by the kidneys through the urine.

Some orally administered drugs are not easily absorbed from the gastrointestinal tract and as a result are significantly excreted in the feces. Excretion can also occur through the bile and certain drugs are removed from the lungs through the expired breath.

The kidneys filter the blood and remove waste (including drugs and metabolites) from it.

As blood flows through a kidney, some of the plasma water is filtered from it into the kidney **nephron** (the functional unit of the kidney) in a process called **glomerular filtration**. As the water moves through the nephron, waste substances are secreted into the fluid, with urine as the end result. Some drugs can be filtered and reabsorbed back into the blood during this process, and some drugs are not filtered at all but are secreted into the urine by specialized processes.

The rate of urinary excretion is much faster than that of fecal excretion.

Drugs that will be excreted through the feces generally take a day to be excreted, whereas drugs may be excreted through the urine within hours of administration.

---

 nephron the functional unit of the kidneys.
glomerular filtration the blood filtering process of the kidneys.

BIOEQUIVALENCE

The amount of a drug that is available to the site of action and the rate at which it is available is called the *bioavailability* of the drug. By FDA definition, it is measured by determining *the relative amount of an administered dose of a drug that reaches the general systemic circulation and the rate at which this occurs.* As a result, it can be measured by a blood concentration-time curve.

Comparing the bioavailability of one dosage form to another determines their *bioequivalency*.

The FDA requires drug manufacturers to perform bioequivalency studies on their products before they are approved for marketing. In such studies, the bioavailability of the active ingredients in a test formulation is compared to that in a standard formulation. Bioequivalency studies are also used to compare bioavailability between different dosage forms (tablets, capsules, etc), different manufacturers, and different production lots.

Bioequivalency is also the goal of compounding or admixing.

In this case, there is no proof of the bioequivalency of the product. For this reason, it is critical that the pharmacist or technician make every effort to make sure the product is correctly compounded or admixed.

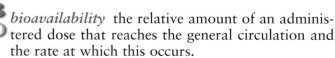

bioavailability the relative amount of an administered dose that reaches the general circulation and the rate at which this occurs.

bioequivalence the comparison of bioavailability between two dosage forms.

BIOEQUIVALENCE

Bioequivalent Drug Products

Bioequivalent drug products are pharmaceutical equivalents or alternatives which have *essentially* the same rate and extent of absorption when administered at the same dose of the active ingredient under similar conditions.

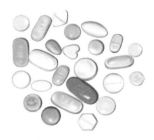

Differences Between Equivalents

Exact bioequivalency between drug products (where blood concentration–time curves for each product are identical) doesn't occur, and is not expected. There are simply too many variables that can contribute to differences between products. In tablets, for example, there can be different amounts or types of fillers, binders, lubricants, and other components. The particle size of the drug itself may be slightly different. The manufacturing process may also produce different results in size, hardness, or other characteristics (especially for different manufacturers, but also for the same manufacturer at different times or different plants). Changes in these or various other factors can affect the bioavailability of a drug. Though there can be differences in the bioavailability of a drug between bioequivalent products because of this, the differences must be slight and not significant.

The following terms are used by the FDA to define the type of equivalency between drug products:

Pharmaceutical Equivalents

Pharmaceutical equivalents are drug products that contain identical amounts of the same active ingredients in the same dosage form, and that meet the same applicable standards of identity, strength, quality, and purity, including potency and, where applicable, content uniformity, disintegration times, and/or dissolution rates. They do not have to contain the same inactive ingredients, or have the same shape, release mechanisms, packaging, or expiration time. Since pharmaceutical equivalents may have different inactive ingredients, different pharmaceutically equivalent products may not be equally suitable for a patient. Some patients may be unusually sensitive to an inactive ingredient in one product that another product does not contain.

➡ same active ingredients
➡ same amounts
➡ same dosage form
➡ inactive ingredients can be different

Pharmaceutical Alternatives

Pharmaceutical alternatives are drug products that contain the identical active ingredients, but not necessarily in the same amount or dosage form. Each such drug product must individually meet the applicable standards of its dosage form. They do not have to contain the same inactive ingredients, or have the same shape, release mechanisms, packaging, or expiration time.

➡ same active ingredients
➡ amounts can be different
➡ dosage form can be different

Therapeutic Equivalents

Therapeutic equivalents are pharmaceutical equivalents which produce the same therapeutic effect in patients.

Note: a related term is **therapeutic alternative**. This refers to drugs that have different active ingredients but produce similar therapeutic effect.

➡ pharmaceutical equivalents that produce the same effects in patients.

ABCD *pharmaceutical equivalent* drug products that contain identical amounts of the same active ingredients in the same dosage form.

pharmaceutical alternative drug products that contain the same active ingredients, but not necessarily in the same amount or dosage form.

therapeutic equivalent pharmaceutical equivalents that produce the same effects in patients.

REVIEW

KEY CONCEPTS

✔ The objective of drug therapy is to deliver the right drug, in the right concentration, to the right site of action at the right time to produce the desired effect.

✔ Only those drugs able to bind chemically to the receptors in a particular site of action can produce effects in that site. This is why specific cells only respond to certain drugs.

✔ Receptor activation is responsible for most of the pharmacological responses in the body.

✔ Agonists are drugs that activate receptors and produce a response that may either accelerate or slow normal cell processes. Antagonists are drugs that bind to receptors but do not activate them. They prevent other drugs or substances from interacting with receptors.

✔ The primary way to monitor a drug's concentration in the body and its related effect is to determine its blood concentrations.

✔ To produce an effect, a drug must achieve a minimum effective concentration (MEC). This is when there is enough drug at the site of action to produce a response.

✔ The range between the minimum effective concentration and the minimum toxic concentration is called the therapeutic window. When concentrations are in this range, most patients receive the maximum benefit from their drug therapy with a minimum of risk.

✔ Blood concentrations are the result of four simultaneously acting processes: absorption, distribution, metabolism, and excretion.

✔ The transfer of drug into the blood from an administered drug product is called absorption.

✔ Besides the four ADME processes, a critical factor of drug concentration and effect is how drugs move through biological membranes. Most drugs penetrate biological membranes by passive diffusion.

✔ Most drugs are given orally and absorbed into the blood from the small intestine. One of the primary factors affecting oral drug absorption is the gastric emptying time.

✔ Many drugs bind to proteins in blood plasma to form a complex that is too large to penetrate cell openings. So the drug remains inactive.

✔ The primary site of drug metabolism in the body is the liver. Enzymes produced by the liver interact with drugs and transform them into metabolites.

✔ The kidneys filter the blood and remove waste (including drugs and metabolites) from it.

✔ The amount of a drug that is available to the site of action and the rate at which it is available is called the bioavailability of the drug.

✔ Bioequivalent drug products are pharmaceutical equivalents or alternatives which have essentially the same rate and extent of absorption when administered at the same dose of the active ingredient under similar conditions.

✔ Pharmaceutical equivalents are drug products that contain identical amounts of the same active ingredients in the same dosage form, but may contain different inactive ingredients.

✔ Pharmaceutical alternatives are drug products that contain the identical active ingredients, but not necessarily in the same amount or dosage form.

SELF TEST

MATCH THE TERMS. *answers can be checked in the glossary*

agonist

antagonist

bioavailability

bioequivalence

enzyme induction

first pass metabolism

passive diffusion

protein binding

receptor

selective (action)

site of action

the location where an administered drug produces an effect.

the cellular material which interacts with the drug.

the characteristic of a drug that makes its action specific to certain receptors.

drugs that activate receptors to accelerate or slow normal cell function.

drugs that bind with receptors but do not activate them.

the movement of drugs from an area of higher concentration to lower concentration.

the attachment of a drug molecule to a protein, effectively making the drug inactive.

the increase in enzyme activity that results in greater metabolism of drugs.

the substantial degradation of a drug caused by enzyme metabolism in the liver.

the relative amount of an administered dose that reaches the general circulation and the rate at which this occurs.

the comparison of bioavailability between two dosage forms.

CHOOSE THE BEST ANSWER. *answers are in the back of the book*

1. Most drugs and their metabolites are excreted by the
   a. liver
   b. kidneys
   c. gall bladder
   d. gastrointestinal tract

2. The percentage or fraction of the administered dose of a drug that actually reaches systemic circulation and the rate at which this occurs is the drug's
   a. bioequivalence
   b. bioavailability
   c. biotransformation
   d. gastric emptying time

3. In metabolism, the breakdown of drugs into metabolites is caused by
   a. passive diffusion
   b. glomerular filtration
   c. enterohepatic cycling
   d. enzymes

4. In the blood concentration-time curve, the range between the Minimum Toxic Concentration (MTC) and the Minimum Effective Concentration (MEC) is called
   a. the onset of action
   b. the concentration at site of action
   c. the duration of action
   d. the therapeutic window

HUMAN VARIABILITY

Human variability in biopharmaceutics and disposition is a significant factor in the outcome of drug activity and effect. Differences in age, weight, genetics, and gender are among the significant factors that influence the differences in response to medication among people.

Age

Human life is a continuous process but it is usually characterized as having stages. The distinctions between the stages are relative and vary among individuals, but they are based on relevant physiological characteristics. The stages are generally considered as:

➡ **Neonate**, up to one month after birth

➡ **Infant**, between the ages of one month and two years

➡ **Child**, between two years and twelve years of age

➡ **Adolescent**, between the ages of 13 and 19 years

➡ **Adult**, between 20 and 70 years

➡ **Elder**, older than 70 years of age

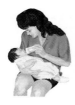

Drug distribution, metabolism, and excretion are quite different in the **neonate** and **infant** than in adults because their organ systems are not fully developed. They are not able to eliminate drugs as efficiently as adults. Older infants reach approximately adult levels of protein binding and kidney function, but liver function and the blood-brain barrier are still immature.

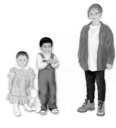

Children metabolize certain drugs more rapidly than adults. Their rate of metabolism increases between 1 year and 12 years of age depending on the child and the drug. Afterwards, metabolism rates decline with age to normal adult levels. Some of the drugs eliminated faster in children include clindamycin, valproic acid, ethosuximide, and theophylline.

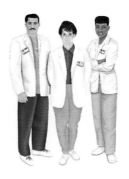

Adults

Adults experience a decrease in many physiological functions from 30 to 70 years of age, but these decreases and their affects on drug activity are gradual.

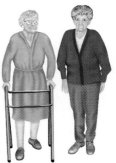

The Elderly

The elderly typically consume more drugs than other age groups. They also experience physiological changes that significantly affect drug action.

➡ Changes in gastric pH, gastric emptying time, intestinal movement, and gastrointestinal blood flow all tend to *slow the rate of absorption.*

➡ Changes in the cardiovascular system (including lower cardiac output) tend to *slow distribution* of drug molecules to their sites of action, metabolism, and excretion.

➡ Though there is probably a decrease in the liver's production of metabolizing enzymes, the metabolism of drugs does not appear to slow.

➡ A decline in kidney function (including glomerular filtration and drug secretion) occurs which tends to *slow urinary excretion* of drugs.

Gender

Gender is generally not considered a major influence on drug action. Most research has involved men, with the findings applied to women. One particular reason has been to avoid exposing a fetus or potential fetus to unknown risks.

However, some gender based differences in drug response appear to be related to hormonal fluctuations in women during the menstrual cycle. For women with clinical depression, for example, higher dosage levels of antidepressant medication may be necessary when menstrual symptoms are worst.

Distribution may also be somewhat different between men and women simply as a result of differences in body composition (males have more muscle, women more fat).

Pregnancy

A number of physiological changes (including delayed gastric emptying and decreased movement in the gastrointestinal tract) occur in women in the latter stages of pregnancy.

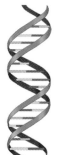

These changes tend to *reduce the rate of absorption.* Drug binding may be reduced. *Urinary excretion increases,* and the rate of excretion for a number of drugs is much greater in pregnant women than in non-pregnant women.

Genetics

Genes determine the types and amounts of proteins produced in the body, with each person being somewhat different. Since drugs interact with proteins in plasma, tissues, receptor sites, and elsewhere, genetic differences can result in differences in drug action.

Genetics can also cause variations in metabolism in which people with certain genetic characteristics will not metabolize a drug that most people metabolize, or will metabolize it at an abnormal rate. In such cases, the individual may experience no therapeutic effect at all, or perhaps even an adverse or toxic effect instead.

Body Weight

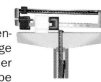

Weight adjustments are generally not made for dosage regimens because the other variability factors tend to be more significant. However, weight adjustments may be needed for individuals whose weight is more than 50% higher than the average adult weight. Weight adjustments are also made for children, or unusually small, emaciated, or obese adult patients.

Psychological

Though the specific reasons are unknown, it is clear that psychological factors can influence individual responses to drug administration. For example, in clinical trials in which placebos are used, patients receiving them often report both therapeutic and adverse effects. This may account for some variability in patient responses to an administered (non-placebo) drug. At a fundamental level, it is a factor in patient willingness to follow prescribed dosage regimens.

ADVERSE EFFECTS

Drugs generally produce a mixture of *therapeutic* (desired) and *adverse effects* (undesired effects).

An adverse effect can be any symptom or disease process and involve any organ. They may be common or rare, localized or widespread, mild or severe depending on the drug and the patient. Some adverse effects occur with usual doses of drugs (often called side effects). Others are more likely to occur only at higher than normal dosages.

COMMON ADVERSE EFFECTS

Central Nervous System Effects

 CNS effects may result from CNS stimulation (e.g., agitation, confusion, delirium, disorientation, hallucinations) or CNS depression (dizziness, drowsiness, sedation, coma, impaired respiration and circulation).

Hepatotoxicity

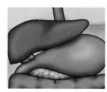 "Hepato" means "of the liver." Hepatotoxity includes hepatitis, hepatic necrosis, and biliary tract inflammation or obstruction. It is relatively rare but potentially life-threatening. Commonly used hepatotoxic drugs include acetaminophen, halothane, isoniazid, chlorpromazine, methotrexate, nitrofurantoin, phenytoin, and aspirin.

Hypersensitivity or Allergy

Almost any drug, in almost any dose, can produce an allergic or hypersensitive reaction in a patient. It generally happens because a patient develops antibodies to a drug he or she has taken. Once this occurs, the drug will interact with the antibodies, releasing histamines and other substances that produce reactions that can range from mild rashes to potentially fatal **anaphylactic shock.**

Allergic reactions can occur within minutes or weeks of drug administration. Anaphylactic shock occurs within minutes. It is a hypersensitivity reaction that can lead to cardiovascular collapse and death if untreated. Its symptoms include severe respiratory distress and convulsions. Immediate emergency treatment with epinephrine, antihistamines, or bronchodilator drugs is required.

Gastrointestinal Effects

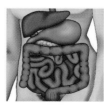 Anorexia, nausea, vomiting, constipation, and diarrhea are among the most common adverse reactions to drugs. More serious effects include ulcerations and colitis (irritable bowel disease).

hepato a prefix meaning "of the liver."

hypersensitivity an abnormal sensitivity generally resulting in an allergic reaction.

anaphylactic shock a potentially fatal hypersensitivity reaction producing severe respiratory distress and cardiovascular collapse.

Nephrotoxicity

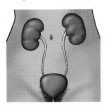

Kidney failure can occur with gentamicin and other amino-glycosides, and with ibuprofen and other nonsteroidal anti-inflammatory drugs.

Idiosyncrasy

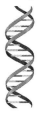

Idiosyncrasy is the unexpected reaction to a drug the first time it is given to a patient. Such reactions are generally thought to be caused by genetic characteristics that alter the patient's drug metabolizing enzymes.

Hematological Effects

Blood coagulation, bleeding, and bone marrow disorders are potentially life threatening and can be caused by various drugs. Anticoagulants can cause excessive bleeding. Antineoplastic drugs may cause bone marrow depression.

Drug Dependence

Chronic usage of narcotic analgesics, sedative-hypnotic agents, antianxiety agents, and amphetamines often results in physiological or psychological dependence. Physiological dependence is accompanied by unpleasant physical withdrawal symptoms when the dose is discontinued or reduced. Psychological dependence involves an emotional or mental fixation on drug usage.

Teratogenicity

This is the ability of a substance to cause abnormal fetal development when given to pregnant women. Drug groups considered teratogenic include analgesics, diuretics, antihistamines, antibiotics, and antiemetics.

Carcinogenicity

This is the ability of a substance to cause cancer. Several drugs are carcinogens, including some hormones and anticancer drugs.

idiosyncrasy an unexpected reaction the first time a drug is taken, generally due to genetic causes.

nephrotoxicity the ability of a substance to harm the kidneys.

carcinogenicity the ability of a substance to cause cancer.

DRUG-DRUG INTERACTIONS

The administration of more than one drug at a time to a patient can cause *drug-drug interactions.*

The probability of a drug-drug interaction increases with the number of drugs a patient takes. Such interactions can affect the disposition of one or more drugs and *result in either increases or decreases in therapeutic effects or adverse effects.* Some drug-drug interactions may not alter drug disposition but will still change the therapeutic effect.

An understanding of the ways drug-drug interactions occur is important. Examples of some common types are on these pages.

Drug-drug interactions that *increase* the therapeutic or adverse effects of drugs:

➥ **Additive effects** occur when two drugs with similar pharmacological actions are taken.

   Example: alcohol + sedative drug = increased sedation

➥ **Synergism** or **potentiation** occurs when two drugs with different sites or mechanisms of action produce greater effects when taken together than either does when taken alone.

   Example: acetaminophen + codeine = increased analgesia

➥ **Interference** by one drug with the elimination of a second drug may intensify the effects of the second drug.

   Example: cimetidine inhibits drug metabolizing enzymes in the liver and therefore interferes with the metabolism of many drugs. When these drugs are given at the same time as cimetidine, their blood concentration increases and they are more likely to cause adverse reactions or toxic effects.

➥ **Displacement** of one drug from protein binding sites by a second drug increases the effects of the displaced drug. This occurs because the blood concentration of the now free displaced drug is increased.

   Example: aspirin + warfarin = increased anticoagulant effect

additive effects the increase in effect when two drugs with similar pharmacological actions are taken.

synergism when two drugs with different sites or mechanisms of action produce greater effects when taken together than when taken alone.

antidote a drug that antagonizes the toxic effect of another drug.

Drug-drug interactions that *decrease* the therapeutic effects of drugs:

➥ An **antidote** to a particular drug is given to **block or reduce its toxic effects.**

Example: naloxone + morphine = relief of morphine induced respiratory depression. Naloxone molecules displace morphine molecules from their receptor sites on nerve cells, preventing the morphine molecules from causing further effect.

➥ **Decreased intestinal absorption** of oral drugs occurs when drugs combine to produce nonabsorbable compounds.

Example: aluminum or magnesium hydroxide + oral tetracycline = binding of tetracycline to aluminum or magnesium. This causes decreased absorption and a decreased antibiotic effect of the tetracycline dose.

➥ When drugs activate metabolizing enzymes in the liver, it **increases the metabolism** of other drugs affected by the same enzymes. Enzyme inducing drugs include some anticonvulsants, barbiturates, and antihistamines.

Example: phenobarbital + warfarin = decreased effects of warfarin

➥ Some drugs **increase excretion** by raising urinary pH and lessening renal reabsorption.

Example: sodium bicarbonate + phenobarbital = increased excretion of phenobarbital. The sodium bicarbonate raises urine pH and ionizes the phenobarbital, increasing its excretion.

Time Course of Drug Interactions

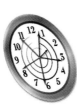

The time it takes for drug-drug interactions to occur can vary substantially. Some interactions occur almost immediately while others may take weeks. Knowing the time course of an interaction allows quick identification and treatment of potential interactions. It also allows clinicians to evaluate the relative importance of an interaction from two drugs compared to their therapeutic effects. For example, if an interaction requires one to two weeks to occur, short term administration over a few days may not cause a significant adverse effect.

DRUG-DRUG INTERACTIONS (cont'd)

ABSORPTION

There are several means by which one drug may affect the gastrointestinal absorption of another:

➡ **drug binding** in the gastrointestinal tract

➡ **alterations in gastrointestinal movement**

➡ **alterations in gastrointestinal pH**

Drug Binding

Some drugs can form nonabsorbable complexes by binding to other drugs, resulting in decreased absorption. For example, iron salts can affect the absorption of several tetracyclines, methlydopa, and levodopa this way.

Gastric Emptying

Certain drugs will affect gastric emptying and therefore the absorption of other drugs. For example, use of propantheline will delay acetaminophen absorption. On the other hand, use of metoclopramide will increase acetaminophen absorption, since metoclopramide increases the rate of gastric emptying. Another problem with reducing gastric emptying time is that drugs that are degraded by gastric acid have a longer time to degrade, resulting in a decreased amount of drug available for absorption from the intestine.

Gastric pH

Drugs that alter the gastrointestinal pH can have a complex effect on other administered drugs. Some of the factors affected by pH are:

➡ the amount of unionized drug available for absorption

➡ the rate of dissolution

➡ gastric emptying

➡ degradation

DISTRIBUTION

Displacement

One drug can displace another from a plasma protein binding site and so increase the amount of the free drug available for distribution. This will increase its pharmacological effect and its elimination, since more of the drug is available for metabolism and excretion.

The biggest consequence of displacement interactions is the *change in pharmacological effect*. If drugs are highly protein bound, displacement tends to have a greater effect than with drugs that are not highly bound. For example, warfarin is 98% plasma protein bound, with only 2% free or unbound. If a drug interaction displaces only 2% of the bound warfarin, then 96% will be bound, but 4% will now be free. That is a 100% increase in the free concentration of warfarin, and it might double its pharmacological effect. By comparison, for a drug that is only 50% bound, displacing 2% will cause only a minor increase in the free concentration.

Such displacement interactions generally occur within the first week or two of administration. When they do occur, many turn out to be self-correcting after a few days, at which point the concentration of displaced drug often returns to pre-interaction levels, even if the patient continues to take both drugs.

METABOLISM

Enzyme Induction

Some drugs are capable of increasing the metabolizing enzymes in the liver. This process is call **enzyme induction**. It increases the metabolism of drugs and usually results in a *reduction in pharmacological effect.* Examples of enzyme inducers include phenobarbital, carbamazepine, phenytoin, and rifampin. Cigarette smoking and chronic alcohol use may also induce metabolism.

The time course of drug interactions from enzyme induction is slower than for many other types of interactions. Though enzyme induction may be dose related, it can also be caused by age, genetics, or liver disease. As a result, it is a difficult type of interaction to predict.

Enzyme Inhibition

The other alteration in metabolism is called **enzyme inhibition,** which usually occurs when two drugs compete for binding sites on the liver's metabolizing enzymes. This generally *increases the plasma concentration (and consequently the pharmacological effect) of at least one of the drugs.* Enzyme inhibition is one of the most common drug interactions. In fact, if a drug is known to be metabolized by the liver, manufacturers often study its potential for enzyme inhibition early in the drug development process.

Unlike enzyme induction, which has a much slower time course, enzyme inhibition has a rapid onset, generally within 24 hours, and tends to disappear quickly once the inhibitor is discontinued. Enzyme inhibition is also easier to predict since it appears to be dose related. It is also true that drugs that share a similar chemical structure often share the potential for enzyme inhibition.

EXCRETION

Filtration

Drug interactions that actually change the filtration rate itself are rare. Changes in the filtration rate are more likely to occur in response to specific drugs, such as those that change the systemic blood pressure, for example. Whatever the cause, changes in the filtration rate will also change the rate of drug excretion.

Kidney Secretion

There are different transport systems in the kidneys for basic drugs and acidic drugs. Basic drugs do not seem to compete for the acidic drug transport system, or visa versa. However, two basic drugs or two acidic drugs may compete for the same transport system and this can cause one or both of the drugs to accumulate in the blood. For example, probenecid competes with penicillin and reduces penicillin's secretion. Probenecid also inhibits the secretion of cephalosporins. An example of such a competition involving basic drugs involves quinidine and digoxin. Quinidine reduces digoxin excretion by 30% to 50%.

Urinary Reabsorption

Urinary reabsorption, a passive transport process, is influenced by the pH of the urine and the extent of ionization of the drug. In acidic urine, acidic drugs tend to be reabsorbed while basic drugs are not. As a result, they are excreted in the urine. In alkaline urine, acidic drugs will not be reabsorbed but will instead be excreted in the urine, while basic drugs will be reabsorbed. An example of these interactions is quinidine, which is a base. The excretion of quinidine is reduced nearly 90% when the urine pH is increased from less than 6.0 to over 7.5.

DRUG-DIET INTERACTIONS

Dietary intakes and patterns vary widely among individuals and can contribute to variability in the disposition of drugs. Differences may be attributed to various factors, including food preferences and availability, diets designed for weight gain or loss, and variations for seasonal, religious, and therapeutic reasons.

ABSORPTION

The physical presence of food in the gastrointestinal tract can alter absorption in several ways:

- ➡ interacting chemically (e.g., certain medications and tetracycline)
- ➡ improving the water-solubility of some drugs by increasing bile secretion
- ➡ affecting the performance of the dosage form (e.g., altering the release characteristics of polymer-coated tablets)
- ➡ altering gastric emptying
- ➡ altering intestinal movement
- ➡ altering liver blood flow.

As a result, some drugs have increased bioavailability and some have decreased bioavailability in the presence of food. For example, the bioavailability of propranolol is enhanced by the presence of food.

The bioavailability of a drug is generally decreased when the presence of food slows absorption. For example, when tablets or capsules are taken with food, they dissolve more slowly, slowing absorption as a result.

Food may also combine with a drug to form an insoluble drug-food complex. This is how tetracycline interacts with dairy products, such as milk and cheese. It combines with the calcium in milk products to form an insoluble, non-absorbable compound that is excreted in the feces.

DISTRIBUTION

The presence of food can also influence drug distribution. For example, high-fat meals can increase fatty acid levels in the blood. The fatty acids bind to the same plasma protein binding sites as many drugs. This displaces previously bound drug and increases the free concentration of that drug, leading to an increased effect.

There are also differences in the plasma protein binding of certain drugs between well-nourished and undernourished people.

ADMINISTRATION TIMES

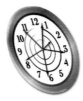

Interactions that alter drug absorption can be minimized by separating the administration of drugs and food intake about 2 hours.

 drug-diet interactions when elements of ingested nutrients interact with a drug and this affects the disposition of the drug.

METABOLISM

Most foods are complex mixtures of carbohydrate, fat, and protein. Research studies designed to determine the influence of diet on drug metabolism have diets in which one of these nutrients is increased, another decreased, and the third nutrient and total caloric intake are kept constant. In general, high-protein (low-carbohydrate) diets are associated with accelerated metabolism while high-carbohydrate (low-protein) diets appear to decrease metabolism. The substitution of fat calories for carbohydrate seems not to affect drug metabolism rates.

In general, mildly or moderately undernourished adults have normal or enhanced metabolism of drugs and severely malnourished adults have decreased drug metabolism. As with any diet, however, there are many variables in malnourishment that can produce an affect on metabolism.

EXCRETION

Reducing dietary protein appears to decrease filtration, increase reabsorption, and increase secretion in the kidney. The total effect of restricted protein intake will depend on the urinary excretion characteristics of the specific drug.

SPECIFIC FOODS

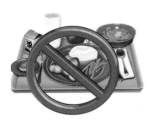

Some foods contain substances that react with certain drugs. For example, eating foods containing tyramine while using monoamine oxidase (MAO) inhibitors may produce severe hypertension or intracranial hemorrhage. MAO inhibitors include isocarboxazid, phenelzine, and procarbazine. Foods containing tyramine include beer, red wine, aged cheeses, yeast products, chicken livers, and pickled herring.

Certain cruciferous vegetables (i.e., brussels sprouts, cabbage) stimulate the metabolism of a few drugs. Other foods that might also have the similar effect are alfalfa, turnips, broccoli, cauliflower, or spinach. Some of the same foods are also involved with an interaction with oral anticoagulants such as warfarin. Spinach and other greens contain vitamin K, and vitamin K inhibits the action of oral anticoagulants. A patient ingesting foods containing vitamin K while taking an anticoagulant would not receive a therapeutic effect from the drug.

DISEASE STATES

The disposition and effect of some drugs can be influenced by the presence of diseases other than the one for which a drug is used. Hepatic, cardiovascular, renal, and endocrine disease all increase the variability in drug response.

HEPATIC

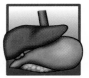

There are a variety of liver diseases that affect hepatic function differently. Some, but not necessarily all, require that special care should be taken when administering drugs to patients with hepatic diseases.

Cirrhosis tends to decrease the hepatic metabolism of drugs. On the other hand, **acute viral hepatitis** decreases metabolism in about half of drugs, but has no affect on the metabolism of the other half. **Obstructive jaundice** appears to diminish drug elimination.

The effect of hepatic disease on drug absorption is not well understood. However, to the extent that liver activity is decreased, it appears that the first-pass effect is also reduced. This results in increased bioavailability for drugs that are usually severely degraded by first-pass metabolism. Another factor that increases bioavailability is that patients with cirrhosis can develop a condition in which a significant amount of the blood coming from the intestine bypasses liver cells and enters the circulatory system directly. When this happens, the bioavailability of drugs that would otherwise be degraded by first-pass metabolism rises substantially.

CIRCULATORY

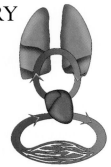

Circulatory disorders are generally characterized by diminished blood flow to one or more organs of the body. Since blood flow influences drug absorption, distribution, and elimination, this may also affect the action of drugs.

Decreased blood flow from cardiovascular disorders can delay or cause erratic drug absorption. As a result, intravenous administration may be needed to obtain a desired effect.

Decreased blood flow can also affect the metabolizing action of the liver. For example, when blood flow to the liver is decreased, the metabolism of lidocaine also decreases.

 hepatic disease liver disease.

cirrhosis a chronic and potentially fatal liver disease causing loss of function and resistance to blood flow through the liver.

acute viral hepatitis a virus caused systemic infection that causes inflammation of the liver.

obstructive jaundice an obstruction of the bile excretion process.

RENAL

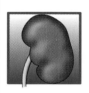

In patients with renal disease, the urinary excretion of drugs decreases in proportion to the decrease in kidney function.

Such decreases can be measured by monitoring the amount of creatinine excreted in the urine. Creatinine is produced by muscle activity in the body and is excreted at a standard rate by healthy kidneys. In diseased kidneys, the rate of creatinine clearance decreases as an indication that kidney function (including glomerular filtration) decreases. In such cases, drug excretion is reduced and to avoid excessive accumulation of the drug in the blood, the dosage must be reduced.

THYROID

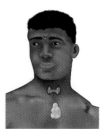

Changes in thyroid function can affect many of the aspects of absorption, excretion, and metabolism.

In **hypothyroidism** (a condition in which the thyroid is underactive), the bioavailability of a few drugs (i.e., riboflavin, digoxin) is increased. In **hyperthyroidism** (an overactive thyroid condition) their bioavailability is decreased because of changes in gastrointestinal movement.

Some other changes affected by thyroid conditions are:

➥ Renal blood flow is decreased in hypothyroidism and increased in hyperthyroidism.

➥ The activity of metabolizing enzymes in the liver is reduced in hypothyroidism and increased in hyperthyroidism.

➥ The metabolism of theophylline, propranolol, propylthiouracil, and methimazole is increased by hyperthyroidism.

 hypothyroidism a condition in which thyroid hormone secretions are below normal, often referred to as an underactive thyroid.

hyperthyroidism a condition in which thyroid hormone secretions are above normal, often referred to as an overactive thyroid.

REVIEW

KEY CONCEPTS

✔ Differences in age, weight, genetics, and gender are among the significant factors that influence the differences in medication responses among people.

✔ Drug distribution, metabolism, and excretion are quite different in the neonate and infant than in adults because their organ systems are not fully developed.

✔ Children metabolize certain drugs more rapidly than adults.

✔ The elderly typically consume more drugs than other age groups. They also experience physiological changes that significantly affect drug action.

✔ A number of physiological changes that occur in women in the latter stages of pregnancy tend to reduce the rate of absorption.

✔ Genetic differences can cause differences in the types and amounts of proteins produced in the body, which can result in differences in drug action.

✔ Almost any drug, in almost any dose, can produce an allergic or hypersensitive reaction in a patient. Anaphylactic shock is a potentially fatal hypersensitivity reaction.

✔ Anorexia, nausea, vomiting, constipation, and diarrhea are among the most common adverse reactions to drugs.

✔ Teratogenicity is the ability of a substance to cause abnormal fetal development when given to pregnant women.

✔ Drug-drug interactions can result in either increases or decreases in therapeutic effects or adverse effects.

✔ Additive effects occur when two drugs with similar pharmacological actions are taken.

✔ Synergism or potentiation occurs when two drugs with different sites or mechanisms of action produce greater effects when taken together than either does when taken alone.

✔ Interference by one drug with the elimination of a second drug may intensify the effects of the second drug.

✔ Displacement of one drug from protein binding sites by a second drug increases the effects of the displaced drug.

✔ Decreased intestinal absorption of oral drugs occurs when drugs combine to produce nonabsorbable compounds.

✔ When drugs activate metabolizing enzymes in the liver, it increases the metabolism of other drugs affected by the same enzymes.

✔ Some drugs increase excretion by raising urinary pH and lessening renal reabsorption.

✔ The physical presence of food in the gastrointestinal tract can alter absorption.

✔ Some foods contain substances that react with certain drugs, e.g., foods containing tyramine can react with monoamine oxidase (MAO) inhibitors.

✔ The disposition and effect of some drugs can be influenced by the presence of diseases other than the one for which a drug is used. For example, decreased blood flow from cardiovascular disorders can delay or cause erratic drug absorption.

SELF TEST

MATCH THE TERMS. *answers can be checked in the glossary*

additive effects

anaphylactic shock

antidote

carcinogenicity

cirrhosis

hepato

hypersensitivity

idiosyncrasy

nephrotoxicity

synergism

teratogenicity

a prefix meaning "of the liver."

the ability of a substance to cause abnormal fetal development when given to pregnant women.

an abnormal sensitivity generally resulting in an allergic reaction.

a potentially fatal hypersensitivity reaction producing severe respiratory distress and cardiovascular collapse.

an unexpected reaction the first time a drug is taken, generally due to genetic causes.

the ability of a substance to harm the kidneys.

the ability of a substance to cause cancer.

the increase in effect when two drugs with similar pharmacological actions are taken.

when two drugs with different sites or mechanisms of action produce greater effects when taken together than taken alone.

a drug that antagonizes the toxic effect of another drug.

a chronic and potentially fatal liver disease causing loss of function and resistance to blood flow through the liver.

CHOOSE THE BEST ANSWER. *answers are in the back of the book*

1. What organ is associated with the adverse effect of nephrotoxicity?
   a. liver
   b. kidney
   c. gall bladder
   d. gastrointestinal tract

2. When two drugs with different sites or mechanisms of action produce greater effects when taken together then when either does when taken alone is called:
   a. an additive effect
   b. a synergestic effect
   c. an interference effect
   d. a displacement effect

3. Enzyme induction and inhibition would be part of which process?
   a. absorption
   b. distribution
   c. metabolism
   d. excretion

4. An unexpected adverse effect to a drug the first time it is given to a patient is considered what type of reaction?
   a. hypersensitivity
   b. anaphylaxis
   c. idiosyncrasy
   d. autoimmune

INFORMATION

The tremendous amount of drug research being done results each year in the appearance of many new drugs on pharmacy shelves. As a pharmacy technician, you may find it difficult to keep up with this constantly changing pharmaceutical information. If you do not, however, your knowledge and skills will become outdated in a very short time. It is therefore essential that you become familiar with the sources of pharmaceutical information that will provide current information to enable you to perform your job as required.

Pharmacy literature can be thought of as a pyramid divided into three sections.

Primary literature sits at the base. It provides the foundation for the development of **secondary** and **tertiary** sources of professional literature that sit on top of it.

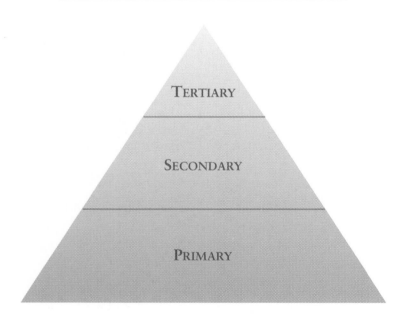

Primary Literature

Primary literature provides direct access to the most current information resulting from contemporary research. It is the largest and most current source of information. This type of literature includes original reports of scientific, clinical, technological, and administrative research projects and studies, and is found in professional and scientific journals such as The Journal of Pharmacy Technology. The need for large storage spaces and the varying quality of journal articles constitute the greatest disadvantage of this type of literature.

PHARMACY LITERATURE

Secondary Literature

Secondary literature primarily consists of general reference works based upon primary literature sources. This type of literature reference includes **abstracting services**, indexing or bibliographic services, and specialized microfiche systems.

Abstracting services (e.g., Drugdex) summarize information contained in a finite number of professional and scientific journals. Indexing or bibliographic services (e.g., Index Medicus) contain a comprehensive listing of current articles that have appeared in professional and scientific international journals. You can usually find these indexing services in hospital or university libraries considering they require large amounts of space for storage. It's important to remember that a lag time (the time between a discovery or idea and the time of publication), varying from one week to twelve months, exists for secondary literature references.

Tertiary Literature

Tertiary literature sources contain condensed and compact information based on primary literature. This type of literature reference includes: textbooks, monographs, standard reference books, and review articles.

Of the three types of literature reference materials, the pharmacist and pharmacy technicians find the tertiary the easiest and most convenient to use. However, no single tertiary reference source contains all the information needed by the pharmacy department. View tertiary references carefully, since authors of the information may misinterpret or misquote the original literature. In addition, remember that these references may be published one or more years after the original literature and no longer current.

LEGAL ASPECTS

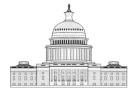

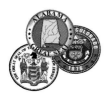

Federal

At present, no federal law exists that mandates the professional literature to be maintained in a pharmacy. The Occupational, Safety, Health Administration (OSHA) does require pharmacies to have Material Safety Data Sheets (MSDS) for each hazardous chemical they use. A pharmacy can obtain these MSDS's from the manufacturer of the hazardous chemical or the local OSHA area office. The MSDS provides information you need to ensure the implementation of proper protective measures for exposure to hazardous chemicals.

State

Many states have laws or State Board of Pharmacy rules and regulations that require pharmacies to maintain specific professional literature references. For example, the Colorado State Board of Pharmacy requires a professional reference library located in the pharmacy area to contain the current edition of the *United States Pharmacopoeia Drug Information Volumes II & III*. They also request a current *ASHP Formulary Service and Guide to Parenteral Admixtures* or *Handbook of Injectable Drugs* if the pharmacy compounds sterile parenteral products.

Legal References

An awareness of the legal aspects of pharmacy protects both the pharmacy technician and the patients. The pharmacy law references described below provide information of laws concerning controlled substances, drug control, and those critical to the practice of pharmacy.

➥ *United States Pharmacopoeia Drug Information (USPDI) Volume III* contains the USP and NF drug standards and dispensing requirements, as well as relevant state and federal legal requirements.

➥ *Handbook of Federal Drug Law* provides an understanding of federal drug law as it affects the practice of pharmacy.

➥ *Pharmacy Law Digest* provides information on controlled substance, pharmacy inspection, drug control, civil liability and business laws. It also contains the addresses of the boards of pharmacy and a survey of the state pharmacy laws compiled and published by the National Association of Boards of Pharmacy (NABP).

 primary literature original reports of clinical and other types of research projects and studies.

secondary literature general reference works based upon primary literature sources.

tertiary literature condensed works based on primary literature, such as textbooks, monographs, etc.

abstracting services services that summarize information from various primary sources for quick reference.

COMMON REFERENCES

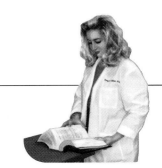

Pharmacists and pharmacy technicians routinely use pharmaceutical reference information in the course of their work.

The nine tertiary literature sources described on these pages are the pharmacy references most commonly available in drug information centers in the United States.

Drug Facts and Comparisons (DFC)

The DFC is a preferred reference for comprehensive and timely drug information, containing information about prescription and OTC products. DFC divides drugs into therapeutic groups. Similar drugs are grouped together with easy-to-use comparative tables. The loose-leaf edition provides the most up-to-date drug reference, with new or revised information sent each month.

Martindale: The Extra Pharmacopoeia

This provides the best source of information on drugs in clinical use internationally. It contains drug monographs that provide information of the properties, actions and uses of drugs. Martindale lists proprietary drug names and their country of origin.

American Hospital Formulary Service (AHFS) Drug Information

The AHFS is accepted as the authority for drug information questions. It groups drug monographs by therapeutic use. Various organizations and programs recognize it as a leading source of drug information for determining reimbursement of prescriptions and as a resource for Drug Utilization Reviews (DUR). The AHFS master volume appears in January. Updates on newly approved uses, new drugs, and other timely information are released periodically.

Handbook on Injectable Drugs

This is a collection of monographs on commercially available parenteral drugs that include concentration, stability, dosage and compatibility information.

Physicians' Desk Reference (PDR)

The PDR is an annual publication intended for physicians that provides prescription information on major pharmaceutical products. You will find that PDR information is similar to the pharmaceutical manufacturer's drug package inserts since manufacturers prepare the essential drug information found in the PDR. The PDR contains five color-coded sections: an alphabetical brand name drug index, a drug classification index by company, a generic and chemical name index, a product identification section, and a product information section of drug monographs. New and revised information is published periodically in supplements. Be aware that the PDR is not a comprehensive source of drug information.

Merck Index

This is an encyclopedic source of chemical substance data, contains monographs referenced by trade, code, chemical, investigational and abbreviated drug names. The index also provides the pharmacy technician with two additional features: an extensive section of tables, and a formulary index.

American Drug Index

This index provides the most exhaustive list of drug products. It contains trade and generic drug names, phonetic pronunciations, indications, manufacturers and schedule information in a dictionary format. The index cross-references drugs by generic, brand, and chemical names.

Drug Topics Red Book and American Druggist Blue Book

These are the pharmacist's guides to products and prices, provide annual price lists of drug products including manufacturer, package size, strength and wholesale and retail prices. The Red Book contains an OTC product interaction guide, a list of HHC products, a product identification chart, an alphabetical arrangement of catalogs of manufacturers, and a list of products available in unit dose. The Blue Book provides the Controlled Substance Act manual and inventory sheets.

United States Pharmacopeia Drug Information (USP DI)

The USP DI provides comprehensive and clinically relevant information on drugs in current use. Divided into three volumes: Volume I is *Drug Information for the Health Care Professional*, Volume II is *Advice for the Patient*, and Volume III is *Approved Drug Products and Legal Requirements.* This volume includes the "Orange Book", which is the common name for the FDA's Approved Drug Products publication.

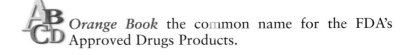

Orange Book the common name for the FDA's Approved Drugs Products.

OTHER REFERENCES

Professional Practice Journals

These journals are official publications of pharmacy organizations and can reflect the political views or policies of these groups. They also reflect changes in standards of practice and indicate trends in the profession. They may publish some original research studies. Examples are The Journal of Pharmacy Technology (PTEC), America's Pharmacist (NCPA), American Journal of Health-System Pharmacy (ASHP) and Journal of the American Pharmaceutical Association (APhA).

Trade Journals

Trade journals are published commercially for pharmacist but are not produced by the profession. They tend to contain large amounts of advertising material. Examples are American Druggist, Pharmacy Times, US Pharmacist, and Community Pharmacist

Primary Literature

Primary literature can be accessed by printed indexes and abstracts or by CD-ROM and online database searching. The continuing development of online and CD-ROM databases has increased the efficiency of the access, retrieval, and storage of information. Micromedix CCIS and MEDLINE are two databases of importance to the pharmaceutical researcher. Micromedix CCIS provides a compilation of full-text databases covering drug information, toxicology and critical care. It includes Drugdex, Poisondex, and Identidex. Index Medicus, online as MEDLINE, contributes the most comprehensive index of international medical literature. Citations are arranged alphabetically by first author and by subject headings.

Newsletters

Newsletters are published rapidly and frequently and provide a useful source of current information. The Medical Letter, FDA Bulletin, PharmIndex and The Green Sheet are a few examples of the many newsletters available to pharmacy personnel.

➡ *The Medical Letter* contains short abstracts from journal articles. It also provides information on clinical trials and profiles on products recently granted New Drug Application (NDA) status.

➡ *FDA Bulletin* contains short, alerting articles on changes in recommended dosages, adverse and side effects and new standards and labeling changes.

➡ *PharmIndex* a cumulative index produced annually that covers new, changed, discontinued and pending products.

➡ The *Weekly Pharmacy Report* or *The Green Sheet* reports relevant legislative issues, professional society information, as well as, company marketing changes and plans.

Textbooks

Textbooks can provide basic information on a particular topic or a range of topics. As with any publications, there is a wide range in the quality, level, and usefulness of textbooks. So it is important to not necessarily accept the information in them as the last word on a subject. However, textbooks are very useful for explaining basic concepts and in refreshing your understanding of a topic. The texts below are noted for their authoritativeness and reliability in providing pharmaceutical information and in including the citations of primary material.

Handbook of Nonprescription Drugs

The Handbook provides the most comprehensive source available for OTC products. It serves both as a textbook for the pharmacy student and an information source for the practicing pharmacist. It is also a useful source for patient education. Infrequent revision is the main drawback of this reference.

Remington's Pharmaceutical Sciences

Published every 5 years since 1885, Remington's is the most comprehensive work in the pharmaceutical sciences. Remington's covers all aspects of pharmacy for students, practitioners and researchers, including evolution of pharmacy, ethics, pharmacy practice, industry and government, drug information and research.

Goodman and Gilman's The Pharmacological Basis of Therapeutics, 9th edition

This is a principal pharmacy text on pharmacology and therapeutics, emphasizing clinical pharmacy practice. It guides the reader to citations in the primary literature.

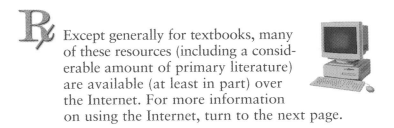

℞ Except generally for textbooks, many of these resources (including a considerable amount of primary literature) are available (at least in part) over the Internet. For more information on using the Internet, turn to the next page.

THE INTERNET

Acomputer network is a series of computers connected by a communication line that allows the computers to exchange information.

The Internet is a "supernetwork," with many networks from around the world all connected to each other by telephone lines, and all using a common "language" (software and rules for communication) that enable them to communicate with each other.

The Internet is the world's largest network.

It has grown from a skeletal experimental network used by scientists to a gigantic commercial "information superhighway" used daily by over fifty million people in 1998. It also contains the world's largest source of information, the **World Wide Web**.

The World Wide Web is a "virtual" library in which electronic information existing on hundreds of thousands of Web sites is accessible to Internet users.

Among this information is a growing amount of pharmacy literature and reference. In addition, patients are increasingly using the World Wide Web to find pharmaceutical and health information.

What It Costs

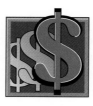

There's a monthly fee for the ISP and whatever the cost is of a local phone call. Most heavy Internet users set up both their ISP and local phone service on an "unlimited" basis. That is, they pay a flat rate for unlimited local calls and unlimited time on the Internet. Otherwise, it's very easy for both phone bills and ISP bills to build up quickly, especially if you have an hourly access plan.

World Wide Web a collection of electronic documents at addresses called Web sites.

modem a piece of hardware that enables a computer to communicate through telephone lines.

browser a software program that allows users to view Web sites on the World Wide Web.

Internet Service Provider (ISP) a company that provides access to the Internet.

URL(uniform resource locator) a web address.

search engine software that searches the web for information related to criteria entered by the user.

GETTING CONNECTED

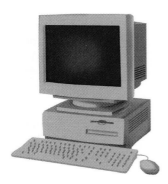

A computer user can connect to the Internet and explore the World Wide Web if they have the following:

➡ **An Internet ready computer:** this is a computer with a **modem**, a small hardware item that can connect the computer to a telephone line.

➡ **A connection:** the modem needs to be connected to a telephone line, the same kind of connection a standard telephone uses.

➡ **Internet software:** Typically, this has been called a **browser**, the most popular of which are Netscape Navigator and Microsoft Explorer. Browsers have many functions that allow you move around the Web, view Web sites, print their contents, save information, and so on. They generally include an Email function that allows you to send messages to anyone on the Internet with an email address.

➡ **An Internet Service Provider (ISP):** America Online, AT&T Worldnet, and Microsoft Network are just some of the popular providers. Generally, people use providers with local area code "access numbers" so their Internet "calls" cost no more than a local phone call.

Web addresses can and do change. If one of the addresses on this page doesn't work, try looking up the address in a search engine.

FINDING WHAT YOU WANT

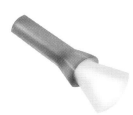

Connecting to the Internet is only a starting point. To find information, you must have the specific addresses of Web sites you want to visit. Web addresses are also referred to as **URLs** (uniform resource locators). For the browser to recognize the address, you first enter the address prefix, **http://**, followed by the address. For example, to go to the USP site, you enter **http://www.usp.org** in the address line of your browser. This is not unlike dialing a "1" before you dial a long distance area code. Note that addresses can use numbers and may begin with "www." or not, but they *always require correct spelling.* If you make a mistake, you may get to a Web site but it won't be the one you wanted.

If you don't know the address you want, you can use a **search engine** to look for it. This is software that will search the Web for specific information you enter. Different search engines have different rules for entering search criteria, but they are very easy to use, and most Internet users rely on them heavily. Here are addresses for a few:

➥ **AltaVista**: www.altavista.digital.com

➥ **Infoseek**: www.infoseek.com

➥ **HotBot**: www.hotbot.com

PLACES TO VISIT

Pharmacy Education and Related Information

➥ www.altimed.com
Alti-Med Pharmacist's Guide to the Internet

➥ pharminfo.com
Pharmaceutical Information Network: drug information and disease discussion groups

➥ www.rxlist.com
RxList: Internet Drug Index, Top 200 drugs

➥ pharm-law.buffalo.edu
Pharmacy law newsletter

➥ 157.142.72.77/pharmacy/pharmint.html
The Virtual Library in Pharmacy

➥ www.geocites.com/~techlectures/
Tech Lectures: continuing education for technicians

➥ ourworld.compuserve.com/homepages/RxTrek/
Rx Trek, information for technicians

Pharmacy Organizations/Publications

➥ www.usp.org
US Pharmacopeia

➥ www.ncpanet.org
National Community Pharmacists Association

➥ www.aphanet.org
American Pharmaceutical Association

➥ www.ashp.org
American Society of Health-System Pharmacists

➥ www.mbnet.mb.ca/ptec
Pharmacy Technician Educators Council

➥ www.ptcb.org
Pharmacy Technician Certification Board

➥ www.merck.com
Merck Manual

➥ www.nabp.net
National Association of Boards of Pharmacy

Government

➥ www.usdoj.gov/dea
Drug Enforcement Agency

➥ www.fda.gov/cder/drug.htm
FDA Drug Information

➥ www.access.gpo.gov
Government Printing Office

➥ www.osha.gov
Occupational Safety & Health Administration

TECHNICIAN REFERENCES

There are various references that provide valuable information on the pharmacy technician profession.

They are useful references for those interested in entering the field, technicians wishing to improve their skills and professionalism, and instructors.

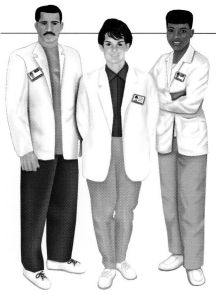

Occupational Information

These references present an overview of the profession for those interested in becoming pharmacy technicians.

➡ Rudman, Jack. Pharmacy Technician (Career Examination Serv.; Vol. C-3822).

➡ The Pharmacy Technician Companion: Your Road Map to Technician Training and Careers. Washington, DC: American Pharmaceutical Association, 1998

➡ Occupational Outlook Handbook. Washington, D.C.: Bureau of Labor Statistics (annual edition).

Occupational Information on the Internet

A considerable amount of information is available on the Internet regarding what a pharmacy technician does, the training required, compensation, job opportunities, and so on. A good first stop for this information is the Educational Testing Service's SIGI PLUS® site: www.ets.org/sigi/pharmtec.html

You can also visit the Bureau of Labor Statistics' Occupational Outlook Handbook site (http://www.bls.gov/ocohome.htm) and use the Index to look up pharmacy technicians and pharmacy assistants.

Another good way to look up job descriptions, training programs, opportunities, and other information is to use a search engine. Just enter "pharmacy technician" and start exploring!

Training Information

These texts present specific pharmacy technician training information. Pharmacy technician training programs utilize these to train pharmacy technician students in general, as well as, specific aspects of pharmacy practice.

➡ Model Curriculum for Pharmacy Technician Training, Bethesda, MD: American Society of Health-System Pharmacists, 1996.

➡ Manual for Pharmacy Technicians. 2nd ed. Bethesda, MD: American Society of Health-System Pharmacists, 1998.

➡ The Pharmacy Technician Workbook: A Self-Instructional Approach. Bethesda, MD: American Society of Health-System Pharmacists, 1994.

➡ The Pharmacy Certified Technician Calculations Workbook. Lansing: Michigan Pharmacists Association, 1997.

➡ Ethical Practices in Pharmacy: A guidebook for Pharmacy Technicians. Madison, Wisconsin: American Institute of the History of Pharmacy, 1997.

➡ The Community Retail Pharmacy Technician Training Manual. Alexandria, Virginia: The NACDS-NARD Community Retail Pharmacy Working Group.

Certification Examination Preparation

In 1995 the Pharmacy Technician Certification Board (PTCB) began administering the National Pharmacy Technician Certification Examination (PTCE). These texts offer information to help individuals prepare for the PTCE.

➥ Pharmacy Technician Certification review and Practice Exam. Bethesda, MD: American Society of Health-System Pharmacists, 1998.

➥ Pharmacy Certified Technician Training Manual, 7th edition. Washington, DC: American Pharmaceutical Association, 1997.

➥ Kocher, Keith. Pharmacy Certified Technician Calculations Workbook. Washington, DC: American Pharmaceutical Association, 1994.

➥ Pharmacy Technician Workbook and Certification Review. Englewood, CO: Morton Publishing, 1999.

Continuing Education and Information

Once certified, the PTCB requires you to obtain 20 hours of continuing education credit every two years to maintain your certification. This publication offers the certified pharmacy technician ten contact hours of continuing education.

➥ C.E. for Pharmacy Technicians. Washington, DC: American Pharmaceutical Assoc., 1997

Tech Lectures®

The Internet site, Tech Lectures, provides continuing education through correspondence and online courses on the pharmacological use of drugs for pharmacy technicians. It will help the technician to better understand disease states and the drug therapies used in their treatment. Examples of topics covered include:

➥ Diabetes Mellitus

➥ Respiratory System—Asthma

➥ Infection Control—Antibiotics

➥ Pain and Analgesics

➥ Total Parenteral Nutrition

Tech Lectures is approved by the American Council on Pharmaceutical Education. For certified technicians (CPhTs), it can also provide the contact hours necessary for recertification.

 Whether you are considering becoming a pharmacy technician, receiving certification or recertification, or simply maintaining your competency and skills, it's always a good idea to research and read about your job. There's a lot you learn on your own, if you make the effort.

REVIEW

KEY CONCEPTS

- ✔ Primary literature provides direct access to the most current information resulting from contemporary research.
- ✔ Secondary literature primarily consists of general reference works based upon primary literature sources.
- ✔ Tertiary literature sources contain condensed and compact information based on primary literature.
- ✔ OSHA requires pharmacies to have Material Safety Data Sheets (MSDS) for each hazardous chemical they use.
- ✔ Many states have laws or State Board of Pharmacy rules and regulations that require pharmacies to maintain specific professional literature references.
- ✔ Drug Facts and Comparisons (DFC) is a preferred reference for comprehensive and timely drug information, containing information about prescription and OTC products.
- ✔ Martindale's "The Extra Pharmacopoeia" provides the best source of information on drugs in clinical use internationally.
- ✔ The Physician's Desk Reference is an annual publication intended for physicians that provides prescription information on major pharmaceutical products.
- ✔ The American Hospital Formulary Service is accepted as the authority for drug information questions. It groups drug monographs by therapeutic use.
- ✔ The USP DI provides comprehensive and clinically relevant information on drugs in current use.
- ✔ The Handbook on Injectable Drugs is a collection of monographs on commercially available parenteral drugs that include concentration, stability, dosage and compatibility information.
- ✔ The Merck Index is an encyclopedic source of chemical substance data, contains monographs referenced by trade, code, chemical, investigational and abbreviated drug names.
- ✔ The American Drug Index provides an exhaustive list of drug products and contains trade and generic drug names, phonetic pronunciations, indications, manufacturers and schedule information in a dictionary format.
- ✔ The Drug Topics Red Book and American Druggist Blue Book are the pharmacist's guides to products and prices, provide annual price lists of drug products including manufacturer, package size, strength and wholesale and retail prices.
- ✔ The "Orange Book" is the common name for the FDA's Approved Drug Products publication.
- ✔ The Internet is a "supernetwork," with many networks from around the world all connected to each other by telephone lines, and all using a common "language."
- ✔ A search engine will search the Web for specific information you enter.

SELF TEST

answers can be checked in the glossary

abstracting services

browser

Internet Service Provider (ISP)

modem

Orange Book

primary literature

search engine

secondary literature

tertiary literature

URL (uniform resource locator)

World Wide Web

original reports of clinical and other types of research projects and studies.

general reference works based upon primary literature sources.

condensed works based on primary literature, such as textbooks, monographs, etc.

services that summarize information from various primary sources for quick reference.

the common name for the FDA's Approved Drugs Products.

a collection of electronic documents at addresses called Web sites.

a piece of hardware that enables a computer to communicate through telephone lines.

a software program that allows users to view Web sites on the World Wide Web.

a company that provides access to the Internet.

a web address.

software that searches the web for information related to criteria entered by the user.

CHOOSE THE BEST ANSWER.   *answers are in the back of the book*

1. This book contains the USP and NF drug standards and dispensing requirements, as well as relevant State and Federal requirements.
   a. USPDI Volume I
   b. USPDI Volume II
   c. USPDI Volume III
   d. Pharmacy Law Digest

2. Which book would you use to find the average wholesale price (AWP) of a drug?
   a. Red Book
   b. Merck Index
   c. Martindale
   d. none of the above

3. Which newsletter contains short, alerting articles on changes in recommended dosage, adverse and side effects and new standards and labeling changes?
   a. The Medical Letter
   b. FDA Bulletin
   c. Pharm Index
   d. The Green Sheet

4. Of the following books, which one is provided in a loose-leaf format and can be updated monthly?
   a. AHFS
   b. USPDI
   c. PDR
   d. DFC

INVENTORY MANAGEMENT

An *inventory* is a listing of the goods or items that a business will use in its normal operation.

Pharmacies generally develop an inventory of medications based upon what they expect to need. Rarely used medications might not be kept in inventory but instead ordered as needed.

The goal of inventory management is to ensure that drugs are available when they are needed.

Because medication needs are often urgent, pharmacies must maintain good control of their stock or inventory. This means that all drugs which are likely to be needed are both on hand and usable—that is, they have not expired or been damaged, contaminated, or otherwise made unfit for use. The technician plays a critical role in inventory management, but there are many participants in the process—the pharmacy, the institution, the wholesaler, the manufacturer, the government, insurers and other third parties.

Inventory management is an integral part of the technician's job responsibility.

Each technician is required to master the specific inventory system in use at their workplace. In some cases, inventory management may be the technician's primary responsibility. At hospitals and other institutions, for example, a **purchasing/inventory technician** is often responsible for obtaining and maintaining the institution's medication and device supply.

Why Use Wholesalers?

The thousands of medications that a pharmacy stocks represent many manufacturers. Obtaining them from individual manufacturers would be a difficult and costly process. Besides the paperwork involved (individual purchase orders, invoices, payments, etc.), there would be many different procedures to learn: how orders could be placed, how they would be shipped, returns policies, and so on.

Wholesalers stock inventories of the most used medications, obtain less-used medications as they are needed, and make frequent deliveries, often on a daily basis. They also provide added-value services such as emergency delivery, automated inventory systems, automated purchasing systems, generic substitution options, private label products, and many others. Obtaining most medications from a single wholesaler greatly simplifies the purchasing process and reduces the staff needed for it.

THE INVENTORY ENVIRONMENT

There are many participants in the inventory process—the pharmacy, the institution, the wholesaler, the manufacturer, the government, insurers and other third parties.

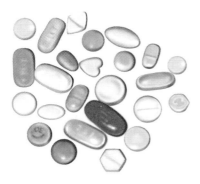

The Formulary

Many hospitals, HMOs, insurers, and other health-care systems maintain a list of medications called a **formulary.** These are the medications that are approved for use in the system.

➡ An **open formulary** is one that allows purchase of any medication that is prescribed.

➡ A **closed formulary** is a limited list of approved medications. A physician must receive permission to use a medication that is not on the list. Closed formularies are generally used as a cost savings tool, in which less expensive substitutes are stocked. Though these substitutes are mainly generic equivalents, in some hospitals a drug in the formulary that is **therapeutically equivalent** (chemically different but with similar actions and effects) may be substituted for a drug not in the formulary.

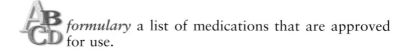

ABCD *formulary* a list of medications that are approved for use.

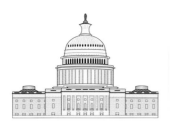

The Government

In the United States, the federal government regulates the distribution of controlled substances and has various distribution, inventory, record keeping, and ordering requirements. Schedule II substances must be stocked separately in a secure place and require a special order form for reordering. Their stock also must be continually monitored and documented.

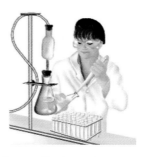

Drug manufacturers

Drugs are not always available from wholesalers due to expense, storage requirements, or other reasons. When this is the case, they can be obtained directly from the manufacturer. When ordering from a manufacturer, a **purchasing account** for the pharmacy must be set up with the manufacturer.

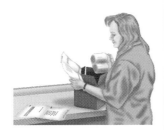

The Pharmacy

Individual pharmacies (whether in community or institutional environments) may use their own inventory system or one provided by another party such as a wholesaler or a corporate parent if they are part of a chain. When drugs need to be purchased, pharmacies buy them directly from wholesalers and sometimes manufacturers, or participate in a large purchasing group which buys the drugs in bulk for its members. Because of the savings that bulk purchasing provides, independent pharmacies often join buying groups that negotiate bulk contracts.

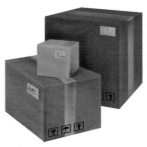

Wholesalers

More than three-quarters of pharmaceutical manufacturers' sales are directly to drug wholesalers*, who in turn resell their inventory to hospitals, pharmacies, and other pharmaceutical dispensers. Wholesalers stock tens of thousands of items from hundreds of manufacturers, everything from disposable razors to Activase, a life saving emergency use drug. They are government-licensed and regulated and offer their customers dependable one-stop-shopping for most of their medication needs. Using wholesalers simplifies the drug purchasing process and saves time, effort, and expense.

*source: National Wholesale Drug Association

INVENTORY SYSTEMS

A pharmaceutical inventory system is able to track inventory, forecast needs, and generate reorders to maintain adequate inventory. This means that neither too many nor too few drugs are on hand at all times. Too many drugs on hand involves unnecessary cost and maintenance and may result in spoilage. Too few drugs means that medications won't be available when needed. The goal of a good inventory system is to have the right amount of stock available at all times.

In order to maintain an adequate supply of medications, pharmacies use a perpetual inventory system.

A perpetual inventory system maintains a continuous record of every item in inventory so that it always shows the stock on hand. This is a requirement for Schedule II substances, but it is also important for many medications since their availability has health consequences.

Spoilage

Time or storage conditions may cause the chemical compounds in medications to break down, resulting in either lost potency or changed function. This is called inventory spoilage. Use of such medications may be dangerous. As a result, medications carry expiration dates and storage requirements that must be honored.

✔ **Note:** As an expiration date approaches, it may already be too late to dispense the medication, since it must be used before the date passes. If an expiration date for a medication has passed, or the medication cannot be completely used before that date, the medication must be appropriately disposed or returned to the supplier for credit. In some cases, wholesalers will not accept expired drugs, but the drug manufacturer will. When returned, packages must generally be unopened.

turnover the rate at which inventory is used, generally expressed in number of days.

point of sale system (POS) an inventory system in which the item is deducted from inventory as it is sold or dispensed.

reorder points minimum and maximum stock levels which determine when a reorder is placed and for how much.

INVENTORY CONCEPTS

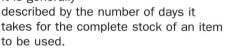

Turnover

Turnover is the rate at which inventory is used. It is generally described by the number of days it takes for the complete stock of an item to be used.

Besides quality and spoilage issues, there's a financial consideration to rapid stock turnover. If a supplier's payment terms are "thirty days net" and stock turnover averages less than thirty days, the stock will be sold before the supplier must be paid for it. The more this is true of the turnover, the lower the cost is of the stock.

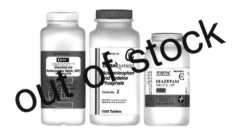

Availability

Besides monitoring stock on hand, it is important to monitor the market availability of medications. At any time, a particular drug may be unavailable due to manufacturing difficulties, raw material unavailability, recalls, etc. This can increase market demand for substitutes for the unavailable drug, sometimes causing shortages in the substitutes as well.

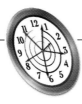

TOOLS FOR PERPETUAL INVENTORY

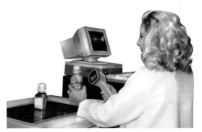

Point of sale (POS)

Pharmacy operations generally use a point of sale system in which the item is deducted from inventory as it is sold or dispensed. The transaction is often triggered by the scanning of a bar code on the medication packaging, though it can also be keyed into the system.

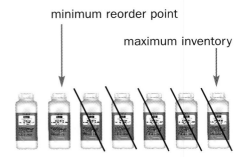

minimum reorder point

maximum inventory

Reorder Points

In order to maintain adequate inventory for their needs, community and institutional pharmacies maintain computer databases of their inventory using drug reorder points. These are **maximum** and **minimum** inventory levels for each drug. As the minimum reorder point of a medication is reached, most computer systems will generate an automatic purchase order for more of it. What medications should be ordered (and how much) is automatically identified on a daily basis. The order amount will be calculated to reach the maximum reorder point. Reorder points for any item can generally be set according to the needs of the facility.

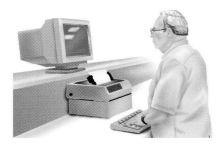

Automated Reports

Computerized inventory systems provide a continuous picture of the inventory situation through automated reports that allow users to analyze and monitor their inventory a variety of ways. They automatically update stock amounts, track turnover, produce purchase orders based on reorder points, and forecast future needs.

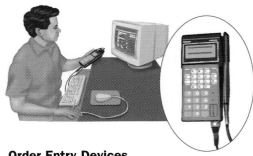

Order Entry Devices

Portable hand held devices are widely used to enter ordering data. When inspection of stock shows that a drug is approaching the minimum inventory level, the reorder can be made using one of these devices. The drug's ID number is entered by hand or scanned into the device using a bar coded shelf tag and the wand attached to the device. A desired quantity, generally enough to reach the maximum inventory level, is then entered to complete the order. The data is sent over a phone line to the institution's ordering computer, which processes the data and sends an order based on it via modem to the supplier's computer.

COMPUTERS & INVENTORY

Computerized inventory systems automatically adjust inventory and generate orders based on maintaining set inventory levels.

The inventory system is often just a component of a comprehensive pharmacy management system that includes elements like patient profiling, management reporting, and so on. In many cases, the drug wholesaler provides the system to its customers as part of the wholesaler service. The customer's system interacts with the wholesaler's so that various types of information (pricing, order information, etc.) can be exchanged automatically between the two systems.

Entering correct information is essential to any computer system.

Computerized systems may automatically create and maintain records based on each inventory transaction. However, many of these transactions are manually entered into the system. So there is always a possibility of error. For this reason, each system produces reports that cover virtually every aspect of the inventory process from stock to turnover to reorders. These reports can be read on screen or in printed form so that errors can be detected.

To protect against possible abuses, users are given passwords to access different features of the system.

This not only protects the employer, but the employee as well. It prevents unauthorized activities and documents who did what and when.

KEY CONSIDERATIONS

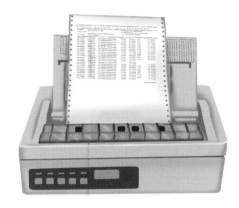

The Importance of Hard Copy

Important reports (especially purchase orders) should be regularly printed out and filed as hard copy both for convenience and as a backup since power disruptions, computer failure, file corruption, or other computer problems can cause information to be lost. Printed reports are also easy to circulate and are required for many uses.

For both business and legal reasons, electronic and hard-copy records are kept for an established amount of time that varies by facility.

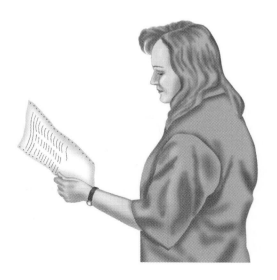

Manual Checking

Checking reports manually is an important step in ensuring that records are correct. Simple data entry errors can result in serious mistakes affecting orders, stock availability, prices, and other issues. For example: If a box containing 150 u/d tablets of Tylenol (R) is set up in the system as one unit, but is incorrectly keyed into the system as 150 units, the system's information will be grossly incorrect.

database a collection of information structured so that specific information within it can easily be retrieved and used.

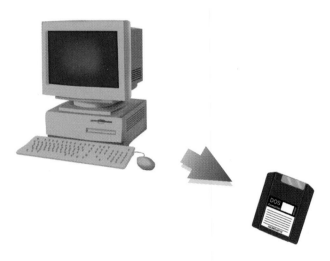

System Backup

Each system's **database** of information is a critical component of the pharmacy or institution in which it functions. These files must be regularly **backed-up** or copied to an appropriate storage media. There are many types of such media, including ordinary "floppy disks." Whatever the media, it is important to know its reliability. Floppy disks, for example, are easily corrupted, and like other types of storage media are vulnerable to erasure by magnetic sources. Therefore, safe back-up may require two different back-ups. Depending on the operation, back up may need to be performed daily.

System Care and Maintenance

Computer systems have become very durable, but they need care and maintenance. It is important to know and follow the operating instructions for any system. Some factors that can cause damage to computers are:

- ✔ temperature;
- ✔ dust;
- ✔ moisture;
- ✔ movement;
- ✔ vibrations;
- ✔ power surges.

The Operation Manual

Computer systems have operation manuals that explain how to use and maintain the system. It is of course necessary that users of the system follow the manual's instructions. It is also important that they store the manual in a safe and accessible location so they can refer to it when they need to.

PC Based Systems

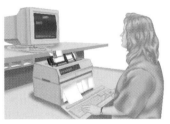

Personal computer-based systems require periodic maintenance, such as **defragmentation** of the files on the system. This is essentially a reorganization of files that have been automatically stored in pieces or fragments on the system. Up to a point, this is not a problem. However, too many fragmented files on a system will slow it down and may cause other problems. Each system contains software that defragments its files. Some work automatically. Some require a user to start the program.

 It is important to know the system care, maintenance, backup, and hard copy requirements that apply to the system you use at your workplace.

ORDERING

Ordering systems involve automated and manual activities.

Much of the work is done by computer systems, both the orderer's and the supplier's. However, manual checking, editing, and confirmation are essential to making such systems work as required.

AUTOMATED ORDERING

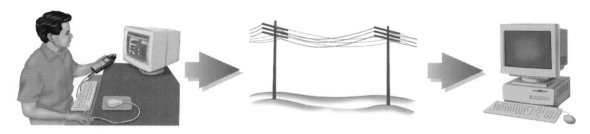

Orders can be generated using an order entry device or automatically generated by the system based on stock levels and reorder points. These reports must then be checked and confirmed. If changes are needed, they can be made manually. The system then produces a revised order, which should again be checked and edited until it is ready for sending to the supplier.

When an order is ready, the ordering system and the supplier's system are connected over phone lines so the order can be "downloaded" from one system to the other.

The supplier's computer system analyzes the order line by line to determine if it can be filled as requested. It checks to see if there is enough of each item in the supplier's inventory to fill the order. If there is more than one warehouse in the system, it may check multiple locations to see if the items are available.

➡ If the order can be filled as ordered, a message will automatically confirm the order to the ordering system. This confirmation can be read onscreen by the orderer but should also be printed for their records.

➡ If the order cannot be filled exactly as ordered, a message containing the **exceptions** will be sent. This report should be printed and appropriate action taken to fill the order. It may be necessary to create a second purchase order, talk with the supplier personally, or find an alternative supplier. Some common reasons for omissions are: temporarily out-of-stocks, back-ordered drugs, or the item may no longer be carried.

ORDER DETAILS

Shipping

When a purchase order is sent to a supplier, the type of shipping is indicated by the orderer. This will determine both the time and cost of shipping.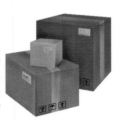

When the order is shipped, it may be a single shipment or multiple shipments. For example, if a single distribution center of a supplier does not have all the items ordered, a partial shipment at a later time or from another distribution center may be needed to fill the order.

Material Safety Data Sheets (MSDS) for hazardous substances such as chemotherapeutic agents indicate when special handling and shipping is required. The Postal Service, Federal Express, United Parcel Service, and others all have specific policies for shipping hazardous substances that must be followed. Some substances are not allowed to be shipped by plane, because the Federal Aviation Administration (FAA) will not allow them onboard. Often these drugs are shipped via a courier.

Credits/Returns

Each supplier has a policy and procedure for returns and credit that must be followed in order to receive the credit. As with orders, the documentation must be carefully checked item by item to make sure it is accurate. A printed copy must be kept on file in addition to any electronic version.

There are companies that specialize in returns to the manufacturer of expired drugs and drugs removed from a formulary. These companies complete each manufacturer's return form, follow their procedures, as well as package, mail and track the drugs. They also return and fill out the paper work for **C-II drugs** and other controlled substances. Their fee is generally a percentage of the return credit, and is deducted automatically from the refund so there is not a separate bill.

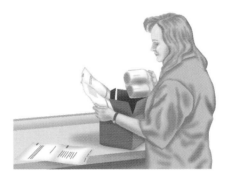

Receiving

Accuracy is essential in checking in the medications received from suppliers. It is important to be alert for drugs that have been incorrectly picked, received damaged, are outdated or missing entirely from the supplier. In many settings, items are stickered with bar codes that can be scanned to do an automatic count.

✔ Shipments, invoices and purchase orders must be reconciled item by item.

✔ The strength and amount of each item must be checked to make sure they are correct. A common mistake is an item sent in bulk instead of unit dose (or the reverse).

✔ Shipment prices on the supplier invoice should match the purchase order exactly. Individual price changes must be identified and may have to be entered into the system manually to make sure the system has the correct information.

✔ If there are any discrepancies, the supplier should generally be notified immediately.

✔ Controlled substances are shipped separately and should be checked in by a pharmacist.

---

 material safety data sheets OSHA required notices on hazardous substances which provide hazard, handling, clean-up, and first aid information.

FORMS

The Online Ordering Screen

Online ordering systems generally contain abbreviated descriptions of drug products in the formulary. The technician uses an "Select" (or similar) function to choose products and may then "Add" it to an order. Quantities may be manually entered or edited—if they have been automatically recorded by the system.

The system automatically assigns to each order a **purchase order number** for identification. Once the order is finished, checked, and ready, it is sent to the supplier's system.

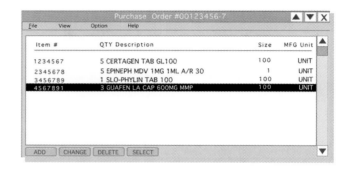

The Confirmation Printout

When an online purchase order is received by the supplier, the supplier's system checks the order to see what items it will be able to ship to the orderer. Once it completes this process, a confirmation of the order is sent back to the orderer's system. This confirmation indicates which items will be shipped, which will not (due to unavailability), and what the cost of the items and any related costs may be. The confirmation comes in the form of a file that is saved on the system, but is also printed out so a hard copy of the confirmation is available for checking.

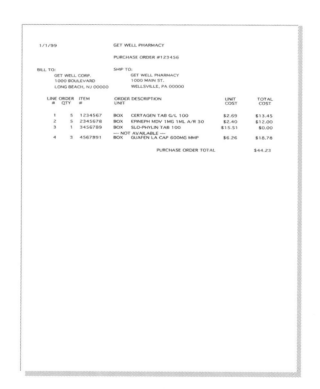

The Shipping Invoice

When the items are shipped, the supplier includes an **invoice** listing the items in the shipment, items that may be shipped separately, items that are unavailable, and the cost of the shipment. The invoice must be checked item by item against the items in the shipment to make certain nothing is missing.

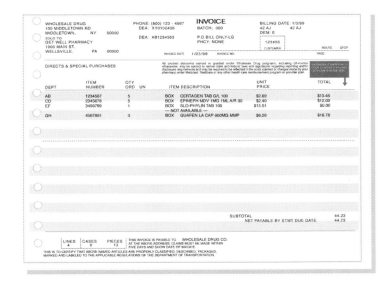

The Returns Form

Preprinted multipart forms are often used for returns, though some computer inventory systems generate their own form. When returning items, the following information is usually required:

➥ original p.o. number
➥ item number
➥ quantity
➥ reason for return

Reasons for returning products can include overshipments, damaged or expired products, or changed needs.

STOCKING & STORING

Most medications are received from the supplier in bulk "stock bottles" that carry FDA required information on the label. This information includes the brand name, generic name, prescription legend, storage requirements, dosage form, quantity, controlled substance mark, manufacturer's name, lot number, expiration date, and NDC number (National Drug code). These bottles often contain bulk quantities from which individual prescriptions will be filled.

Some medications, particularly in hospitals, are packaged in individual doses called "unit/dose" packaging.

Unit dose packaging allows the dispensing of individual doses to patients in hospitals and other settings. Because the dose information is on each dose, it is easily checked before leaving the pharmacy to the nursing unit. In many settings, technicians prepare unit-dose packaging under the supervision of a pharmacist as part of their job.

Drugs must be stored according to manufacturer's specifications.

Most drugs are kept in a fairly constant room temperature of 59°-86°F (and not below, unless stated by the manufacturer to do so). The storage room must have adequate ventilation or proper air distribution. Drug shelves should be sturdy and allow proper air flow around the medications and room.

PACKAGING

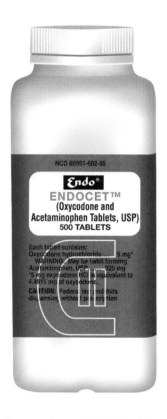

bulk container with 500 tablets of Endocet

 unit-dose packaging a package containing a single dose of a medication.

Unit-Dose Packaging

Unit-dose packaging can take many forms: plastic packs, vials, tubes, ampules, etc. Some unit-dose drugs are packaged in individual bubbles on cards containing ten doses. A box of one hundred unit doses would contain ten such cards. Each unit dose package contains the name of the drug, its strength, and the expiration date. In some settings, technicians are hired specifically to create unit-dose packaging from bulk supplies.

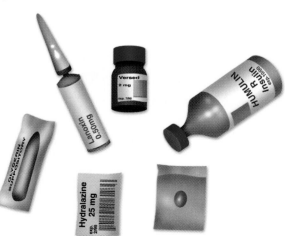

STORAGE

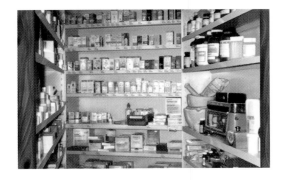

Physical Organization

Drugs may be organized by various methods. Storing by manufacturer would locate the drug using its brand name and is often done in a retail pharmacy. Storing **alpha-generically** organizes drugs alphabetically by their generic names. For example, if the generic name "cimetidine" is on the shelf, Tagamet may be placed there along with the generic.

Whatever the overall organization, the following basic guidelines should be met:

✔ Each medication should be organized in a way that will dispense the oldest items first so that the medications will remain fresh.

✔ The location of each drug should be quickly identifiable through a locator system in which each drug is assigned a location number that is stored in the computer system. This allows quick retrieval of any drug.

✔ Enough space should be provided for each medication to minimize breakage and to make it difficult to accidentally select the wrong medication.

Refrigeration

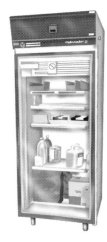

Some drugs must be stored at a constant temperature in a controlled commercial refrigerator designed for medications. If refrigerated or frozen medications are left out for a period of time longer than stated in the literature, they may begin to break down chemically or lose potency. Commercial refrigerators and freezers have gauges on the outside that indicate the internal temperature and allow it to be monitored. The temperature of refrigeration should generally be 40-42°.

The refrigerator or freezer should be plugged into a wall receptacle that is marked for emergency use and will switch to emergency power generators if there is a power failure. If any medication is left out of refrigeration beyond the recommendations of the manufacturer, it should be discarded.

Point of Use Stations

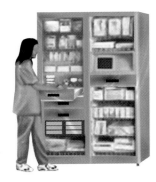

In hospitals and other settings, medications are stocked in dispensing units throughout the facility that may be called supply stations or med-stations. Since they are at the **point of use**, they greatly simplify the dispensing of medications to patients.

Supply Station, courtesy of Pyxis

Items stocked in these stations differ based upon the needs of the patients. For example, a station in an operating room would contain many anaesthetics.

All withdrawals and restocks of stations are recorded just as they would be from a central dispensary, and stations may be linked into the facility computing system so the information can be automatically communicated to it.

℞ Stock that has expired, been damaged, recalled, or has otherwise been targeted for return or disposal must be segregated and clearly marked to avoid contamination and/or mix-up with the good stock.

REVIEW

KEY CONCEPTS

✔ Good inventory management ensures that drugs which are likely to be needed are both on hand and usable—that is, not expired, damaged, contaminated, or otherwise unfit for use.

✔ An open formulary is one that allows purchase of any medication that is prescribed. A closed formulary is a limited list of approved medications.

✔ Schedule II substances must be stocked separately in a secure place and require a special order form for reordering. Their stock must be continually monitored and documented.

✔ More than three-quarters of pharmaceutical manufacturers' sales are directly to drug wholesalers, who in turn resell their inventory to hospitals, pharmacies, and other pharmaceutical dispensers.

✔ A perpetual inventory system maintains a continuous record of every item in inventory so that it always shows the stock on hand.

✔ Turnover is the rate at which inventory is used.

✔ Pharmacy operations generally use a point of sale system in which the item is deducted from inventory as it is sold or dispensed.

✔ Drug reorder points are maximum and minimum inventory levels for each drug.

✔ Important reports (especially purchase orders) should be regularly printed out and filed as hard copy both for convenience and as a backup record-keeping system.

✔ Some factors that can damage computer systems are temperature, dust, moisture, movement, vibrations, power surges.

✔ Pharmacy computer files must be regularly backed-up or copied to an appropriate storage media.

✔ In a computerized inventory system, orders can be generated using an order entry device or automatically generated by the system based on stock levels and reorder points.

✔ In an online ordering system, if an order can be filled as ordered, a message from the supplier will automatically confirm the order to the ordering system. The system automatically assigns to each order a purchase order number for identification.

✔ Material Safety Data Sheets (MSDS) for hazardous substances such as chemotherapeutic agents indicate when special handling and shipping is required.

✔ Controlled substances are shipped separately and should be checked in by a pharmacist.

✔ Most medications are received from the supplier in bulk "stock bottles."

✔ Drugs must be stored according to manufacturer's specifications.

✔ Most drugs are kept in a fairly constant room temperature of 59°-86°F. The temperature of refrigeration should generally be 40-42°.

✔ Medications should be organized in a way that will dispense the oldest items first.

✔ In hospitals and other settings, medications are stocked in dispensing units throughout the facility that may be called supply stations or med-stations.

SELF TEST

closed formulary	a system that allows purchase of any medication that is prescribed.
database	a limited list of approved medications.
material safety data sheets	the rate at which inventory is used, generally expressed in number of days.
open formulary	an inventory system in which the item is deducted from inventory as it is sold or dispensed.
perpetual inventory	minimum and maximum stock levels which determine when a reorder is placed and for how much.
point of sale system (POS)	a collection of information structured so that specific information within it can easily be retrieved and used.
purchase order number	OSHA required notices on hazardous substances which provide hazard, handling, clean-up, and first aid information.
reorder points	number the number system assigned to each order for identification.
turnover	a package containing a single dose of a medication.
unit-dose packaging	a system that maintains a continuous record of every item in inventory so that it always shows the stock on hand.

1. Material Safety Data Sheets (MSDS) provide
   a. protocols for fire hazards in the pharmacy setting
   b. safety codes by OSHA in the storage of inventory
   c. information concerning hazardous substances
   d. none of the above

2. Which of the following concepts involves the deduction of an item as it is sold or dispensed?
   a. spoilage
   b. availability
   c. point of sale system
   d. reorder points

3. If a supplier's terms are thirty days net,
   a. it would be best to have a turnover less than thirty days
   b. it would be best to have a turnover equal to thirty days
   c. it would be best to have a turnover greater than thirty days
   d. none of the above

4. Most drugs are kept fairly in a constant room temperature of
   a. 32 to 59 degrees Farenheit
   b. 59 to 70 degrees Farenheit
   c. 59 to 86 degrees Farenheit
   d. none of the above

FINANCIAL ISSUES

Financial issues have a substantial influence on health care and pharmacy practice.

In 1985, the average prescription price was approximately $10. By 1999, that had tripled. The increase is due to a number of reasons, including inflation and the aging of the population. It is also due to the use of new medications that enhance the quality of health care, but which are often costly.

The use of third party programs to pay for prescriptions has also increased dramatically.

Third party programs are simply another party besides the patient or the pharmacy that pays for some or all of the cost of medication: essentially, an insurer. Although many individuals are uninsured, most people have some form of private or public health insurance. These include both public programs such as Medicaid and Medicare and private programs such as HMOs and basic health insurance. Many but not all such programs include prescription drug coverage. While the growth of these programs is largely a response to the rising costs of health care, in many cases third party programs allow patients to benefit from new and often more expensive drug therapies than they would otherwise be able to afford.

Because of the pharmacy technician's role in the prescription filling process, he or she must understand the different types of health insurance and how drug benefits differ among the programs.

A patient's prescription drug program determines important considerations for filling their prescription. Generic substitution may be required. There may be limits on the quantity dispensed (tablets, capsules, etc.) per fill, or on the frequency and number of refills, and so on.

PHARMACY BENEFITS MANAGERS

Regardless of how the claims are submitted and processed, participating pharmacies must sign contracts with insurers or pharmacy benefit managers before patients can get their prescriptions filled at that pharmacy and billed to their insurer or pharmacy benefit manager. A pharmacy benefit manager (PBM) is a company that administers drug benefit programs. Many insurance companies, HMOs, and self-insured employers use the services of more than 75 PBMs to manage drug benefit coverage for employees and health plan members. The following are the names of some pharmacy benefit managers (PBMs).

- ➥ Aetna Pharmacy Management
- ➥ Caremark Prescription Services
- ➥ Diversified Pharmaceutical Services
- ➥ Express Scripts
- ➥ Medco Containment Services
- ➥ National Prescription Administrators
- ➥ PCS Health Systems

pharmacy benefits managers companies that administer drug benefit programs

online adjudication the resolution of prescription coverage through the communication of the pharmacy computer with the third party computer.

co-insurance an agreement for cost-sharing between the insurer and the insured.

co-pay the portion of the price of medication that the patient is required to pay.

dual co-pay co-pays that have two prices: one for generic and one for brand medications.

maximum allowable cost (MAC) the maximum price per tablet (or other dispensing unit) an insurer or PBM will pay for a given product.

U&C or UCR the maximum amount of payment for a given prescription, determined by the insurer to be a usual and customary (and reasonable) price.

COMPUTERS AND THIRD PARTY BILLING

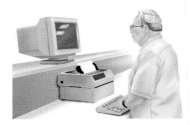

Procedures used by pharmacies to submit third party claims vary. Most insurers or pharmacy benefit managers mail checks to pharmacies (or their accounts receivable departments) at regular intervals along with listings of the prescriptions covered and those not covered (i.e., rejected).

Before the computer age, prescriptions were billed to third parties using paper claims. Although paper claims are still used, most claims are now filed electronically by online claim submission and **online adjudication** of claims. This electronic submission and adjudication process benefits both third party programs as well as pharmacies. The online communication between the prescription-filling computer in the pharmacy and the claim-processing computer of the insurer or pharmacy benefit manager results in improved accuracy and control. It is also much faster and more direct than processing paper claims. The benefits of computerizing the claims process have also been a factor in the rise of third party programs.

CO-PAYS

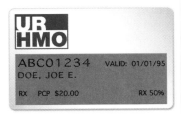

One of the common aspects of many third party programs is **co-insurance**, which is essentially an agreement between the insurer and the insured to share costs. One aspect of this is the requirement for the patient to **co-pay** for the filled prescription. That is, the patient must pay a portion of the price of the medication and the insurance company is billed for the remainder.

The amount paid by the insurer is not equal to the retail price normally charged, but is determined by a formula described in a contract between the insurer and the pharmacy. There is a **maximum allowable cost (MAC)** per tablet or other dispensing unit that an insurer or PBM will pay for a given product. This is often determined by survey of the **usual and customary (U&C)** prices for a prescription within a given geographic area. This is also referred to as the **UCR (usual, customary, and reasonable)** price for the prescription.

Many third party plans have **dual co-pays**, which means that a lower co-pay applies to prescriptions filled with generic drugs and a higher co-pay applies to prescriptions filled with brand name drugs that have no generic equivalent. Some plans have three different co-pays: the lowest co-pay applies to prescriptions filled with generic drugs, a higher co-pay applies to prescriptions filled with brand name drugs which have no generic equivalent, and a third higher co-pay applies to prescriptions filled with brand name drugs which have a generic equivalent.

THIRD PARTY PROGRAMS

PRIVATE HEALTH INSURANCE

Basic private health insurance policies may pay for prescribed expenses (such as prescriptions) when the patient is covered by a supplementary **comprehensive major medical policy** or when the patient's coverage includes an additional prescription drug benefit. Patients covered by comprehensive major medical policies pay out-of-pocket for their prescriptions. Once a **deductible** is met, the insurer may pay a portion of the cost of prescriptions filled the rest of the year. In other words, once a patient has paid a certain dollar amount for prescribed medical expenses (usually including prescriptions), the insurance company will reimburse a portion of the cost of filled prescriptions for the rest of the year. Whether or not a patient is required to get generic drugs when they are available is determined by individual plans and may not be obvious before filling the prescription. Major medical claims frequently involve paper claims. However, the use of electronic claim processing for major medical claims is growing.

Prescription Drug Coverage

Some traditional health insurance policies have the added benefit of prescription drug coverage. Patients with prescription drug coverage through a private insurance company are issued **prescription drug benefit cards** to carry in their wallets. These cards contain necessary billing information for pharmacies, including the patient's identification number, group number, and co-pay amount.

As with other prescription plans, there may be various types of co-pays and patients may be required to get generic drugs (when available). However, basic private health insurance policies often do not require generic substitution because the patient or their employer pays a higher premium for coverage.

Most prescription claims are processed through online adjudication: the pharmacy computer communicates with the insurer's or PBM's computer to determine the prescription drug benefit. When the claim is adjudicated or processed by the insurer or pharmacy benefit manager it becomes obvious if generic substitution is mandatory.

ABCD *deductible* a set amount that must be paid by the patient for each benefit period before the insurer will cover additional expenses.

prescription drug benefit cards cards that contain third party billing information for prescription drug purchases.

MANAGED CARE PROGRAMS

Managed care programs include health maintenance organizations (HMOs), point-of-service programs (POS), and preferred provider organizations (PPOs). Managed care programs provide all necessary medical services (usually including prescription coverage) in return for a monthly premium and co-pays. Most managed care prescription drug plans require generic substitution when a generic is available. Some managed care plans have single co-pays, some have dual co-pays, and some have three types of co-pays.

HMOs

HMOs are made of a network of providers who are either employed by the HMO or have signed contracts to abide by the policies of the HMO. HMOs usually will not cover expenses incurred outside their participating network. *HMOs often require generic substitution.*

POSs

POS programs are made of a network of providers contracted by the insurer. Patients enrolled in a POS choose a primary care physician (PCP) who is a provider in the insurer's network. Patients may receive care outside of the POS network, but the primary care physician is required to make referrals for such care. POSs often partially reimburse expenses incurred outside of their network. *POSs usually require generic substitution.*

PPOs

PPOs are also a network of providers contracted by the insurer. Of the managed care options, PPOs offer the most flexibility for their members. PPOs often partially reimburse expenses incurred outside of their participating network and do not require a primary care physician within their network to make referrals. *PPOs usually require generic substitution.*

Patients with prescription drug coverage through managed care organizations are issued prescription drug benefit cards with billing and co-pay information. Most claims for these programs are processed through online adjudication. Many HMOs, POS, and PPOs use pharmacy benefit managers (PBMs) to manage drug benefit coverage.

HMOs a network of providers for which costs are covered inside but not outside of the network.

POSs a network of providers where the patient's primary care physician must be a member and costs outside the network may be partially reimbursed.

PPOs a network of providers where costs outside the network may be partially reimbursed and the patient's primary care physician need not be a member.

THIRD PARTY PROGRAMS

PUBLIC HEALTH INSURANCE

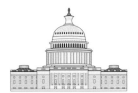

The largest public health insurance plans in the United States are Medicare and Medicaid.

Medicare

Medicare covers people over the age of 65, disabled people under the age of 65 and people with kidney failure. Medicare benefits do not typically cover prescription drugs, although **Qualified Medicare Beneficiaries (QMBs)** may be eligible for state administered prescription assistance. QMB patients may qualify for prescription drug coverage after spending a predetermined out-of-pocket amount on prescribed medical expenditures (including prescriptions). Whether or not QMB patients qualify for prescription drug coverage is determined on a month-to-month basis (similar to a "monthly deductible").

Medicaid

Medicaid is a federal-state program. **ADC (Aid to Dependent Children)** is one type of Medicaid program. State welfare departments usually operate Medicaid. Each state decides who is eligible for Medicaid benefits and what services will be covered. A prescription drug formulary is a listing of the drugs that are covered by Medicaid. Prescription drug formularies for Medicaid recipients are determined by each state. *Medicaid programs do not automatically cover drugs that are not on the state formulary.* Completion of a prior authorization form is sometimes required to justify the need for a medication that is not on the state Medicaid formulary. Completion of the form does not imply the drug will be covered. Medicaid recipients can also qualify for HMO programs.

Medicare a federal program providing health care to people with certain disabilities over age 65; it includes basic hospital insurance and voluntary medical insurance.

Medicaid a federal-state program, administered by the states, providing health care for the needy.

Qualified Medicare Beneficiaries Medicare patients who may at times qualify for prescription drug coverage through a state administered program.

OTHER PROGRAMS

Workers' Compensation

In the United States, the federal government and every state have enacted workers' compensation laws. Under workers' compensation legislation, procedures for *compensation for employees accidentally injured on-the-job* are established. Administrative guidelines require that accidents be reported to a public board that grants compensation awards to injured workers.

In recent years, state workers' compensation programs have been broadened to provide for coverage of occupational diseases. Prescriptions related to the occupational injury or disease can be billed to the state's bureau of workers' compensation or to the employer (if the employer is self-insured). Many workers' compensation claims can be processed through online adjudication. However, some claims require paper claims. It is important to realize the billing procedure can be slightly different for self-insured claims. Pharmacy benefit managers (PBMs) may administer workers' compensation prescription drug benefits.

Patient Assistance Programs

Patient assistance programs are programs offered by some pharmaceutical manufacturers to help needy patients who require medication they cannot afford and do not have insurance coverage. Patient assistance programs require patients and their physicians to complete applications and submit them to the pharmaceutical manufacturer offering the program. Patients who qualify for patient assistance programs are often given cards issued by pharmacy benefit managers.

 workers' compensation an employer compensation program for employees accidentally injured on the job.

patient assistance programs manufacturer sponsored prescription drug programs for the needy.

ONLINE ADJUDICATION

In online adjudication, the technician uses the computer to determine the exact coverage for each prescription with the appropriate third party. The pharmacy computer communicates with the insurer's or pharmacy benefit manager's computer to determine this. Most community pharmacy computer programs are designed so the prescription label does not print until confirmation of payment is received from the insurer or PBM.

THE ONLINE PROCESS

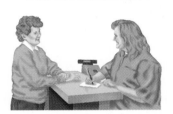

While non-patient information (NABP number, prices, co-pay, etc.) is provided by the computer system, it is generally the pharmacy technician's responsibility to obtain the patient, prescription, and billing information. In a typical community pharmacy, a patient presents a prescription (and often a prescription drug card) to a technician who must then obtain all of the patient and billing information required to enter the prescription and claim. If the patient has had prescriptions filled previously at the pharmacy, much of this information will be in the system already (though it is important for the technician to verify that this information is still correct).

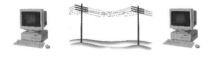

Once the necessary information is obtained, the pharmacy technician enters it into the pharmacy computer. Billing information for the prescription is then transmitted to a processing computer for the insurer or PBM. If all information has been entered correctly and is in agreement with data on-file with the insurer, the prescription claim is processed using online adjudication and an online response is received in less than one minute in the pharmacy. The claim-processing computer instantly determines the dollar amount of the drug benefit and the appropriate co-pay.

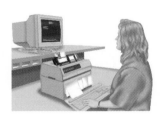

The pharmacy technician usually has an opportunity to review the data provided by the claim-processing computer before giving the OK for the prescription label and receipt to print in the pharmacy. The receipt indicates how much of the price of the prescription the patient must pay as determined by the insurer. The prescription can then be filled. The pharmacy technician should carefully review this adjudication information before proceeding to make sure the claim was processed properly. The pharmacy may be underpaid if the drug dispensed has a generic equivalent. The pharmacy technician should also look for claim processing messages such as drug or disease interaction alerts.

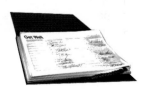

When prescriptions are billed online, pharmacies must keep records to verify prescriptions that prescriptions were actually dispensed. Insurers or PBMs require pharmacies to maintain hard copies of each prescription that must be readily retrievable upon request. Insurers or PBMs also require pharmacies to maintain signature logs for all claims submitted electronically that must be readily retrievable upon request.

ONLINE CLAIM INFORMATION

Although there are many different types of health care insurance, the information required for online processing of claims is remarkably similar. The following information is usually required for online claim processing:

➥ cardholder identification number (usually the social security number of the employee or a variation of this number)

➥ group number (a number assigned by the insurer to the employer of the cardholder)

➥ name of patient

➥ birthdate

➥ sex (M or F)

➥ relationship to cardholder (cardholder (C), spouse (S), dependent (D), other (O))

➥ date RX written

➥ date RX dispensed

➥ is this a new or refill prescription

➥ national drug code (NDC) of drug

➥ DAW indicator

➥ amount or quantity dispensed

➥ days supply

➥ identification number of prescribing physician

➥ identification of the pharmacy (pharmacies are often identified by the NABP Number which has been assigned by the National Association of Boards of Pharmacy or NABP)

➥ ingredient cost

➥ dispensing fee

➥ total price

➥ deductible or co-pay amount

➥ balance due

Dispense As Written (DAW)

When entering patient and prescription information, it is important to verify whether the patient's plan covers the brand name of a particular drug or if the patient is required to get generic drugs. When brand name drugs are dispensed, numbers corresponding to the reason for submitting the claim with brand name drugs are entered in a DAW (Dispense as Written) indicator field. Most health plan members have a choice between brand and generic drugs.

In some programs, if a patient receives a brand name drug when a generic is available, the patient must pay the difference between the cost of the brand and the cost of the generic. The following lists DAW indicators.

0 No DAW (No Dispense As Written)

1 DAW handwritten on the prescription by the prescriber

2 Patient requested brand

3 Pharmacist selected brand

4 Generic not in stock

5 Brand name dispensed but priced as generic

6 N/A

7 Substitution not allowed; brand mandated by law

8 Generic not available

Billing special medications such as compounded prescriptions requires somewhat different procedures. These procedures are different for each insurer or PBM. When billing compounded medications or special medications the pharmacy technician should refer to informational booklets provided to the pharmacy by the insurer or PBM or call the pharmacy help desk as listed on the prescription drug card.

REJECTED CLAIMS

In the online adjudication process, the insurer sometimes rejects the claim as submitted.

This occurs before the prescription is dispensed and provides an opportunity to resolve the problem before it becomes larger. There are various reasons for rejections, and most problems can be resolved by telephoning a representative of the insurer or discussing the rejection with the patient. Rejections are best resolved during normal business hours.

REJECTIONS

At right are common reasons for rejection of pharmacy third party claims and suggestions on how to correct such rejections.

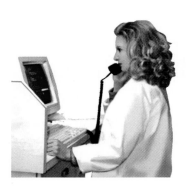

Resolving Rejections

When there is a question on coverage, the pharmacy technician can telephone the insurance plan's **pharmacy help desk** to determine if the patient is eligible for coverage. Pharmacy help desk personnel are often very helpful in resolving problems. If an employer has changed insurers, sometimes pharmacy help desk personnel can advise the pharmacy technician who the new insurer is. Many pharmacies maintain a list of phone numbers for insurers and their processors. If the prescription drug card is not available, the pharmacy technician can obtain the phone number of the insurer from this list.

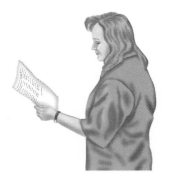

Handling Paper Claim Rejects

When paper claims are rejected by third parties, rejections often do not appear for several weeks after the claim was submitted. Rejections of paper claims are almost always accompanied by an explanation of the rejection and give details on what the technician can do to obtain successful payment of the claim. In many cases, the paper claim form was not completed correctly, information is missing, and the technician needs to only complete the missing information and resubmit the claim. Sometimes a telephone call must be made to the patient and/or the insurer to resolve the problem.

Dependent exceeds age limit as specified by plan

Many prescription drug plans have age limitations for children or dependents of the cardholder. Often, full-time college students are eligible for coverage as long as appropriate paperwork is on file with the insurer.

Invalid birthdate

The birthdate submitted by the pharmacy sometimes does not match the birthdate in the insurer's computer. To solve this problem, first double-check that you have the correct birthdate for the patient.

Invalid person code

The person code (e.g. 00,01,02,03) does not match the person code for the patient with the same sex and birthdate information in the insurer's computer.

Invalid sex

The sex (M or F) submitted by the pharmacy does not match the sex in the insurer's computer for the patient. To solve this problem, change the sex code (if M change to F) and resubmit the claim.

Prescriber is not a network provider

This type of reject is common to Medicaid programs and is sometimes seen with HMO programs. Simply stated, only prescriptions issued by network prescribers are covered by the insurer.

Unable to connect with insurer's computer

Sometimes, due to computer problems, an insurer's computer may be unavailable for claim processing. Under these circumstances, the technician must follow the guidelines of their employer.

Patient not covered (coverage terminated)

This can occur when a patient has a new insurance card, whether the new card is issued by the same insurer or a new one. If the insurer has not changed, perhaps billing numbers have changed (new cardholder identification number, group number, etc.).

Refill too soon

Most third party plans require that most of the medication has been taken before the plan will cover another dispensing of the same medication. Early refills should always be brought to the attention of the pharmacist. If the pharmacist thinks it is appropriate to dispense a refill early (for example, if a patient is going on vacation), the next step is to contact the insurer to determine if it will pay for an early refill.

Refills not covered

Many managed care health programs require mail order pharmacies to fill prescriptions for maintenance medications. Patients often are not aware of mail order requirements of their prescription drug coverage. Ideally the employer is responsible to explain mail order requirements if their employees are required to use mail order for maintenance medications. Sometimes, patients do not realize this restriction until prescription claims are rejected at their community pharmacy. In such cases, the pharmacy technician will have to contact the insurer to determine if emergency refills are covered at the community pharmacy.

NDC not covered

This type of rejection is common with state Medicaid programs and managed care programs with closed formularies. Ideally, the patient is aware that the insurer has a limited formulary for prescription drug coverage. However, often patients are not aware of how this works. The pharmacy technician can determine by calling the pharmacy help desk of the insurer the requirements of the patient's plan. Sometimes, the insurer will consider prior authorization to cover medications that are not on the formulary. Sometimes, the insurer will not cover the prescribed medication and a pharmacist may determine what should be done next.

OTHER ISSUES

PAPER CLAIMS

Processing paper claims usually involves the pharmacy and the patient completing a form that has been issued by the insurer. Most insurers require completion of a form that they provide. A **universal claim form (UCF)** is a standardized form accepted by many insurers. Before online claim submission, most pharmacy third party claims were submitted on universal claim forms. Instructions for completing paper claims (insurer provided forms as well as universal claim forms) are printed on the claim forms so that anyone can complete the forms as long as they have access to the required information. Usually there is a requirement for signature by the patient and the pharmacist or health care provider. Incomplete forms or forms that have not been completed following directions printed on the forms are returned to the pharmacy for correction before the insurer will consider paying the claim. Generally, the same type of information required for online claims is also required for paper claim processing.

IN-HOUSE BILLING PROCEDURES

Pharmacy billing is not limited to billing insurers. Some pharmacies have in-house billing procedures. For example, the finances of an elderly or disabled patient may be handled by a family member or legal representative who does not live with the patient. In these cases, a monthly bill is mailed to the family member or legal representative, who then pays the pharmacy. Most pharmacies do not have in-house billing. When a pharmacy does do in-house billing, the pharmacy technician must carefully follow the policies and procedures of the employer.

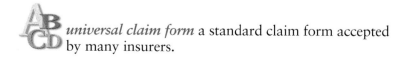 *universal claim form* a standard claim form accepted by many insurers.

PBM AUDITS

Pharmacy benefit managers are responsible to their clients to pay only for legitimate claims. PBMs audit pharmacies to confirm billing practices are proper. Reports that 3% of prescription claims submitted to third party plans are fake give PBMs good reason to audit pharmacies. Also, PBMs sometimes overpay on certain claims, not due to pharmacy fraud but due to technological flaws. About 67 NDCs have package sizes that cannot be expressed by whole numbers. This causes potential discrepancies in how the pharmacy computer recognizes the package size and how the PBM or insurer computer recognizes the package size (for example a 7.5ml bottle of eye drops may be considered as 8ml in the pharmacy computer and 7ml in the insurer's or PBM's computer).

When PBM auditors visit pharmacies they usually give advance notice. Pharmacy technicians can prepare for PBM audits by:

➡ having good filing systems and record keeping systems.
➡ maintaining good filing for patient signature logs.
➡ efficiently filing hard copies of prescriptions.
➡ making sure DAW indicators are properly done.
➡ making sure there are hard copies that can be easily found for all prescriptions filled.

Often it is a good idea to have a highly trained pharmacy technician work with the auditor to locate all items the auditor is looking for.

DISEASE MANAGEMENT SERVICES

Disease management services are evolving as a component of pharmaceutical care. PBMs are selling disease management services to employers and health plans. Conditions most often targeted for disease management include: diabetes, hypertension, asthma, arthritis, and gastroesophageal reflux disease/ulcer. Electronic and paper billing systems can be used for billing disease management services.

REVIEW

KEY CONCEPTS

✔ Third party programs are simply another party besides the patient or the pharmacy that pays for some or all of the cost of medication: essentially, an insurer.

✔ A pharmacy benefit manager (PBM) is a company that administers drug benefit programs for insurance companies, HMOs, and self-insured employers.

✔ Most prescription claims are now filed electronically by online claim submission and online adjudication of claims.

✔ Co-insurance is essentially an agreement between the insurer and the insured to share costs. One aspect of it is the requirement for patients to co-pay a potion of the cost of prescriptions.

✔ The amount paid by insurers for prescriptions is not equal to the retail price normally charged, but is determined by a formula described in a contract between the insurer and the pharmacy.

✔ Prescription drug benefit cards contain necessary billing information for pharmacies, including the patient's identification number, group number, and co-pay amount.

✔ HMOs usually will not cover expenses incurred outside their participating network and often require generic substitution.

✔ POSs often partially reimburse expenses incurred outside of their network and usually require generic substitution.

✔ PPOs usually require generic substitution.

✔ Workers' compensation is compensation for employees accidentally injured on-the-job.

✔ Medicare covers people over the age of 65, disabled people under the age of 65 and people with kidney failure.

✔ Medicaid is a federal-state program for the needy.

✔ In online adjudication, the technician uses the computer to determine the exact coverage for each prescription with the appropriate third party.

✔ When brand name drugs are dispensed, numbers corresponding to the reason for submitting the claim with brand name drugs are entered in a DAW (Dispense as Written) indicator field in the prescription system.

✔ Many prescription drug plans have age limitations for children or dependents of the cardholder.

✔ Most third party plans require that most of the medication has been taken before the plan will cover a refill of the same medication.

✔ Many managed care health programs require mail order pharmacies to fill prescriptions for maintenance medications.

✔ When a claim is rejected, the pharmacy technician can telephone the insurance plan's pharmacy help desk to determine if the patient is eligible for coverage.

✔ Pharmacy benefits managers audit pharmacies to confirm that their billing practices are proper.

SELF TEST

co-insurance

co-pay

maximum allowable cost (MAC)

Medicaid

Medicare

online adjudication

pharmacy benefits

Qualified Medicare Beneficiaries

U&C or UCR

universal claim form

companies that administer drug benefit programs

the resolution of prescription coverage through the communication of the pharmacy computer with the third party computer.

a standard paper claim form accepted by many insurers.

the portion of the price of medication that the patient is required to pay.

the maximum price per tablet (or other dispensing unit) an insurer or PBM will pay for a given product.

the maximum amount of payment for a given prescription, determined by the insurer to be a usual and customary (and reasonable) price.

a federal program providing health care to people with certain disabilities over age 65.

a federal-state program, administered by the states, providing health care for the needy.

Medicare patients who may at times qualify for prescription drug coverage through a state administered program.

a cost-sharing agreement between the insurer and the insured.

---

1. Which of the following information is generally not required in online claim processing?
   a. birth date
   b. weight
   c. sex
   d. group number

2. Which of these is not a reason for disallowing a refill?
   a. too early
   b. C-II drug
   c. DAW
   d. no refills prescribed

3. Medicaid
   a. is a federal/state program for the needy.
   b. is a federal program for people over 65.
   c. offers a completely open formulary.
   d. none of the above.

4. Pharmacies receive payment from third parties equal to
   a. the retail price of the drug
   b. the manufacturer's cost.
   c. a wholesaler's price.
   d. none of the above.

COMMUNITY PHARMACY

Community or retail pharmacy practice is the practice of providing prescription services to the public.

In addition to prescription drugs, community pharmacies sell over-the-counter medications as well as other health and beauty products. A pharmacy may be owned independently or by a chain. Chains may specialize in pharmacy or be part of a broader mass merchandise or food store business.

One of the key characteristics of community pharmacy is the close interaction with patients.

The patient is a customer with alternatives as to where they can bring their business. So good customer service is a requirement, and for this, good interpersonal skills are needed.

Almost two thirds of all prescription drugs in the U.S. are dispensed by community pharmacies.

As a result, more pharmacists and technicians are employed in community pharmacy than any other area. An additional factor in employment is that the role of the community pharmacist in counseling and educating patients has been steadily increasing. This in turn has increased the role of the pharmacy technician in assisting pharmacists to dispense prescriptions. As a result, community pharmacy practice provides great opportunity for pharmacy technicians to find employment and serve the community.

Types of Community Pharmacies

There are about 60,000 community pharmacies in the United States which provide convenient access to medications and medication information. They can be found in a variety of business settings:

➠ **Independent Pharmacies**
   Individually owned local pharmacies.

➠ **Chain Pharmacies**
   Regional or national pharmacy chains such as CVS and Eckerd.

➠ **Mass Merchandiser Pharmacies**
   Regional or national mass merchandise chains such as Walmart, KMart, and Costco that sell various mass merchandise and have in-store pharmacies.

➠ **Food Store Pharmacies**
   Regional or national food store chains such as A&P, Giant Eagle, and Kroger's that have in-store pharmacies.

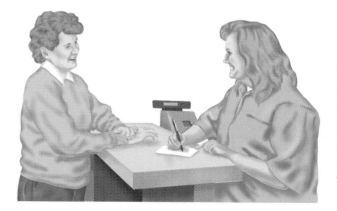

Customer Service

In contrast to institutional and other environments, technicians in the community pharmacy constantly interact with patients as customers. As a result, customer service is a major area of importance in the community pharmacy and technicians employed there must have strong interpersonal skills.

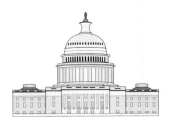

OBRA '90 and Counseling

In the United States, the 1990 Omnibus Budget and Reconciliation Act (OBRA) required community pharmacists to offer counseling to Medicaid patients regarding medications, effectively mandating what was already common practice. Specifically, it required pharmacists to offer counseling and instruction in these areas:

➡ the name and description of the medication, including its generic name;

➡ dosage form, dosage, route of administration, and duration of administration;

➡ special directions and precautions for preparation, administration and use by the patient;

➡ common severe side affects or interactions and therapeutic contraindications, how to avoid them, and what to do if they occur;

➡ techniques for patients to monitor their drug therapy;

➡ proper storage of the medication;

➡ what to do if a dose is missed;

➡ refill information.

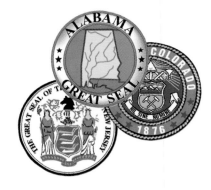

State Regulations

Community pharmacies are most closely regulated at the state level. For example, many states have mandated OBRA '90 counseling requirements for all patients, not just those on Medicaid. States also regulate such things as:

➡ the ratio of pharmacists to technicians (generally one pharmacist for no more than two technicians);

➡ scope of technician practice;

➡ record keeping;

➡ equipment;

➡ work areas.

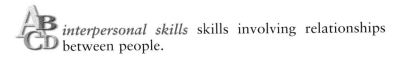

interpersonal skills skills involving relationships between people.

ORGANIZATION

Prescription processing areas among community pharmacies may be organized differently, but they generally contain the same elements.
A number of space and equipment requirements are dictated by State regulations.

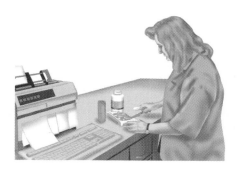

Prescription Counter

The prescription area of a pharmacy must have a counter area on which to prepare prescriptions. This counter should be kept orderly at all times.

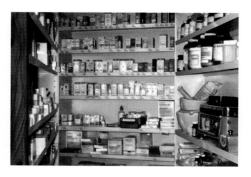

Storage

There must be adequate shelving, cabinets, or drawers for storage of medications. It is common to see several bays with shelving to hold bottles of medications. The medications may be arranged on the shelves alphabetically according to generic name or they may be arranged according to brand, or trade name.

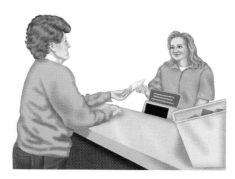

Transaction Windows

Pharmacies often have counter areas (sometimes separate) designated for taking prescriptions and for delivering them to patients.

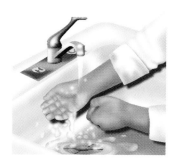

Sink

There must be an easily accessible sink that also must be kept clean at all times.

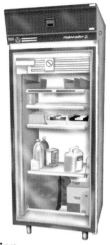

Refrigeration

There must also be a refrigerator in which to store medication that requires storage in temperatures between 2 and 8 degrees Celsius. The refrigerator must be designated for drugs only. No food products are allowed to be stored in the same refrigerator.

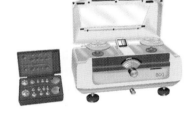

Equipment

Equipment that must be available for use in the pharmacy includes a prescription balance, a set of metric weights, a glass mortar and pestle, glass funnels, stirring rods, graduates for measuring liquids, spatulas, counting trays and or counting devices, ointment board or parchment paper for compounding creams, ointments, etc., prescription labels, and auxiliary or precautionary labels.

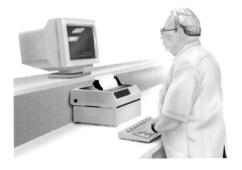

Computer System

There is an area for the computer monitor, keyboard, and printer.

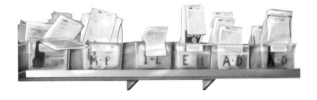

Prescription Bins or Shelves

Completed prescriptions that are not being immediately picked up are generally placed in bins or shelves alphabetized by customer.

CUSTOMER SERVICE

Customer satisfaction is the goal of customer service.

Good customer service requires presenting yourself to customers in a calm, courteous, and professional manner. It requires listening to and understanding customer requests for service and fulfilling those requests accurately or explaining to the customer's satisfaction why the request cannot be serviced.

The health of customers is a significant factor in their experience of community pharmacy service.

Customers may often feel sick or irritable and need their medication quickly. Having to wait in a line may be physically difficult or emotionally upsetting. The cost of the medication may be an additional worry. Consequently, though customer service is important in any type of retail store, it is particularly important in the community pharmacy setting.

It is important to respond to customers in a positive way at all times.

In any situation where a customer is angry, frustrated, or otherwise dissatisfied, it is especially important to give a positive response. This can be done in part by listening intently and making eye contact with the customer. Restating what the customer has said is also important, since it demonstrates that you have listened to their complaint. Use positive, not negative terms to tell the customer what you can do, not what you can't do to solve their problem.

Involve the pharmacist in all difficult situations.

If after spending some time with the customer, you have been unable to resolve the problem, you should inform the pharmacist. This should be done immediately for serious complaints regarding problems with prescriptions. Remember that employees that possess well developed interpersonal skills are good for business and will be appreciated by employers.

AT THE COUNTER

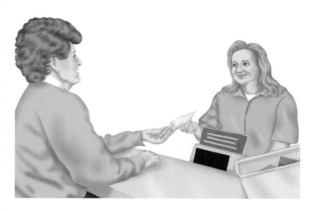

Since pharmacy technicians are generally responsible for handling the pharmacy counter, they have direct contact with customers and play a key role in assisting customers with their needs.

This involves taking in new and refill prescriptions, but also includes directing customers to requested over-the-counter products or answering other questions that do not require the pharmacist's judgment. The technician should be familiar with the layout of the store and must know where various types of products are located so that they may help customers find products quickly.

 A pharmacy technician must know when to refer a customer to the pharmacist. It is a good idea to discuss such situations with the pharmacist regularly.

ON THE TELEPHONE

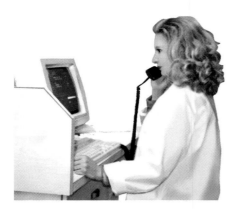

A significant part of the pharmacy technician's responsibilities includes answering the telephone. Calls must be answered in a pleasant and courteous manner, following a standard format that should be indicated by the store manager or pharmacist. Generally, this begins with stating the name of the pharmacy and your name. An example:

"Main Street Pharmacy, Joan speaking, may I help you?"

Many calls will concern the price or stock availability of prescription and over-the-counter products. Some will be to place refill requests. In that case, the same process is followed as when taking refill requests at the counter (see pp.263), except that the technician should also ask the patient when they plan to pick up the prescription.

Some calls will require the pharmacist's judgment. These should be directed immediately to the pharmacist. This applies to questions regarding medication or general health related questions. When patients raise such questions, politely ask them to hold on the line while you get the pharmacist.

INTERPERSONAL TECHNIQUES

At the Counter

Techniques for interacting with customers at the counter include:

➡ listening carefully;

➡ making eye contact;

➡ repeating what the customer has said;

➡ using positive rather than negative language to describe what you can do.

On the Phone

Techniques for interacting with customers on the telephone include:

➡ using a pleasant and courteous manner;

➡ stating the name of the pharmacy and your name;

➡ following the standard procedure indicated for your pharmacy;

➡ referring all calls that require a pharmacist's judgment to the pharmacist.

 Any time you are uncertain of whether a question requires the pharmacist's judgment, refer the question to the pharmacist.

PROCESSING PRESCRIPTIONS

A major responsibility of the pharmacy technician is to process new and refill prescriptions.

This is done using the pharmacy's computerized prescription system. Different pharmacies will use different systems. The pharmacist or another pharmacy technician will usually provide training on the system that is used. Learning to process prescriptions efficiently and accurately on the system is essential and will take some time and commitment.

PATIENT INFORMATION

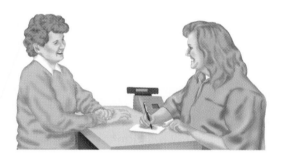

When taking in a new prescription, always ask whether the patient has ever had prescriptions filled at the pharmacy in the past. If the patient had not been to the pharmacy in the past, be sure to get the following information which will be needed for the patient profile information that must be entered into the computer:

- **full name of the patient**
- **address**
- **telephone number**
- **date of birth**
- **any allergies to medication.**

If a patient requests a prescription refill, **be sure to get the patient's name and the prescription number** which appears on the prescription bottle. If the prescription number is unavailable, ask for the name of the medication. Whether the patient is requesting a new or refill prescription, ask if they would like to wait or if they prefer to pick up the prescription later.

PRESCRIPTION INFORMATION

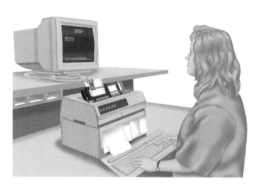

When entering a new prescription into the pharmacy prescription system, the pharmacy technician needs to enter the following information into the appropriate fields on the computer's dispensing screen:

- **correct drug and strength**
- **correct physician's name** (and physician's **DEA number** for prescriptions for controlled substances or for prescriptions being billed to a third party that requires it)
- **directions for use** (the signa)
- **quantity** (i.e. the number of tablets or the metric quantity if dispensing a liquid, cream, inhaler, etc.)
- **number of authorized refills**
- **DAW code** which indicates that a brand name or a generic product is being dispensed.
- **initials of the dispensing pharmacist**

ONLINE BILLING

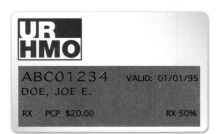

A major feature of computerized prescription systems is online billing of a prescription to a patient's insurance company or other third party. Since the majority of patients today have an insurance plan or third party coverage that will pay for the cost of their prescriptions, the technician must be familiar with all of the private and state administered prescription plans that are accepted by the pharmacy. So entering a prescription also involves entering a code identifying the plan that will be billed. This generally includes:

➥ a **group number**, which identifies the patient's employer;

➥ a **patient or policy identification number**, which is usually, but not always, the patient's social security number;

➥ a **patient code**, which indicates the specific patient covered under the plan (the primary card holder is usually 01, spouse is 02, and so on).

Once all third party billing information is entered, the technician can proceed with online billing. The third party will respond within a few moments by either stating that the claim has been paid or otherwise has been rejected. If a co-payment by the patient is required, the amount is indicated. If a rejection occurs, there will be a general message regarding why the claim has been rejected. If it is due to incorrect number entry, it can be easily corrected. Sometimes however, a call to the third party will be necessary to get the claim paid.

REFILLS

In the case of entering refill prescriptions, most pharmacy computer programs allow looking up a refill either by prescription number or through screening the patient profile for the medication. When processing a refill prescription, be sure to check that there are refills available. Most systems will indicate when no refills are available. If there are no refills, alert the pharmacist so that he or she can call the patient's physician for a new prescription. Prescriptions can be called in by a physician over the phone, but these calls should be handled by the pharmacist.

Note that when refilling prescriptions, be sure it is not too early to refill the medication. If it is more than a week early, many third parties will reject the claim. Also, refills for controlled medications should not be refilled early since they have the potential for abuse. In the case of a patient requesting an early refill of a controlled substance, involve the pharmacist right away.

SAFETY

Another important aspect of entering new and refill prescriptions has to do with screening for safety of prescription medication. Many computer software systems will flag drug interactions and allergy conflicts. When these flags occur, always alert the pharmacist so that he or she can evaluate the significance of the flag. The pharmacist may tell the pharmacy technician this is okay to proceed or will otherwise stop the process and may need to make a call to the patient's physician.

PREPARING THE PRESCRIPTION

The prescription system will print a prescription label based on the patient and prescription information that has been entered into it. Once the label is generated, it is time to prepare the prescription. This begins with locating the medication and its container.

MEASURING

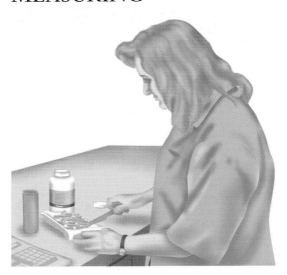

If it is a tablet or capsule, find the stock bottle on the shelf and count the correct number of pills using a **counting tray**. A counting tray is a tray that allows a pharmacist or pharmacy technician to count pills from the tray into a side container-like area. This special tray allows for the pills remaining on the tray to be easily slid back into the stock bottle. The pills that will be dispensed will slide easily into a prescription vial.

Other counting devices also exist that are intended for larger volume use. A "Kirby Lester" machine automatically counts pills as they are dropped into it. Other devices automatically fill cells or compartments with tablets or capsules and have a control panel that allows the pharmacist or technician to order a given number of a certain medication.

When necessary, solutions are measured using a graduate, and ointments are weighed using a balance.

CONTAINERS

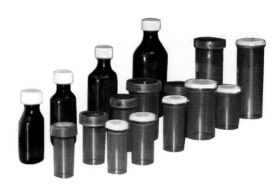

There are various size containers for tablets and capsules from which to choose an appropriate one. If preparing a liquid medication, select the appropriate size bottle and pour the correct volume of liquid into the bottle. For creams and ointments, find a tube of the correct metric quantity. If the cream or ointment is not pre-packaged in the appropriate size tube or perhaps was compounded at the pharmacy, it will be necessary to transfer the product with a spatula to an ointment jar of the correct size. It may be necessary to use a balance to weigh out the correct amount.

SAFETY CAPS

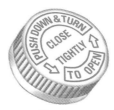

All dispensed prescription vials and bottles must have a safety cap or child resistant cap, *unless the patient requests an easy-open or non-child resistant cap.* Most computer software programs have a field in which to record the patient's preference regarding this. It is important to pay attention to which cap is indicated as some elderly or arthritic patients have extreme difficulty opening child-resistant caps.

LABELS

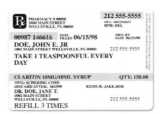

Once the desired pills or other product is put in an appropriate container, the finished prescription label is placed on the product along with any **auxiliary labels** that may be necessary. These labels identify important usage information, including specific warnings or alerts on:

➡ administration
➡ proper storage
➡ possible side effects
➡ potential food and drug interactions

Examples include "take with food", "may cause drowsiness", and others shown at right. Some computer systems automatically identify which auxiliary labels are needed. If this is not the case, ask the pharmacist which labels should be applied.

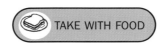
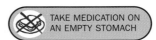
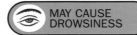
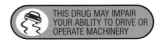
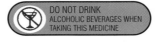
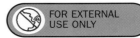
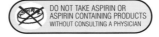
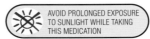

sample auxiliary labels

FINAL CHECK BY THE PHARMACIST

As a final step of the preparation process, organize the final product and all paperwork, including the original prescription, for the pharmacist's final check. Also, leave stock bottles, or other packaging next to the final product so the pharmacist can see that the correct product was used. After the pharmacist has checked the prescription, it is a responsibility of the pharmacy technician to return any products used to their proper place on the shelf, cabinet, or drawer.

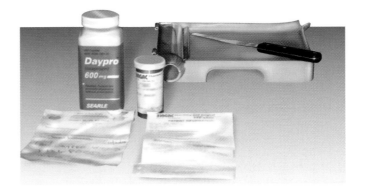

counting tray a tray designed for counting pills.
auxiliary labels labels regarding specific warnings, foods or medications to avoid, potential side effects, and so on.

CUSTOMER PICK-UP

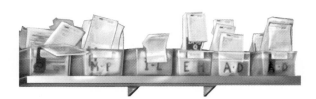

alphabetized prescription bins

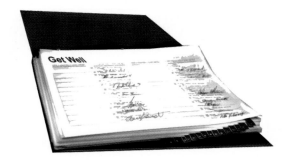

a signature log

Picking Up the Prescription

When the customer is picking up a prescription, locate the prescription, which will usually be filed alphabetically by the last name of the patient either in bins or another storage area. For confidentiality reasons, when a prescription is located for a family member, do not ask for instance, "Would you also like to pick up your daughter's prescription while you're here?" Though this may seem helpful, it is a breach of confidentiality. Find only the prescription that was requested.

Signature Logs

Most community pharmacies will have customers sign a log which records that the prescription was picked-up. Signatures are required for Medicaid and most third party insurer or HMO prescriptions, along with Schedule V controlled substances, poisons, and certain other prescriptions (depending upon the state).

The log may serve a dual purpose of also recording that patient medication counselling was offered. The usual process is to ask the patient if they would like the pharmacist to speak with them regarding their prescription. The patient is then asked to sign that they have either accepted the offer of medication counselling, or that they have declined the offer.

Always be sensitive to the confidential nature of prescription information. While customers may wish to hear prescription information themselves, they may not want others to.

signature log a book in which patients sign for the prescriptions they receive, for legal and insurance purposes.

USING A CASH REGISTER

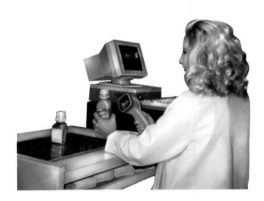

scanning a price

It is often a responsibility of the pharmacy technician to ring up prescriptions and over the counter products into the register and accept payment for them. Cash registers are integrated into the pharmacy's computerized system so prices for products can be automatically entered by using bar code scanners. Scanners can be hand-held or built into the counter. The scanner beam is targeted at the bar code and identifies the product for the register. The product's price (or discounted price if there is a prescription plan discount) is automatically entered into the register. If a mistake is made between the pricing on the product or shelf and the amount in the system, changes can be made manually, though each system is different, and technicians need to know and follow the procedures used at their pharmacy.

Operating a cash register also requires handling payments properly. When cash payment is made, it is it is important to count the payment within the customer's line of sight and to confirm the amount orally to the customer. This will avoid misunderstandings over what the customer thought they gave you. If change is necessary, the amount should be counted out loud and placed into the customer's hand. An example of such a transaction would be:

> A twenty dollar bill is given as payment for a bill of $14.50.

> ➥ The bill should be held or placed within the customer's line of sight and the amount confirmed as "That's Twenty dollars."

> ➥ The amount is then entered into the register and a receipt is produced.

> ➥ The change is counted out as it is placed into the customer's hand, i.e. "fifty cents makes fifteen dollars, and five dollars makes twenty dollars".

> ➥ After the customer has received their change and is given the receipt, the twenty dollar bill is placed into the register drawer.

Following this general procedure will avoid disputes, either out of confusion or intent to deceive, over whether a larger bill was tendered or the correct change given.

The pharmacy technician must also be able to handle checks and credit cards appropriately. It is very important to follow the store policy and procedure regarding handling of these transactions. Be sure to check the identification of the customer as instructed by the store manager or pharmacist

OTHER DUTIES

The pharmacy technician should know the names and locations of the various over-the-counter products carried in the pharmacy. When asked, the technician should be able to direct customers to an OTC product. Some of the many OTC products that are available will include cough and cold preparations, laxatives and antidiarrheals, medications for the treatment of indigestion, analgesics, vitamins, first aid supplies, dental and denture care products, and infant care products.

The technician should not recommend OTC products to pharmacy customers, however.

Though OTC products may be bought freely by customers, they are not without risks. Incorrect dosages and drug-drug interactions with OTC products can produce significant adverse effects. For example, many cough and cold preparations contain ingredients that may increase blood pressure and worsen a diabetic condition. Therefore, the technician should *refer patients asking about OTC products to the pharmacist.* As always, the technician must involve the pharmacist whenever judgement is needed.

Ordering stock is another responsibility of the pharmacy technician.

As stock diminishes, it is important to reorder. The technician must know which products are used more frequently than others and reorder in appropriate quantities. For instance, popular anti-hypertensive medication should be kept well stocked, while medications that are not as popular do not need to be available in large quantities.

The pharmacy technician is also generally responsible for keeping the pharmacy clean, neat, and in proper working order.

Periodically, the counting trays, and the pharmacy counter should be wiped with alcohol. Pharmacy supplies, such as prescription bags, prescription vials and bottles, prescription labels and computer paper should be available at all times and thus, must be stocked regularly. The stock bottles of drugs on the shelves should periodically be readjusted so that they are neatly arranged with all labels facing front. At least monthly, the pharmacy technician should check all bottles for outdated expiration dates as it is unlawful to dispense outdated medications. Expired drugs must be sent back to the wholesaler or be destroyed.

RETAIL CONCEPTS

Community pharmacies do not just dispense prescriptions. They are **retail businesses** that sell over-the-counter medications and various other products. Retail businesses resell consumer ready products that they have purchased from wholesalers or manufacturers. To make a profit, the retailer sells the products at a **mark-up** from their purchase price. The mark-up is the amount of the retailer's sale price minus their purchase price. For example, if an over-the-counter medication is purchased at $5.00 a package, and the mark-up is 50%, the retailer's price to the consumer will be: $5.00 plus a $2.50 markup ($5.00 times 50%), or $7.50.

The mark-up represents the portion of sales that the retailer will clear after paying suppliers. This is what pays for the costs of doing business (building, equipment, salaries, etc.) and generates profits. So calculating the mark-up is very important to retailers. It is generally calculated by the pharmacy computer system and based on business costs and profit goals. They will differ by pharmacy and can differ by product. That is, some product lines may have lower or higher mark-ups than the standard products in the pharmacy. Each price that the technician stickers on a product includes the cost of the product and its mark-up.

Shelf Stickers

OTC products have shelf-stickers that can be scanned for inventory identification. They also indicate **unit price** information for consumers. A unit price is the price of a unit of medication (such as an ounce of a liquid cold remedy), rather than the price of the entire package. Unit prices protect the consumer from packaging and pricing that suggests that more is contained in the item than actually is.

STOCK DUTIES

Ordering

Ordering stock in most pharmacies is done by transmitting the order to a drug wholesaler via a telephone line. Every product has a stock number which is entered, either into a computer with a modem or into a device that connects to a phone line and transmits the order to the drug wholesaler.

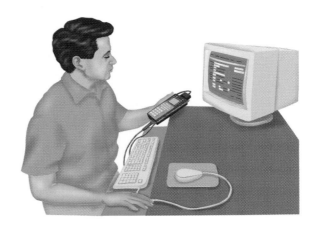

Receiving

When an order from a drug wholesaler is received, it is generally the pharmacy technician's responsibility to unpack the order and check that all items on the invoice have, in fact been received. Items must be checked to make sure the following are as ordered:

- ✔ **drug product**
- ✔ **strength**
- ✔ **packaging**
- ✔ **quantity**

In addition items must be inspected for:

- ✔ **damage**
- ✔ **expiration dates**

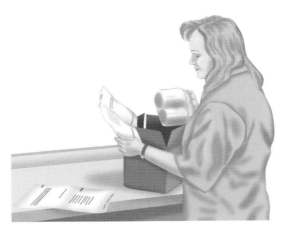

Stickering

Products are often stickered with pricing information and reorder numbers for each item. These stickers may be applied with a stickering gun or by hand. They are placed on each item. Once this process is complete, the items will need to be put on the shelves in their proper places. The invoices will also need to be filed for reference purposes.

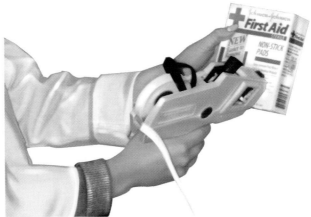

℞ Schedule II controlled substances must be checked and signed for by the pharmacist.

REVIEW

KEY CONCEPTS

- ✔ In addition to prescription drugs, community pharmacies sell over-the-counter medications as well as other health and beauty products.
- ✔ Almost two thirds of all prescription drugs in the U.S. are dispensed by community pharmacies.
- ✔ The role of the community pharmacist in counseling and educating patients has been steadily increasing.
- ✔ Customer service is a major area of importance in the community pharmacy, since technicians constantly interact with patients as customers.
- ✔ In the United States, the 1990 Omnibus Budget and Reconciliation Act (OBRA) required community pharmacists to offer counseling to Medicaid patients regarding medications. Many states have expanded this requirement to apply to all customers.
- ✔ Technicians should always respond to customers in a positive and courteous way.
- ✔ Telephone calls must be answered in a pleasant and courteous manner, following a standard format that should be indicated by the store manager or pharmacist.
- ✔ When processing a refill prescription, it is necessary to check that there are refills available.
- ✔ In the case of a patient requesting an early refill of a controlled substance, involve the pharmacist right away.
- ✔ Whenever the prescription system flags drug interactions and allergy conflicts, alert the pharmacist so that he or she can evaluate the significance of the flag.
- ✔ All dispensed prescription vials and bottles must have a safety cap or child resistant cap, unless the patient requests an easy-open or non-child resistant cap.
- ✔ Auxiliary labels identify important usage information, including specific warnings or alerts on: administration, proper storage, possible side effects, and potential food and drug interactions.
- ✔ As a final step of the preparation process, the final product and all paperwork, including the original prescription, is organized for the pharmacist's final check.
- ✔ Customer signatures in a log are required for Medicaid and most third party insurer or HMO prescriptions, along with Schedule V controlled substances, poisons, and certain other prescriptions (depending upon the state).
- ✔ Mark-up is the amount of the retailer's sale price minus their purchase price.
- ✔ OTC products may be bought freely by customers, but they are not without risks, and the technician should not recommend them to pharmacy customers.
- ✔ Ordering stock is often a responsibility of the pharmacy technician.
- ✔ The pharmacy technician is generally responsible for keeping the pharmacy clean, neat, and in proper working order.

SELF TEST

MATCH THE TERMS.   *answers can be checked in the glossary*

auxiliary labels

counting tray

interpersonal skills

mark-up

safety cap

shelf-stickers

signature log

transaction windows

unit price

skills involving relationships between people.

counter areas designated for taking prescriptions and for delivering them to patients.

a child resistant cap

the price of a unit of medication (such as an ounce of a liquid cold remedy).

a tray designed for counting pills.

specific warnings that are placed on filled prescriptions.

a book in which patients sign for the prescriptions they receive, for legal and insurance purposes.

the amount of the retailer's sale price minus their purchase price.

stickers with bar codes that can be scanned for inventory identification.

CHOOSE THE BEST ANSWER.   *answers are in the back of the book*

1. When reviewing a prescription for a C-II substance, which of these is not required:
   a. NDC number
   b. patient street address
   c. DEA number
   d. DAW information

2. When the prescription system warns of a potential interaction:
   a. tell the patient
   b. get the correct auxiliary label
   c. include it on the sig
   d. inform the pharmacist

3. The pharmacist always checks the prescription
   a. after it is filled by the technician.
   b. when the patient signs the log.
   c. after it is rung on the cash register.
   d. as it is given to the patient.

4. The difference between the price the customer pays and the price the pharmacy pays for a product is called
   a. profit.
   b. overhead.
   c. margin.
   d. mark-up.

HOSPITAL PHARMACY

Though they may be organized differently, hospitals generally contain the same elements.

Patient rooms are divided into groups called nursing units or patient care units. Patients with similar problems are often located on the same unit. This allows for specialized nursing care based on similar issues, problems, or disease states. An example of this would be an area for patients who are in labor or about to deliver a baby (OB Unit), or an intensive care unit specifically for cardiology patients (CCU). Intensive care units are for patients who are more severely ill and require close monitoring and nursing attention.

The work station for medical personnel on a nursing unit is called the nurses' station.

In this area, various items required for care of the patients on the unit will be stored, including patient medications.

There are several other areas of the hospital, called ancillary areas, that also provide patient care.

These areas use certain medications and are serviced by the pharmacy department. Each hospital has different ancillary areas, but some common ones that may be seen are: radiology, the cardiac catheterization lab, and the emergency room.

Every hospital has a center responsible for distributing supplies to all areas of the facility.

This is often referred to as central supply or materials management. This department supplies the pharmacy with several items required for daily operations including paper towels, soap, needles, syringes, etc. Central supply does not, however, handle storage or delivery of any medications.

THE HEALTH CARE TEAM

It takes a team of many different types of health care professionals to meet the needs of patients, and individual patients generally receive care from a variety of these professionals. Most health care personnel are identified by abbreviations that indicate their discipline. Each individual profession plays a part on the multidisciplinary healthcare team. Their common objective is to care for patients and assist in their recovery.

Around the Clock Care

Since hospitals are open 24 hours a day, 7 days a week, there are a lot of shifts that must be covered. This allows for a great deal of variability in scheduling. Standard eight hour shifts in the hospital are: 7am to 3:30pm; 3:00pm to 11:30pm; and 11:00pm to 7:00am. Other combinations of work times are possible using four, six, and twelve hour shifts. At smaller hospitals, the pharmacy may not be open 24 hours a day. In these situations, a pharmacist can be contacted by phone in the case of any pharmacy or medicine related questions. The nurse manager or other authorized personnel may have access to pharmacy areas during these times for emergency medication needs. State laws mandate what is acceptable in these situations.

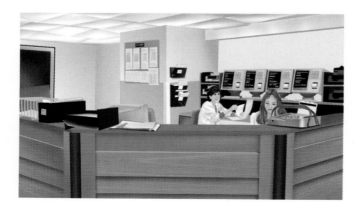

The nurses' station is a central storage and communication center for patient care in the hospital.

Medical Staff

M.D., Medical Doctor

A physician examines patients, orders and interprets lab tests, diagnoses illnesses, and prescribes and administers treatments for people suffering from injury or disease. A M.D. may be a general or a specialty doctor.

P.A., Physician's Assistant

A specially trained medical care provider who coordinates care for patients under the close supervision of a medical doctor. They are allowed to prescribe certain medications.

Therapy and Other Staff

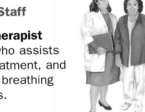

R.T., Respiratory Therapist

A trained individual who assists in the evaluation, treatment, and care of patients with breathing problems or illnesses.

P.T., Physical Therapist

A healthcare worker providing services that help restore function, improve mobility, relieve pain, and prevent or limit permanent physical disabilities of patients .

O.T., Occupational Therapist

A therapist who works with patients who have conditions that are mentally, physically, developmentally, or emotionally disabling, and helps them to develop, recover, or maintain daily living and work skills.

M.S.W., Master's of Social Work

A healthcare provider who is concerned with patient social factors such as child protection, ability to pay for medications, and coping capacities of patients and their families.

R.D., Registered Dietitian

A dietitian helps prevent and treat illnesses by assessing and scientifically evaluating patients' nutritional needs and recommending appropriate modifications.

Nursing

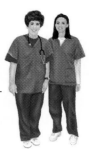

N.P., Nurse Practitioner

A registered nurse with additional training who can provide basic primary health care. The N.P. may work closely with doctors and can prescribe various medications in most states.

R.N., Registered Nurse

A nurse who provides bedside care, assists physicians in various procedures, and administers medical regimens to patients.

L.P.N., Licensed Practical Nurse

A nurse who provides basic bedside care under the supervision of an R.N. The LPN is not allowed to perform all functions of an R.N. and may not administer medication to patients.

Pharmacy

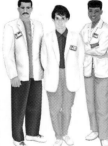

Pharm.D., Doctor of Pharmacy

A registered pharmacist with advanced training in providing pharmaceutical care.

R.Ph., Registered Pharmacist

A pharmacist who is licensed to work by the state. Duties include reviewing patient drug regimens for appropriateness, dispensing medications, and advising the medical staff on the selection of drugs.

Pharmacy Technician

Pharmacy technicians in the hospital work under the direct supervision of a pharmacist and play a vital role in the preparation, storage, and delivery of medications to patients. Technicians assist the pharmacist but are often given specific duties, such as "inventory technician." Training requirements may vary by state and hospital, but hospitals are increasingly seeking technicians that have already received certification (CPhT).

UNIT DOSE SYSTEM

Oral medications are commonly provided to the nursing unit in medication carts containing 24 hour dosages for specific patients.

These carts have an individual drawer or tray for each patient on the nursing unit. Medications in the cart are packaged in individual containers holding the amount of drug required for one dose. This system is referred to as **unit dose** medication packaging. By preparing medication this way, nurses are not required to select medication from large bulk bottles, decreasing the chance of making an error.

Each individual drawer in a medication cart is filled daily to meet patient medication needs.

Technicians play a large role in this type of dispensing by either manually filling the carts or by operating equipment designed for that function. Computer generated drug profiles are prepared daily for each patient, and the appropriate amount of medications for the 24 hour period are placed manually or mechanically onto each patient's tray. The trays are labeled with the patient's name and room number. The filled carts are checked by the supervising pharmacist before being delivered to the nursing units.

At various times throughout the day adjustments in the patient trays are necessary to account for changes in medication orders.

This may require removing discontinued medications and adding new drugs where needed. Pharmacy computer systems are usually capable of providing this information, but in some hospitals a manual recording system for these changes is still in use.

The final step in the cart filling process is the delivery of the completed medication carts to the nursing units and retrieving the used carts.

All medication returned in the previous day's trays must be credited to the patient, and then the carts are prepared to go through the entire process again on the following day.

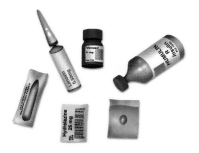

typical unit dose packaging

Packaging

There are a number of different types of packages that are used in unit dose medications. They include:

plastic blister	tablets/capsules
foil blister	tablets
paper	tablets
packet	powder
tube	ointment
foil cup	oral liquid
cartridge	syringe
vial	injection

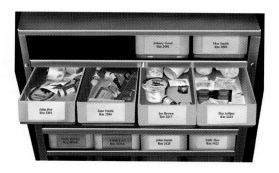

patient-specific trays

 unit dose a package containing the amount of a drug required for one dose.

Technicians often "pre-pack" medications that have been supplied in bulk into unit doses.

Machines that automate this process are generally used for pre-packing oral solid medications. Such systems restrict access by password or other means to authorized users and label each package with the information required by the institution. In cases where manual preparation is necessary (e.g., parenterals), technicians must follow institutional requirements exactly.

Unit dose packages are labeled with some of the same information found on multiple dose packages.

When packaged by the manufacturer, each unit dose is labeled with the name of the drug, its dosage form and strength, lot number, expiration date, and other identifying information. When pre-packed, labels must meet state and institutional requirements. Pre-packing equipment includes a label creation and application function.

Unit dose labels contain bar codes for identification and control.

If the bar code is to be applied at the hospital, technicians may do this using a bar code printer. Bar codes enable the item to be scanned into the dispensing and inventory system at various stages up to dispensing. This reduces the chances of medication errors and improves documentation and inventory control.

a medication cart

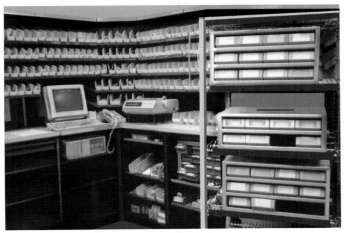

the cart filling area of a hospital pharmacy

Cart Filling Robots

Several machines referred to as robots have been developed to assist in the cart fillling process. While this reduces the manual filling responsibilities of technicians, there is still a requirement for some medications, such as those stored in the refrigerator, to be hand filled. Additionally, there is a large amount of special packaging required to stock these robots, and technicians who would traditionally be hand filling trays often perform these duties. Cart-filling robots are very expensive and require a large amount of space within the pharmacy area, therefore, the machines are usually seen only in larger hospitals.

MEDICATION ORDERS

Several different people have the ability to write medication orders in the hospital setting.

The most obvious of these is the doctor. However, both nurses and pharmacists may write orders if they are directly instructed to do so by a doctor. These are referred to as verbal orders and must be cosigned by the physician who approved them. Other specialized healthcare providers with advanced training can write orders without the signature of a physician. These people include physician's assistants and nurse practitioners.

In the hospital, all drugs ordered for a patient are written on a medication order form and not a prescription blank as seen in a community pharmacy.

Medication order forms are an all-purpose communication tool used by the various members of the healthcare team. Orders for various procedures, laboratory tests, and x-rays may be written on the form in addition to medication orders. Several medication orders may be written on one medication order form unlike pharmacy prescription blanks seen in the retail setting. These forms are traditionally prepared in duplicate so the original may always remain in the medical chart while copies are sent to appropriate areas of the hospital for processing.

There are several different types of orders that can be written.

One is a standard medication order for patients to receive a certain drug at scheduled intervals throughout the day, sometimes called a standing order. Orders for medications that are administered only on an as needed basis are called PRN medication orders. A third type of order is for a medication that is needed right away and these are referred to as STAT orders.

---

standing order a standard medication order for patients to receive medication at scheduled intervals.

PRN order an order for medication to be administered only on an as needed basis.

STAT order an order for medication to be administered immediately.

medication administration record (MAR) a form that tracks the medications administered to a patient.

ORDER PROCESSING

Once a medication order is written, it is removed from the chart and processed. Order processing involves many steps including:

✔ entry of the medication order into the pharmacy computer system;

✔ verification of the medication order by a pharmacist;

✔ dispensing of medication (including 1st doses and those required to complete the 24 hour supply);

✔ checking of medications;

✔ delivery of medications to the nursing units.

DOCUMENTATION

sample medication
order form

sample medication
administration record

There are also several ways an order can be processed.

Order entry may be performed by a nursing unit clerk, pharmacy technician, pharmacist, nurse, or even physician. For technicians to perform order entry, however, requires specialized training in the interpretation of medical orders.

Only a pharmacist may verify orders in the computer system and check medications being sent to the nursing floors.

Delivery, however, is varied and may be done by pharmacy technicians, hospital delivery staff, a pneumatic tube system, or a special robot that is designed to deliver medications to patient care areas. Often, these deliveries, or rounds, are done on an hourly basis.

Nurses record and track medication orders on a patient specific form called the medication administration record (MAR).

On this form every medication ordered for a patient is written down as well as the time it is administered and the person who gave the dose. These forms may be handwritten by the nursing staff or generated by the pharmacy computer system. The MAR is an important document in tracking the care of the patient as it give a 24 hour picture of a patient's medication use. The accuracy of this document as well as the pharmacy computer system from which it is generated is crucial.

INVENTORY CONTROL

Another responsibility that may be assigned to the hospital pharmacy technician is inventory control.

Ensuring adequate supplies of medications is the primary responsibility for staff in this area. Without an adequate supply of medication, the pharmacy will be unable to meet patient medication needs. This is especially important in the hospital setting where several of the drugs are needed in emergency situations.

A primary area of concern for inventory control is narcotics, or controlled substances, which require an exact record of the location of every item to the exact tablet or unit.

There are several systems for controlling narcotics, some are manual and others involve electronic equipment (e.g. PYXIS). In some institutions pharmacy technicians are not allowed to handle narcotics or may require special training. In contrast, some pharmacy departments assign all controlled substance management to technicians.

All patient care areas are required to have *code carts* which are used in the case of a medical emergency on the floor.

They contain different medications commonly used in these situations. Each code cart has a special lock that can be broken when the cart needs to be used. Once a lock is broken, it cannot be reused and the medication drawer must be replaced. The pharmacy is responsible for maintaining these carts. It may be the job of the technician to refill the cart and charge the missing medications to the appropriate patient. As with all medications leaving the pharmacy, the pharmacist must first verify the work of the technician filling the carts.

 See Chapter 13 for more information on inventory systems.

 code carts a locked cart of medications designed for emergency use only.

INVENTORY

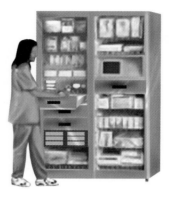

an automated Pyxis Medstation®

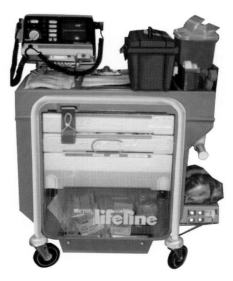

a code cart—note that the plastic yellow tie-lock must be broken to use the cart.

STERILE PRODUCTS

STERILE PRODUCTS

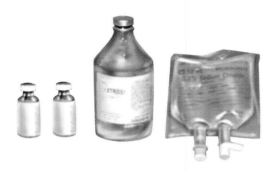

parenterals

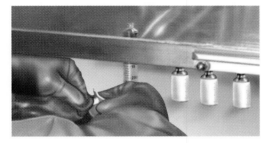

preparing parenteral admixtures on a laminar flow hood

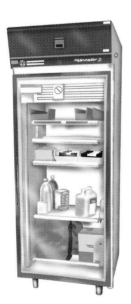

refigerator used for storing parenterals

A large portion of the medication used in the hospital is administered intravenously.

The hospital pharmacy technician plays a large role in preparing these products. I.V. admixtures may include small and large volume parentals, enteral nutrition therapy, or chemotherapy. This requires special safety training and the use of a vertical flow hood.

A supply of some large volume parenterals may be kept on the nursing unit.

These medications are referred to as **floor stock** and do not require patient specific labeling by the pharmacy.

A daily supply of other, scheduled intravenous medications will also be prepared with patient specific labels and delivered to the floor.

These products are stored in the refrigerator when required or other designated areas on the nursing unit since there is not enough room to store them in the medication carts.

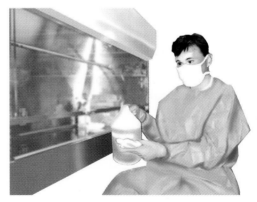

cleaning a laminar flow hood

 See Chapter 8 for more information on sterile products and parenterals.

 floor stock stock (such as large volume parenterals) that does not require patient specific labeling.

HOSPITAL PHARMACY AREAS

There are two basic organizational models for pharmacy departments within a hospital: centralized and decentralized.

In the centralized system, all pharmacy activities are conducted from one location within the hospital: the inpatient pharmacy. In a decentralized system, there are several pharmacy areas located throughout the hospital, each performing a specific function in order to provide pharmaceutical care to the entire hospital.

In the decentralized model, there is a central pharmacy which is generally responsible for the preparation and delivery of patient medication carts.

The central pharmacy also may conduct a variety of packaging functions in order to keep other areas within the department supplied with drugs they need. Medication order processing occurs at several decentralized locations throughout the hospital called pharmacy **satellites**. Satellites are responsible for providing first doses of medications, any emergency medications, and replacing missing or lost doses. Although not a primary focus of the satellite work load, a laminar flow hood may be used to prepare parenteral products as needed. There are usually several satellites located throughout the hospital, each serving a fraction of the patient care units in the hospital and each may have a specialized focus (i.e. pediatrics, oncology).

In the decentralized system, a separate area for preparation of parenteral products may be established.

This area could be a separate room or zone within the central pharmacy or exist in a separate location in the hospital. These areas, called sterile product areas, frequently contain specialized **clean rooms** for the preparation of sterile products. Laminar flow hoods will be located here since this is where the majority of parenterals will be made.

---

centralized pharmacy system a system in which all pharmacy activities in the hospital are conducted at one location, the inpatient pharmacy.

inpatient pharmacy the hospital pharmacy in a centralized system.

decentralized pharmacy system a system in which pharmacy activities occur in multiple locations within a hospital.

CENTRALIZED

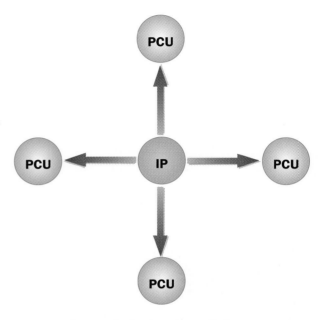

In a centralized system, all pharmacy activities are conducted at a single location, the inpatient pharmacy (IP). Medications are provided from there to the patient care units (PCU).

DECENTRALIZED

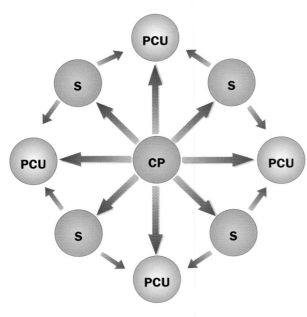

In a decentralized system, a central pharmacy (CP) is still responsible for many operations but satellite pharmacies (S) also operate at multiple locations throughout the hospital.

A centralized area for storage of drug product may also be a part of the pharmacy department.

In larger hospitals this area requires an entire staff of its own that deals only with the order and delivery of drug products for the other pharmacy areas. Technicians often make up a large portion of this staff and may be entirely in charge of running the area. In smaller institutions, however, the functions of inventory room personnel may be only a part of the pharmacy technician's duties during their scheduled shift.

A number of hospitals have an investigational drug service which is a specialized pharmacy subsection that deals solely with clinical drug trials.

These drug studies require a great deal of paperwork and special documentation of all doses of medication taken by patients. Technicians are frequently used in this area to assist the pharmacist with the large amount of documentation required and in preparing individual patient medication supplies. The investigational drug service may provide drugs to both patients located in the hospital and those receiving study medication at home.

Hospitals frequently have doctor's offices or clinics attached to them along with an outpatient or clinic pharmacy.

These pharmacies provide prescription medications to patients visiting their doctor. They are run very similarly to a retail pharmacy, but hospital technicians may be required to staff in these areas in addition to their inpatient responsibilities. Although an outpatient or clinic pharmacy may be located within a hospital, it does not supply inpatients with medications. It only provides patients who have obtained prescriptions from their doctors at the clinic or upon leaving the hospital.

 satellites pharmacy locations in a decentralized sytems that operate outside the central pharmacy.

clean rooms areas designed for the prepartion of sterile products.

outpatient pharmacy a pharmacy attached to a hospital servicing patients who have left the hospital or who are visiting doctors in a hospital outpatient clinic.

COMMUNICATION

In order to coordinate patient care, there must be communication between the various departments within the hospital.

Written medication orders are the routine method for letting the pharmacy know a medication is needed, but it is not the only way that pharmacy personnel interact with staff from other departments. The pharmacy technician needs to understand the variety of ways that healthcare professionals communicate with the pharmacy department.

The telephone is an important tool for communication with patient care areas, but it is limited to oral communication.

Some information must be written or printed. Fax machines are often used to quickly transmit written information such as drug orders from one area to another, but delivery of medication to these areas still requires someone to transport the drug.

Two systems are frequently used that allow both the transfer of written communication and the delivery of drugs without anyone having to leave their assigned work area.

The first of these is the dumbwaiter. A dumbwaiter is like a small elevator that moves vertically, in a straight path, between different floors of the hospital.

Another system, the pneumatic tube, gives more flexibility in the areas of the hospital it can serve.

Tube stations are located throughout the hospital and the tube system is placed within the walls of the building allowing users to send items around corners, between floors, and in some advanced systems even between buildings using compressed air. The item that is desired to be sent is placed in a plastic shuttle and the destination is programmed into the tube station. Within a matter of minutes the shuttle will arrive at the desired location. Both of the dumbwaiter and pneumatic tube allow orders to be sent to the pharmacy and the rapid return of drug to the patient care areas.

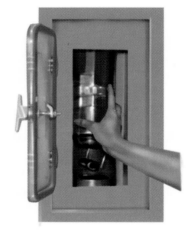

pneumatic tube and capsule

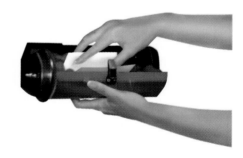

pneumatic capsule with document and medications

dumbwaiter a small elevator that carries objects (but not people) between floors of a building.

pneumatic tube a system which shuttles objects through a tube using compressed air as the force.

COMPUTER SYSTEMS

Most hospital information and documentation are computerized.

Information systems can integrate patient information, care and medication records, laboratory data, billing and many other types of information. However, each hospital system is customized to its own needs and therefore different. Individual systems may or may not integrate various areas of the hospital.

Hospital pharmacies rely heavily on computerized systems.

Knowledge of the hospital's pharmacy information system will be a large part of the initial training for a hospital pharmacy technician, since they must rely on it to perform many of their daily tasks.

An important responsibility for the pharmacist is to provide information on medications and their use to patients and other healthcare professionals.

Previously, much of this information was found in written form (e.g., Facts and Comparisons) or on disk. Newer hospital information systems link drug information directly with the pharmacy computer system allowing information on patients' specific medications to be viewed online.

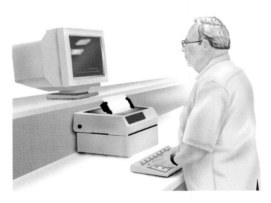

A technician using a hand held entry device for a computerized inventory system.

Among their many functions, hospital information systems provide quick access for the pharmacist to medication information for patients and care providers.

Confidentiality and Security

The information contained on a hospital information system is *highly confidential.* In many cases (especially with patient information), it is illegal to give the information to anyone except those who are authorized to have it. As a result, access to the computer system is limited by password or other security measures. It is essential that all staff follow security and confidentiality rules. Technicians should never provide information about medications or patients to anyone unless specifically directed to do so by the pharmacist in charge.

 It is important for the pharmacy technician to be aware of the various sources of drug information available. For more information on sources, see chapter 13.

GENERAL HOSPITAL ISSUES

Hospitals are a unique work environment.

There are some conditions that all hospital employees are required to complete that are not likely to be encountered in other pharmacy settings. First of all, instead of just interviewing with the pharmacy department, an interview with the Human Resources department is usually required. This department oversees the hiring of all employees in the hospital and usually manages the advertisement of available positions. Human resources accepts applications for employment and conducts and initial interview before providing pharmacy with a list of potential candidates. The pharmacy department then conducts its own interview before the final decision is made.

After being hired for a position in a hospital pharmacy new employees are required to attend a hospital wide orientation.

In this session, information is given about the benefits available to employees, rules and regulations of the hospital that all employees are expected to follow, and safety training for various situations such as fires and chemical spills. This will be in addition to the program that the pharmacy department will have planned.

All hospital employees are required to undergo a physical exam and often drug testing as a condition of employment.

At the medical screening vaccinations and immunizations such as the flu shot and the vaccine for hepatitis B may be offered. Hepatitis B is a severe infection that is carried in the blood. All employees who may be exposed to blood products, which may or may not be the case for a pharmacy technician, are encouraged to receive this vaccination. Many hospitals will give the vaccine free of charge and all personnel should seriously consider taking advantage of this opportunity.

POLICY & PROCEDURES

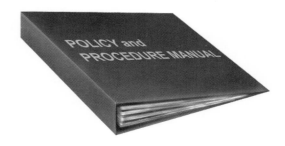

The Policy and Procedure Manual

All departments within the hospital are required to maintain a policy and procedures manual by regulating agencies.

This document contains information about every aspect of the job from dress code to disciplinary actions and step by step directions on how to perform various tasks that will be required of technicians. The pharmacy technician should become familiar with this document as all employees are expected to follow the rules and directions as described in the manual.

REGULATORY AGENCIES FOR HOSPITAL PHARMACY

Several different regulatory bodies oversee all aspects of hospital operations including the pharmacy department.

➡ **The Joint Commission on Accreditation of Healthcare Organizations (JCAHO)**

JCAHO surveys and accredits healthcare organizations. Healthcare Organizations must undergo this survey every 3 years. JCAHO lays out specific guidelines for every department within the hospital. Although this survey is not required, Medicare and several insurance providers now require JCAHO accreditation for reimbursement.

➡ **Health Care Financing Administration (HCFA)**

HCFA inspects and approves hospitals to provide care for Medicaid patients. Approval by this organization is required to receive reimbursement for any of these patients.

➡ **The Department of Public Health (DPH)**

The DPH is a state run organization that oversees hospitals including the pharmacy department. Hospitals undergo inspections by the DPH in order to assure compliance with laws concerning hospital practice.

➡ **The State Board of Pharmacy (BOP)**

The BOP is the agency that registers pharmacists and technicians. While their authority does not allow them to govern hospital pharmacy departments, they do regulate the registration of the pharmacists and technicians that work in this setting.

 It is absolutely essential that technicians know what they must and must not do in their job as outlined in their institution's policy and procedure manual.

 policy and procedure manual documentation of required policies, procedures, and disciplinary actions in a hospital.

LONG-TERM CARE

Long-term care facilities provide care for people unable to care for themselves because of mental or physical impairment.

Patients may be of any age and include chronically ill elderly, impaired children, and permanently disabled adults whose families can no longer care for their needs. Nursing homes make up the majority of long-term care facilities, but others include mental retardation and psychiatric institutions, and chronic disease and rehabilitation facilities. The amount of time a patient may need long-term care can extend from months to years or even a lifetime.

Because of limited resources, most long-term care facilities will contract out dispensing and clinical pharmacy services.

This means that they will pay for another company to take care of the majority of patient medicines. The licensed professional pharmacy or practice that provides medications and/or clinical services to long-term care facilities and their residents is called a long-term care pharmacy organization. Although a pharmacist or pharmacy technician does not have to physically be present at the facility during all hours, pharmacy services must be made available 24 hours a day.

Pharmacists perform two types of functions for long-term care: distributive and consultant.

The distributive pharmacist is responsible for making sure the patients are receiving the correct medicines that were ordered. This job is mainly done outside of the long-term care facility itself.

The consultant pharmacist is responsible for developing and maintaining an individualized pharmaceutical plan for every long-term care resident.

This is done by reviewing patient charts, assessing how a patient may receive optimal benefits from their medicines, and monitoring for drug-related problems. They interact with doctors, nurses, and other health professionals. An individual consultant pharmacist is usually responsible for several different nursing homes or other facilities and so may only visit each on certain weekly or monthly intervals. It is important to make the distinction between these types of responsibilities because the pharmacy technician working for a long-term care pharmacy organization may be assisting in these different tasks.

ENVIRONMENT

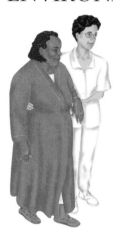

Nursing Homes

Most long-term care facilities are nursing homes that provide daily nursing care. Patients in this setting are generally referred to as **residents.**

Residents' Rights

Because residents of nursing homes were often victimized by people who were supposed to provide their care, federal and state laws were enacted in the U.S. designed to ensure residents' basic quality of life. These laws guarantee residents' rights to the following:

➥ safe and adequate care in a decent environment.
➥ privacy and confidentiality.
➥ personal property and clothing.
➥ personal privacy.
➥ freedom from abuse.

 distributive pharmacist makes sure long-term care patients receive the correct medications ordered.

consultant pharmacist develops and maintains an individual pharmaceutical plan for each long-term care patient.

Training

The orientation process at a long-term care pharmacy organization is comparable to the hospital setting. There is an initial orientation and training regarding performance of assigned functions and special requirements in the long-term care setting. Also, there is a written job description of the functions the pharmacy technicians may perform in accordance with specific regulations in the state. It is important to be aware of what the pharmacy technician is able to do or not do according to the law.

Changing Responsibilities

In addition to typical duties such as preparing, packaging, stocking, and delivering medications, new opportunities are emerging for pharmacy technicians in the long-term care environment. These include working closer with the consultant pharmacist to assist in the collection of data for patient assessment, compiling quality improvement data, maintaining computerized information between dispensing and consultant pharmacists, performing reviews of drug use in individual long-term care facilities, and preparing pharmacy reports.

Automated Dispensing Systems

When a medication is needed suddenly, the time it takes for delivery from an ouside supplier can present problems. Because of this, many nursing homes are turning to point-of-use automated dispensing systems. The medication order is communicated by computer to a central pharmacy system which then sends a confirmation of the order to the unit at the point of use. As soon as the unit receives this confirmation, a nurse can get the medication from the unit.

Many of the duties of pharmacy technicians in the long-term care pharmacy organization are similar to those in the hospital. These include filling medication carts, packaging prescriptions, mixing intravenous solutions, ordering medication stock, maintaining **automated dispensing systems** and emergency medication carts, and crediting returned medications. As in the hospital environment, the technician works under supervision of the pharmacist and must understand the limitations set forth by law.

In some facilities, the medication cart may be filled with enough medications to last for a week.

This is different from the hospital setting as there is much less medication and patients' drug therapies are not changed as frequently. However, if a patient receives a new medication order, there must be a system in place to make sure the appropriate drugs are received. To handle this, the pharmacy organization in charge of the facility may make arrangements with an alternative pharmacy or use an automated dispensing system. Copies of new medication orders may be faxed to an alternative pharmacy that will deliver the appropriate drugs. Some facilities may have a limited drug inventory stored in a secured location where only authorized personnel may obtain access, and pharmacy technicians may be required to keep track of inventory in these locations.

Emergency kits, or code carts, similar to those in hospitals are also located in long-term care facilities for emergency situations.

As in hospitals, if these emergency kits are opened, the appropriate patient must be charged for the medications used and the cart must be refilled. The technician is responsible for these duties and the pharmacist makes a final check before the cart is re-sealed. A pharmacy technician working with the pharmacist may also be responsible for the inventory of controlled substances stored in the long-term care facility.

 automated dispensing system a system in which medications are dispensed from an automated unit at the point of use upon confirmation of an order communicated by computer from a central system.

REVIEW

KEY CONCEPTS

✔ Patient rooms are divided into groups called nursing units or patient care units with patients having similar problems are often located on the same unit.

✔ The work station for medical personnel on a nursing unit is called the nurse's station. Various items required for care of patients are stored there, including patient medications.

✔ Ancillary areas (such as the emergency room) also use medications and are serviced by the pharmacy department.

✔ Pharmacy technicians in the hospital work under the direct supervision of a pharmacist.

✔ Computer generated drug profiles are prepared daily for each patient, and the amount of medications for the 24 hour period are placed in patient trays that are loaded into carts.

✔ Medications in the cart are packaged in individual containers holding the amount of drug required for one dose, called a unit dose.

✔ In the hospital, all drugs ordered for a patient are written on a medication order form and not a prescription blank as in a community pharmacy. Physicians write medication orders for hospital patients, though both nurses and pharmacists may also write orders if they are directly instructed to do so by a doctor. In addition, physician's assistants and nurse practitioners may sometimes write orders, depending upon the institution.

✔ Only a pharmacist may verify orders in the computer system and check medications being sent to the nursing floors.

✔ Nurses record and track medication orders on a patient specific form called the medication administration record (MAR).

✔ A primary area of concern for inventory control is narcotics, or controlled substances, which require an exact record of the location of every item to the exact tablet or unit.

✔ All patient care areas are required to have code carts which are used in the case of a medical emergency on the floor.

✔ A large portion of the medication used in the hospital is administered intravenously.

✔ In the centralized pharmacy system, all pharmacy activities are conducted from one location within the hospital: the inpatient pharmacy. In a decentralized system, there are several pharmacy areas located throughout the hospital, each performing a specific function.

✔ All departments within the hospital are required to maintain a policy and procedures manual by regulating agencies.

✔ The Joint Commission on Accreditation of Healthcare Organizations (JCAHO) surveys and accredits healthcare organizations. Organizations undergo this survey every 3 years.

✔ Because of limited resources, most long-term care facilities will contract out dispensing and clinical pharmacy services.

✔ The distributive pharmacist in long-term care is responsible for making sure patients receive the correct medicines that were ordered. The consultant pharmacist develops and maintains an individualized pharmaceutical plan for every long-term care resident.

SELF TEST

automated dispensing system

clean rooms

code cart

consultant pharmacist

distributive pharmacist

medication administration record

PRN order

satellites

standing order

STAT order

a standard medication order for patients to receive medication at scheduled intervals.

an order for medication to be administered only on an as needed basis.

an order for medication to be administered immediately.

a form that tracks the medications administered to a patient.

a locked cart of medications designed for emergency use only.

pharmacy locations in a decentralized sytems that operate outside the central pharmacy.

areas designed for the prepartion of sterile products.

makes sure long-term care patients receive the correct medications ordered.

develops and maintains an individual pharmaceutical plan for each long-term care patient.

a system in which medications are dispensed from an automated unit at the point of use upon confirmation of an order communicated by computer from a central system.

---

1. Which order allows a patient to receive medication at scheduled intervals?
   a. standing order
   b. prn order
   c. stat order
   d. multiple order

2. Which of the following is required by regulatory agencies of each hospital department?
   a. Facts and Comparisons
   b. laminar flow hood
   c. policy and procedures manual
   d. none of the above

3. In the hospital, each medication drawer in a medication cart is generally filled with a
   a. 12 hour supply of medications
   b. 24 hour supply of medications
   c. 36 hour supply of medications
   d. 48 hour supply of medications

4. A code cart is:
   a. a cart of medications designed to be used by nursing stations when the pharmacy is closed.
   b. a locked cart of medications on a nursing unit designed to be used in an emergency.
   c. a locked cart of controlled substances to be used by a designated registered nurse.
   d. none of the above.

MAIL ORDER PHARMACY

Mail order pharmacy is one of the fastest growing areas in pharmacy.

A mail order pharmacy sends medications to patients through mail or other delivery services. They have staffs of pharmacists, registered nurses, and technicians and can offer all the services of a community pharmacy, including compounding.

Because mail order medications involve a delivery time of at least 24-48 hours, they are used in situations where the need for the medication is known in advance.

This is true of chronic conditions like diabetes, high blood pressure, or depression, where the need for medication can be predicted and the supply can be easily maintained by mail delivery. This type of medication is called a maintenance medication, because it is used to maintain the patient with a chronic condition. By comparison, if a patient has an acute condition, such as a sudden infection, they would go to their community pharmacy to obtain the prescribed medication immediately after diagnosis.

Because they use the mail, mail order pharmacies can serve broad geographic areas.

In the U.S., for example, they can provide services to all states. This means that they can operate at a high volume. In addition to high volume discounts, this provides mail order pharmacies with economies of scale. These and other factors allow them to sell their medications at lower costs than community pharmacies. For this reason, mail order pharmacies are increasingly popular with third party insurers, a major source of their growth.

Chronic Conditions

Mail order pharmacy is used for maintenance therapy with chronic conditions that include:

- depression
- gastrointestinal disorders
- heart disease
- hypertension
- diabetes
- arthritis
- HIV/AIDS

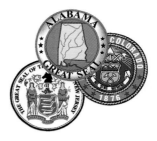

Regulation and Licensing

Though mail order pharmacies must follow federal and state requirements in processing prescriptions, they are not necessarily licensed in each state to which they send medications. As a condition for doing business there, some states now require that mail order pharmacies employ pharmacists licensed to practice in that state. However, not all do.

 acute condition a sudden condition requiring immediate treatment.

chronic condition a continuing condition that requires ongoing treatment for a prolonged period.

maintenance medication a medication that is required on a continuing basis for the treatment of a chronic condition.

Automation and Quality Control

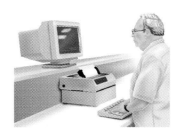

Mail order pharmacies are generally large scale operations that are highly automated. They use assembly line processing in which each step in the prescription fill process is completed or managed by a person who specializes in that step. For example, one technician may be responsible for entering prescriptions into the system, another for running an automated dispensing machine to fill prescriptions, and another for preparing the prescription for shipping. There are also steps for pharmacists to review the prescription before and after filling. Bar-coding of each prescription is used so that the prescription may be checked continually throughout the process against the information in the system. This ensures a high level of quality control. In fact, the increasing ability of automated systems to deliver a high quality product is one of the key contributing factors in the growth of mail order pharmacy.

Counseling and Information

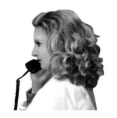

Mail order pharmacies have help desk or customer service numbers that patients can call when in need of counseling. Since calls may be related to medications, billing or other issues, these areas can be staffed with a mix of pharmacists, nurses, and technicians. As in the community pharmacy, technicians may not answer any questions related to medications, but of course can answer questions regarding forms, claims, and other non-medication issues.

Mail Order and Community Pharmacy

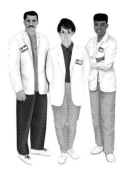

Much of the growth of mail order pharmacy has come at the expense of community pharmacy, which has historically served all patients, including those with chronic conditions. The large scale and sophistication of mail order pharmacies gives them many advantages (price being an extremely important one) which will undoubtedly help them to continue growing. At the same time, the personal availability of the pharmacist in the community pharmacy is an advantage that is likely to ensure the continuation of their vital role in the health of their communities. Both areas offer excellent career opportunities to pharmacy technicians.

HOME INFUSION

Home care provides health care in a patient's home that might otherwise be provided in an institutional setting or physician's office. The primary providers of such care are home care agencies. Care is supervised by a registered nurse who works with a physician, pharmacist, and others to administer a care plan that involves the patient or another care giver. The primary advantage of home care over institutional care is a better quality of life, though in many cases it may also be less expensive.

The fastest growing area of home health care is home infusion.

Advances in infusion pump technology have made the infusion process more accurate and easier to administer and have been a major factor in the growth of home infusion. Pumps are available for specific therapies or multiple therapies. There are ambulatory pumps that can be worn by patients and allow freedom of movement compared to being restricted to an infusion pump attached to an administration pole.

Pumps are chosen for therapy based on various factors.

These include the type of therapy or therapies, the ambulatory status of the patient, the involvement of caregivers, and so on. The supervising nurse and the pharmacist consult on the patient's care plan and choose the appropriate pump.

One of the fundamental activities of home care is patient education.

That is, the patient is educated about their therapy: how to self-administer, monitor, report problems, and so on. The supervising nurse is the primary person responsible for personally educating the patient or their care giver about therapy. However, the pharmacist is responsible for providing medication information to the supervising nurse and the patient or care-giver. Patients or care givers are generally required by law to sign a form indicating that they have received the appropriate information.

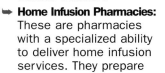

Primary Providers

The primary providers of home infusion services are:

➡ **Home Care Agencies:** These are essentially home nursing care businesses that provide a range of home health care services, which can include infusion.

➡ **Home Infusion Pharmacies:** These are pharmacies with a specialized ability to deliver home infusion services. They prepare admixtures, provide infusion pumps, and are involved in various aspects of the patient's care plan.

➡ **Hospitals:** Many hospitals offer home infusion therapies as a way to ensure continued therapy outside the hospital after patients are released.

Primary Home Infusion Therapies

The primary therapies provided by home infusion services are:

➡ **Antibiotic Therapy:** Antibiotic therapy is a common home infusion service used in treating AIDS related and other infections.

➡ **Parenteral Nutrition:** Parenteral nutrition is often required for patients with various intestinal disorders or AIDS.

➡ **Pain Management:** This generally applies to the infusion of narcotics for patients with painful terminal illnesses or other types of severe chronic pain.

➡ **Chemotherapy:** In certain situations, chemotherapy is provided in the home, generally in conjunction with an oncology program at a hospital or clinic.

 home care agencies home nursing care businesses that provide a range of health care services, including infusion.

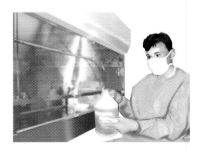

Compounding

The same rules apply to preparing parenteral admixtures in the home infusion setting as in the hospital. Compounding such admixtures requires the use of clean rooms, special equipment such as laminar flow hoods, and the use of aseptic practices. As with other parenteral admixtures, stability of the admixture for its intended use is a primary issue and storage a major concern. A complicating factor is that storage cannot be monitored as closely in a patient's home as an institutional setting. This results in short stability time limits that along with storage conditions require special attention. It also sometimes results in the on site preparation of certain therapies by the patient or care giver. In addition, automated devices that mix parenteral nutrition formulations at the time of administration are sometimes used. (See "Ready to mix systems," p.139.)

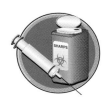

Hazardous Waste

Chemotherapy, the treatment of AIDS patients, and other infusion therapies involve the transportation, storage, and disposal of hazardous materials and is a primary area of concern. Home infusion personnel, patients and care givers must comply with all regulations governing such material. Compliance is a fundamental responsibility of home infusion personnel and is monitored by various regulatory agencies.

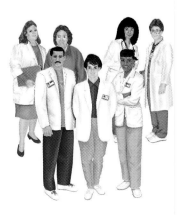

Home Care Team

The team that provides home health care includes the following:

physician: The patient's physician orders the infusion therapy.

registered nurse: The nurse is responsible for coordinating and monitoring the care plan and the home care team, and for educating the patient.

pharmacist: The pharmacist works with the supervising nurse to develop a pharmaceutical care plan which includes selection of the infusion device, identification of potential adverse reactions and interventions, and monitoring practices.

pharmacy technician: The technician works under the pharmacist's supervision and may be involved with compounding, labeling, delivery, and other non-consulting activities.

home care aide: Aides are non-professional staff employed by the home care agency who work under the supervision of the registered nurse. They assist in various aspects of a patient's care, but generally not in medication therapy.

REVIEW

KEY CONCEPTS

✔ Mail order pharmacy is used for maintenance therapy with chronic conditions that include depression, gastrointestinal disorders, heart disease, hypertension and diabetes.

✔ Mail order pharmacies must follow federal and state requirements in processing prescriptions, but are not necessarily licensed in each state to which they send medications.

✔ Mail order pharmacies are generally large scale operations that are highly automated. They use assembly line processing in which each step in the prescription fill process is completed or managed by a person who specializes in that step.

✔ Pharmacists review mail order prescriptions before and after filling.

✔ Home care is supervised by a registered nurse who works with a physician, pharmacist, and others to administer a care plan that involves the patient or another care giver.

✔ The fastest growing area of home health care is home infusion.

✔ Infusion pumps are available for specific therapies or multiple therapies, and include ambulatory pumps that can be worn by patients.

✔ In home infusion, the patient or their care giver is educated about their therapy: how to self-administer, monitor, report problems, and so on.

✔ The primary therapies provided by home infusion services are: antibiotic therapy, parenteral nutrition, pain management and chemotherapy.

✔ The same rules apply to preparing parenteral admixtures in the home infusion setting as in the hospital.

SELF TEST

MATCH THE TERMS.   *answers can be checked in the glossary*

acute condition

a continuing condition that requires ongoing treatment for a prolonged period.

antibiotic therapy

a medication that is required on a continuing basis for the treatment of a chronic condition.

chronic condition

a sudden condition requiring immediate treatment.

a common home infusion service used in treating AIDS related and other infections.

home care agencies

businesses that provide a range of home nursing care services, including infusion.

maintenance medication

infusion of nutrition solutions for patients with various intestinal disorders or AIDS.

pain management

generally the infusion of narcotics for patients with painful terminal illnesses or other types of severe chronic pain.

parenteral nutrition

ANSWERS TO SELF TEST

Chapter 1
1. b
2. d
3. b
4. d

Chapter 2
1. d
2. c
3. d
4. c

Chapter 3
1. d
2. c
3. a
4. a

Chapter 4
1. e
2. f
3. b
4. h
5. i
6. a
7. g
8. c
9. d
10. q
11. k
12. m
13. l
14. n
15. j
16. p
17. o
18. r
19. u
20. v
21. w
22. t
23. s

Chapter 5
1. c
2. c
3. c

Chapter 6
p. 81-Conversions
a. 1.5
b. 0.15
c. 0.1
d. 1.0
e. 0.81
f. 1.5
g. .065
h. 121%
i. 150%
j. 7%
k. 75%
l. 11.5%
m. 10%
n. 2.6%

p. 81-Roman Numerals
a. XVIII
b. LXIV
c. LXXII
d. CXXVI
e. C
f. VII
g. XXVIII
h. 33
i. 110
j. 1,100
k. 1.5
l. 19
m. 24
n. 14 capsules
o. 1,000 drops
p. 48 tablets
q. 21 tablets

page 85
a. mcg
b. L
c. ml
d. g (gm)
e. mg
f. Kg
g. 1,000 gm
h. 1,000 mcg
i. 130 mg
j. 1,000 ml
k. 0.001 L
l. 0.01 g
m. 7,000 mcg

n. 3,200 mg
o. 0.065 g
p. 30 ml
q. 300 ml
r. 7,000 g
s. 437.5 gr
t. 1.1 lb
u. 2 tsp.
v. 1 tbs.
w. 32°
x. 0.25 L

page 95
a. 2 ml
b. 8 ml
c. 75 ml
d. 2.08 ml/mn
e. 4.8 ml

page 97
a. 60%
b. 80%
c. 12%
d. .5
e. .125
f. .99
g. 35 g
h. 52.5 g
i. 14 g
j. 50 ml
k. 70 ml
l. 20 ml
m. 0.12%

page 102
a. 73.5 ml Amin. 8.5%
b. 37.5% ml Dex. 50%
c. 2 ml KCl
d. 0.45 ml Ca Gl.
e. 5 ml Ped MVI
f. qsad 131.55 ml sterile water

page 108
a. 500,000 mg
b. 10,000 g
c. 0.25 L
d. 0.325 g
e. 0.12 mg
f. 224.4 lb
g. 3560 g

h. 0.473 L
i. 65.9 Kg
j. 30,000,000 mg
k. 7.8°
l. 3 ml
m. 2.5 ml
n. 142.85 dext 70% and 357 ml sterile water
o. b
p. c
q. c
r. d
s. d
t. a
u. a
v. b
w. b

Chapter 7
1. d
2. d
3. c
4. b

Chapter 8
1. a
2. d
3. c
4. a

Chapter 9
1. b
2. a
3. d
4. b

Chapter 10
1. b
2. b
3. d
4. d

Chapter 11
1. b
2. b
3. c
4. c

Chapter 12
1. c
2. a
3. b
4. d

Chapter 13
1. c
2. c
3. a
4. c

Chapter 14
1. b
2. c
3. a
4. d

Chapter 15
1. a
2. d
3. a
4. d

Chapter 16
1. a
2. b
3. b
4. b

RUG NAMES & CLASSES

When a drug compound is first synthesized or isolated, it is known by its atomic composition: the types and numbers of atoms contained in it. For example, the compound $C_{14}H_{19}Cl_2NO_2$ has 14 carbon atoms, 19 hydrogen atoms, 2 chlorine atoms, 1 nitrogen atom, and 2 oxygen atoms. Besides being awkward to pronounce, this kind of identification does not really describe the structure of the molecule.

A drug's name begins with a chemical name that describes its structure and its components.

These names identify a specific compound, but they are long and complicated and not useful for general communication. As a result, highly specific chemical names are shortened to less descriptive but more easily pronounceable ones.

While a potential drug is under development, the developer gives it a code number or a "suggested nonproprietary name."

Once a suggested nonproprietary name is officially approved, it becomes the generic name of the drug compound. Many pharmaceutical companies will assign code numbers to their compounds in the earliest development stages, and then a suggested nonproprietary name if the compound shows promise of being effective as a drug. At that point, the sponsor will apply for a proprietary or trademark name from both the U.S. Patent Office and foreign agencies. If approved, the proprietary name will have the ® symbol next to it when used in interstate commerce.

When a drug is under patent protection, it has one nonproprietary name and one proprietary or brand name, and both of these belong to the sponsor.

When a drug goes off-patent, other companies may market the same compound under their own brand names. For example, ampicillin is a generic drug that has been off patent for many years. It is available as Polycillin®, Principen®, D-Amp®, Omnipen®, or Totacillin®. Each name is a brand name used by a different company. But Viagra® (which has the generic name sildenafil) is available only under one brand name because the compound is still under patent protection. The point to remember is that there is only one nonproprietary (generic) name for a drug, but it may be sold under many different brand names once its patent protection has expired.

296

WHAT'S IN A NAME

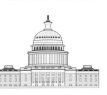

USAN

The United States Adopted Names Council (USAN) designates nonproprietary names for drugs. This council was organized in the early 1960s at the joint recommendation of the American Medical Association and the United States Pharmacopeial (USP) Convention. Other organizations, the American Pharmaceutical Association and the FDA, were included in the Council during the latter part of the 1960s. There are publications that list "official" nonproprietary and proprietary names, as well as drug code designations, empirical names, chemical names, and show the molecular structures. The USP Dictionary of USAN and International Drug Names is such a reference.

Applying for a name

To apply for a name, the sponsoring company initiates a request for a name. The USAN and the sponsor will arrive at a "Proposed USAN" that is suitable to both. This proposed name is then submitted for consideration to US and foreign drug regulatory agencies. When approved by these different agencies, the name becomes the "official" name of the drug. The USAN guidelines for the recommendation of names include that the name should:

➡ be short and distinctive in sound and spelling and not be such that it is easily confused with existing names

➡ indicate the general pharmacological or therapeutic class into which the substance falls or the general chemical nature of the substance if the latter is associated with the specific pharmacological activity

➡ embody the syllable or syllables characteristic of a related group of compounds.

STEMS & CLASSES

Following are the USAN approved stems and the drug classes associated with them.

Stem	Drug Class
-alol	Combined alpha and beta blockers
-andr-	Androgens
-anserin	Serotonin 5-HT$_2$ receptor antagonists
-arabine	Antineoplastics (arabinofuranosyl derivatives)
-ase	Enzymes
-azepam	Antianxiety agents (diazepam type)
-azosin	Antihypertensives (prazosin type)
-bactam	Beta-lactamase inhibitors
-bamate	Tranquilizers/antiepileptics
-barb	Barbituric acid derivatives
-butazone	Anti-inflammatory analgesics (phenylbutazone type)
-caine	Local anesthetics
-cef	Cephalosporins
-cillin	Penicillins
-conazole	Anti-fungals (miconazole type)
-cort-	Cortisone derivatives
-curium	Neuromuscular blocking agents
-cycline	Antibiotics (tetracycline type)
-dralazine	Antihypertensives (hydrazine-phthalazines)
-erg-	Ergot alkaloid derivatives
estr-	Estrogens
-fibrate	Antihyperlipidemics
-flurane	Inhalation anesthetics
-gest-	Progestins
-irudin	Anticoagulants (hirudin type)
-leukin	Interleukin-2 derivatives
-lukast	Leukotriene antagonists
-mab	Monoclonal antibodies
-mantadine	Antivirals
-monam	Monobactam antibiotics
-mustine	Antineoplastics
-mycin	Antibiotics
-olol	Beta-blockers (propranolol type)
-olone	Steroids
-oxacin	Antibiotics (quinolone derivatives)
-pamide	Diuretics (sulfamoylbenzoic acid derivatives)

Drug classes are group names for drugs that have similar activities or are used for the same type of diseases and disorders.

The assignment of a drug to a drug class is proposed when the sponsor makes an application to the USAN Council for an adopted name. The USAN Council and the sponsor then agree to a pharmacological or therapeutic classification. Unlike the generic and brand names, this classification is not an "official" one, however, and the drug may be listed in different classifications by different sources. For example, drugs classified one way in this chapter may appear in other classifications in other reference works.

There are common stems or syllables that are used to identify the different drug classes.

The USAN Council approves the stems and syllables and recommends using them in making new nonproprietary names. There are always new stems and syllables being approved by the Council, so the list is ever changing. On this page is a list of some common stems and syllables and the drug class associated with them.

Stem	Drug Class
-pamil	Coronary vasodilators
-parin	Heparin derivatives
-peridol	Antipsychotics (haloperidol type)
-poetin	Erythropoietins
-pramine	Antidepressants (imipramine type)
-pred	Prednisone derivatives
-pril	Antihypertensives (ACE inhibitors)
-profen	Anti-inflammatory/analgesic agents (ibuprofen type)
-rubicin	Antineoplastic antibiotics (daunorubicin type)
-sartan	Angiotensin II receptor antagonists
-sertron	Serotonin 5-HT$_3$ receptor antagonists
-sulfa	Antibiotics (sulfonamide derivatives)
-terol	Bronchodilators (phenethylamine derivatives)
-thiazide	Diuretics (thiazide derivatives)
-tiazem	Calcium channel blockers (diltiazem derivatives)
-tocin	Oxytocin derivatives
-trexate	Antimetabolites (folic acid derivatives)
-triptyline	Antidepressants
-vastatin	Antihyperlipidemics (HMG-CoA inhibitors)

COMMON DRUGS

There are a number of generic and brand name drugs that are commonly prescribed and whose names should be remembered.

Below is a compilation of the most commonly prescribed drugs in the United States. Both the proprietary (brand name) and the nonproprietary (generic) name are shown.

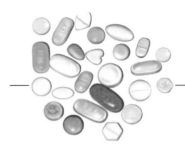

Brand Name	Generic Name
Accupril	quinapril
Adalat	nifedipine
Advil	ibuprofen
Altase	ramipril
Ambien	zolpidem
Amoxil	amoxicillin
Ativan	lorazepam
Atrovent	ipratropium
Augmentin	amoxicillin and clavulanic acid
Axid	nizatidine
Azmacort	triamcinolone
Bactrim, Septra	cotrimoxazole
Bactroban	mupirocin
Beconase AQ	beclomethasone
Beepen-VK	penicillin V potassium
Biaxin	clarithromycin
Bumex	bumetanide
BuSpar	buspirone
Calan SR	verapamil
Capoten	captopril
Carafate	sucralfate
Cardec DM	carbinoxamine, pseudoephedrine, and dextromethorphan
Cardizem CD	diltiazem
Cardura	doxazosin
Ceclor	cefaclor
Ceftin	cefuroxime
Cefzil	cefprozil
Cipro	ciprofloxacin
Claritin	loratadine
Compazine	prochlorperazine
Contuss XT	guaifenesin and phenyl-propanolamine
Coumadin	warfarin
Cycrin	medroxyprogesterone
Darvocet-N 100	propoxyphene napsylate with acetaminophen
Daypro	oxaprozin
Deltasone	prednisone
Demulen 1/35-28	ethinyl estradiol and ethynodiol diacetate
Depakote	valproic acid
Desogen	ethinyl estradiol and desogestrel
Diflucan	fluconazole
Dilantin	phenytoin
Duricef	cefadroxil

Brand Name	Generic Name
Dyazide	triamterene and hydrochlorothiazide
DynaCirc	isradipine
Elocon	mometasone
Entex LA	guaifenesin and phenyl-propanolamine
Erythrocin	erythromycin
Estrace	estradiol
Estraderm	estradiol (patch)
Fiorinal	butalbital, caffeine and aspirin
Floxin	ofloxacin
Glucotrol	glipizide
DiaBeta	glyburide
Hismanal	astemizole
Humulin	insulin
Hytrin	terazosin
Imitrex	sumatriptan
Intal	cromolyn sodium
K-Dur, Micro-K, Slow K	potassium chloride
Keflex	cephalexin
Klonopin	clonazepam
Lanoxin	digoxin
Lasix	furosemide
Levoxyl	levothyroxine
Lo/Ovral-28	ethinyl estradiol and norgestrel
Lodine	etodolac
Loestrin-FE 1.5/30	ethinyl estradiol and norethindrone
Lopressor	metoprolol
Lorabid	loracarbef
Lorcet Plus	hydrocodone and acetaminophen
Lotrisone	betamethasone dipropionate and clotrimazole
Lozol	indapamide
Macrobid	nitrofurantoin
Mevacor	lovastatin
Naprosyn	naproxen
Nasacort	triamcinolone
Nitrostat, Nitro-Dur	nitroglycerin
Nizoral	ketoconazole
Nolvadex	tamoxifen
Norvasc	amlodipine
Ogen	estropipate
Ortho-Cept 28	ethinyl estradiol and desogestrel
Ortho-Novum 7/7/7-28	norethindrone and ethinyl estradiol
Oruvail	ketoprofen
Paxil	paroxetine
Penicillin VK, Pen-Vee K, Veetids	penicillin V potassium

Brand Name	Generic Name	Brand Name	Generic Name
Pepcid	famotidine	Tegretol	carbamazepine
Percocet	oxycodone and acetaminophen	Tenormin	atenolol
Peridex	chlorhexidine	Terazol	terconazole
Phenergan	promethazine	Timoptic	timolol (ophthalmic)
Pravachol	pravastatin	TobraDex	tobramycin and dexamethasone
Premarin	conjugated estrogens	Toradol	ketorolac
Prilosec	omeprazole	Trental	pentoxifylline
Principen	ampicillin	Tri-Levlen 28, Triphasil	ethinyl estradiol and levonorgestrel
Prinivil	lisinopril	Tussionex	hydrocodone and chlorpheniramine
Procardia	nifedipine	Tylenol with Codeine	acetaminophen with codeine
Propacet	propoxyphene and acetaminophen	Valium	diazepam
Propulsid	cisapride	Vancenase AQ, Vanceril	beclomethasone
Proventil, Ventolin	albuterol	Vantin	cefpodoxime
Provera	medroxyprogesterone	Vasotec	enalapril
Prozac	fluoxetine	Vicodin	hydrocodone with acetaminophen
Relafen	nabumetone	Voltaren	diclofenac
Retin-A	tretinoin	Xanax	alprazolam
Ritalin	methylphenidate	Zantac	ranitidine
Slo-Bid, Theo-Dur	theophylline	Zestril	lisinopril
Sumycin	tetracycline	Zithromax	azithromycin
Suprax	cefixime	Zocor	simvastatin
Synthroid	levothyroxine	Zoloft	sertraline
Tagamet	cimetidine	Zovirax	acyclovir

Common Drug Abbreviations

There are many abbreviations and short forms that are used to identify drugs. Below is a list of common ones:

5-FU	5-fluorouracil	INH	isoniazid	NTG	nitroglycerin
6-MP	6-mercaptopurine	ISDN	isosorbide dinitrate	OC	oral contraceptive
6-TG	6-thioguanine	K	potassium	PABA	p-aminobenzoic acid
$Al(OH)_3$	aluminum hydroxide	KCl	potassium chloride	PAS	p-aminosalicylic acid
APAP	acetaminophen	LD	levodopa	PCN	penicillin
Ara-C	cytarabine	MAOI	monoamine oxidase	PCP	phencyclidine
ASA	aspirin (acetylsalicylic acid)		inhibitor	PDN	prednisone
		Mg	magnesium	PTH	parathyroid hormone
AZT	zidovudine	MgO	magnesium oxide	PZI	protamine zinc
B&O	belladonna and opium	$MgSO_4$	magnesium sulfate	SSKI	saturated solution of potassium iodide
C	ascorbic acid	Mn	manganese		
Ca	calcium	MOM	milk of magnesia	T_3	triiodothyroxine, liothyronine
Cl	chloride	MS	morphine sulfate		
DA	dopamine	MTX	methotrexate	T_4	Levothyroxine
DDAVP	desmopressin acetate	MV	multiple vitamin	TCN	tetracycline
DES	diethylstilbestrol	Na	sodium	TMP	trimethoprim
DIG	digoxin	NaCl	sodium chloride	TMP/SMX	trimethoprim/sulfamethoxazole
Fe	iron	$NaHCO_3$	sodium bicarbonate		
FeGluc	ferrous gluconate	NO	nitrous oxide	t-PA	tissue plasminogen activator
$FeSO_4$	ferrous sulfate	NPH	neutral protamine Hagedorn (insulin)		
HCTZ	hydrochlorothiazide			U	ultralente insulin
I	iodine	NSAIDs	nonsteroidal anti-inflammatory drugs		

RECEPTORS & CLASSES

Most organs in the body are influenced by both the parasympathetic and sympathetic nervous systems.

The parasympathetic system is made up of nerves coming from the cranial and sacral levels of the spinal cord. When these nerves are activated, the body conserves energy and maintains organs at lower activity levels. The sympathetic nervous system is made up of nerves that come from the thoracic and lumbar levels of the spinal cord. When these nerves are activated, the body is in a "fight or flight" state: heart rate and blood pressure increase, circulation to skeletal muscles increases, blood glucose increases, and so on. Generally, these two systems stimulate opposing responses in the organs, and in a normal state of **homeostasis**, there is a balance between sympathetic and parasympathetic effects.

The nerves in these systems interact with other nerves and body organs by releasing chemicals called neurotransmitters.

Neurotransmitters interact with cell receptors to produce an effect. Drug products can act on the same receptors to enhance or block the normal action of the neurotransmitter.

Classifications of drugs that influence the autonomic nervous system are based on whether they influence the parasympathetic or sympathetic system.

Acetylcholine is the neurotransmitter of the parasympathetic nervous system and drugs that act on this system are called **cholinergic**. Drugs that act on the sympathetic nervous system are known as **adrenergic**. That's because **norepinepherine** and **epinepherine**, the neurotransmitters for this system, are secreted from the adrenal glands and are also known as **noradrenaline** and **adrenaline**.

Classifications are also named for the type of interaction with the receptor.

Agonist or **antagonist** interaction is the primary basis for classification, but there are others. For example, cholinergic receptor responses are categorized as **muscarinic** and **nicotinic**. Adrenergic receptor responses are categorized as **alpha** (α) and **beta** (β). For the purposes of this appendix, it's not necessary to know exactly why these categories exist, but only that they are based on specific types of receptor action.

THE NERVOUS SYSTEM

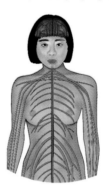

The human nervous system has two main parts: the **central nervous system (CNS)** and the **peripheral nervous system.** The CNS is essentially the brain region. The CNS controls the processes necessary for survival and coordinates sensory and motor function, emotional state, and reflexive acts. The peripheral nervous system consists of nerves that exit the spinal cord at different locations all along its length. There are two subdivisions of the peripheral nervous system: the **autonomic nervous system** and the **somatic nervous system.**

The autonomic nervous system influences the heart, blood vessels, visceral organs, glands, and a number of other organs. This system functions automatically, i.e., without conscious control, which is why it is sometimes called the "involuntary" or "automatic" nervous system.

Nerves that control the skeletal muscles are termed **somatic** nerves, and they are functionally and anatomically different from autonomic nerves. These nerves are involved with many of the "voluntary" actions of the person. There are two major divisions of the autonomic nervous system: **parasympathetic** and **sympathetic.**

ANTAGONISTS, AGONISTS, AND RECEPTORS

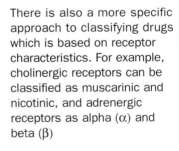

antagonists block action

———

agonists activate receptors

Antagonists

Antagonists are drugs that bind to cell receptors but do not activate them. They block the receptor's action by preventing neurotransmitters and other drugs from interacting with them.

Agonists

Agonists are drugs that activate receptors and produce a response that may either accelerate or slow normal cell processes, depending on the type of receptor involved. They imitate the effect of a neurotransmitter.

Receptor Based Classifications

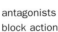

Besides classifying drugs as agonist or antagonist, they are classified by which nervous system (sympathetic or parasympathetic) they affect.

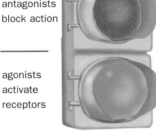

There is also a more specific approach to classifying drugs which is based on receptor characteristics. For example, cholinergic receptors can be classified as muscarinic and nicotinic, and adrenergic receptors as alpha (α) and beta (β)

Parasympathetic	**Sympathetic**
cholinergic receptor antagonists	adrenergic receptor antagonists
cholinergic receptor agonists	adrenergic receptor agonists

This classification approach can be broken down even further into these subclassifications:

Parasympathetic	**Sympathetic**
muscarinic cholinergic receptor antagonist	α-adrenergic receptor antagonists
muscarinic cholinergic receptor agonist	α-adrenergic receptor agonists
nicotinic cholinergic receptor antagonist	β-adrenergic receptor antagonists
nicotinic cholinergic receptor agonist	β-adrenergic receptor agonists

For the purposes of this appendix, it is not necessary to know the scientific basis for these subcategories, other than that they are based on differences in receptor characteristics. It's these specific receptor characteristics that allow for the development of drugs that have specific therapeutic effects.

 neurotransmitter chemicals released by nerves that interact with receptors to cause an effect.

homeostasis the state of equilibrium of the body.

CLASSIFICATION SCHEMES

Classification schemes have been significantly enlarged as subgroups of different types of receptors have been discovered.

Each new type of receptor has been found to be responsible for a specific pharmacological effect. As these effects are related to these receptors, drugs specifically designed to interact with the receptors are developed. As a result, there is an increased complexity in the naming of drugs that affect these receptors.

There are also other factors which complicate classifications schemes.

A complicating factor for drugs that affect the autonomic nervous system is the use of prefixes or suffixes such as **blocker, -lytic,** or **anti-** to mean antagonist and **-mimetic** to mean agonist.

Another factor is the presence of neurotransmitters other than acetylcholine, norepinephrine, and epinephrine.

Other neurotransmitters include serotonin (5-hydroxytryptamine or 5-HT), dopamine, histamine, gamma-amino butyric acid (GABA), glutamate, glycine, and aspartate. Each has subtypes, and each has agonists and antagonists that act by a variety of mechanisms.

The classifications used in this appendix are at right.

Each classification includes information on the therapeutic uses of the drugs in that classification, the diseases for which they are used, important side effects or interactions, and the names of various drugs in the classification.

NOMENCLATURE

Classification schemes for drugs can be highly complex. It is important to recognize that there is no standard nomenclature used in published medical and pharmaceutical literature. Therefore, any combination of terms or nomenclature schemes might be used. *Drugs will be idenitified in this chapter as either adrenergic or cholinergic, and agonist or antagonist.* "Lytic" or "mimetic" will not be used. "Blocker" will be used when it is a recognized part of a drug's classification name.

blocker another term for an antagonist drug, because antagonists block the action of neurotransmitters.

mimetic another term for an agonist, because agonists imitate or "mimic" the action of the neurotransmitter.

CLASSIFICATIONS

The classifications used in this appendix are:

Anticonvulsants (antiepileptics)
Antidiabetics
  Insulin
  Sulfonylureas
  Biguanides
  Thiazolidinedione
Antiemetics
  Dopamine antagonists
  Serotonin antagonists
Agents for Gout
Antihyperlipidemic
  Bile acid sequestrants
  HMG-CoA-reductase inhibitor
  Fibric acid derivatives
  Miscellaneous
Antihypertensive
  β_1-blockers and peripherally acting α_1-blockers
  Diuretics (thiazide, loop, potassium-sparing, carbonic anhydrase inhibitors, osmotic)
  ACE inhibitors; AT_1 antagonist
  Calcium channel blockers
  Orally active direct vasodilators
  Centrally acting α-adrenergic agonists
Anti-infectives
  Antibiotics
  Antimycobacterial drugs
  Antifungals
  Anti-protozoal drugs
  Antimalarials
  Antihelminthic agents
  Urinary tract anti-infectives
Antineoplastics
  Alkylating agents
  Antimetabolites
  Antibiotics
  Hormonal agents
  Plant alkaloids
  Miscellaneous
Anti-Parkinson's Disease

Antivirals
  Uncoating blockers
  Inhibitors of DNA/RNA synthesis
  Protease inhibitors
Corticosteroids
Dermatologicals
Gastrointestinal Drugs
  Therapy Associated with Stomach Acid Production
  Prokinetics
  Antidiarrheals
  Laxatives and Stool Softeners
  Pancreatic Enzymes (Digestants)
Heart Drugs
  Antianginals
    Nitrates
    β-blockers
    Calcium channel blockers
  Antiarrhythmics
    Classes I, II, III, and IV
  Heart Failure
    Digitalis glycosides
    Adrenergic receptor agonists
    Phosphodiesterase inhibitors
Hematological Agents
  Coagulation enhancers
  Hematopoietic agents
  Anticoagulants
    Heparins, Coumarins, Thrombin inhibitors, Antiplatelet agents, Thrombolytic enzymes, Hemostatic agents
Hormone Related Agents
  Oral contraceptives and Ovulation stimulants
  Thyroid hormones
  Oxytocic and tocolytic agents
  Androgens and antiandrogens

Immunological Agents
  Immunoglobulins and antigen binding fragments, and monoclonal antibodies
  Immunosuppressives
Muscle and Bone Related
  Neuromuscular blockers
  Skeletal muscle relaxants
  Bone disorders
Ophthalmic Drugs
  Antiglaucoma agents
  Ophthalmic mydriatics
  Other Ophthalmic Conditions
Pain Related Agents
  Analgesic Agents
    NSAIDs
    Salicylates
    Opiates
  Migraine Headaches
  Anesthetic Agents
    Local
    General
Psychotropic Agents
  Antidepressants
    Tricyclic antidepressants
    MAOIs
    SSRIs
    Heterocyclic antidepressants
  Antipsychotics
  Sedatives — Hypnotics
    Anxiolytic drugs
    Hypnotics
Respiratory Drugs
  Asthma
  Antihistamines
  Decongestants
  Antitussives
  Expectorants
Vasopressors
Miscellaneous New Drugs

CLASSIFICATIONS

Epilepsy is a chronic disorder characterized by recurring seizures with symptoms such as fainting and muscle spasms.

It is believed that one cause of seizures may be an excessive firing of neurons in the brain. The table below shows the two general classes of seizures. A partial seizure occurs in just one cerebral hemisphere and involves a focal point of neuron activity. A generalized seizure involves both cerebral hemispheres and a general area of activity.

Partial Seizures	Clinical Signs
Simple partial	conscious, but impaired motor, sensory, or speech ability.
Complex partial	unconscious, in dream like state.

General Seizures	Clinical Signs
Grand mal	unconscious with falling at onset; muscle spasms, verbal cries.
Petit mal (absence)	primarily in children and disappear at puberty; conscious is briefly impaired, with and without motor involvement
Atypical	shock-like contractions, loss of muscle tone

The recurrence of seizures interferes with a person's ability to function normally. When treated with the appropriate anticonvulsant, however, most epileptic patients are able to remain seizure free. **Anticonvulsant (antiepileptic) drug therapy reduces the seizure frequency by reducing the excitability of the brain's neurons.**

The primary anticonvulsant drugs are:

➡ phenytoin,
➡ carbamazepine,
➡ valproic acid.

Additional antiepileptic drugs include phenobarbital and primidone, and the benzodiazepines clorazepate and clonazepam. Newer compounds approved by the FDA since 1993 include lamotrigine, felbamate, gabapentin, topiramate, and tiagibine. Topiramate was approved to be used in combination with other antiepileptic drugs. Tiagabine was approved in 1997. Inorganic magnesium salts are given orally as laxatives but parenterally as anticonvulsants. **Nearly all anticonvulsants can cause side effects ranging from minor to severe, including drug-induced seizures if serum concentrations are too high.**

ANTIDIABETICS

Diabetes is a common disorder that is caused by a deficiency of the hormone insulin or an inability of the body to use it effectively.

Diabetic symptoms include abnormally high levels of blood glucose, increased urination, thirst, and weight loss.

Insulin is produced by the pancreas. It controls the ability of the body's cells to absorb glucose from the blood. Since the cells of diabetic patients don't absorb glucose efficiently, glucose concentrations in their blood are abnormally high. Glucose concentrations can be determined through a simple test using a glucometer. Other symptoms include increased urination, thirst, fatigue, and weight loss in spite of normal caloric intake.

There are two types of diabetes, **diabetes insipidus** and **diabetes mellitus,** which is by far, the most common. Diabetes mellitus in turn has two types:

➡ **Type 1 (insulin dependent diabetes mellitus, IDDM)**
Type 1 is characterized by decreased production of insulin and so must be treated with insulin. It is most often found in children and adolescents.

➡ **Type 2 (non-insulin dependent diabetes mellitus, NIDDM)**
Type 2 is caused by either decreased insulin production or abnormal cell sensitivity to the insulin that is present. It may be treated with diet alone, with oral hypoglycemic agents, or with insulin. It is more commonly diagnosed in adults.

Insulin does not cure diabetes. It is merely a treatment for the disease. Over time, many complications can occur in diabetic patients taking insulin. Some of these are coronary heart disease, peripheral vascular disease, eye disorders, renal failure, and limb amputations. Because of reduced circulation and nerve damage, diabetic patients are especially prone to developing foot ulcers, a major cause of amputations. They are less able to feel a foot infection, which allows it to grow and cause permanent damage. Proper foot care is essential and includes avoiding injures or restricting circulation, cleaning wounds, controlling infection, relieving weight from the ulcer area, and improving circulation. A new genetically engineered drug, becaplermin, promotes the healing process in diabetic foot ulcers.

Diabetic patients are prone to heart disease, circulatory problems, eye disorders, and infections of the feet.

INSULIN

There are many types of insulin and many salt forms of it.

Insulins are derived synthetically or from different animal sources such as beef and pork. There is now a genetically engineered human insulin available. **Different insulins differ in the onset of action and the duration of action.** Some are mixed together to achieve a desired effect such as a quick onset but a longer duration of action. The most common mixture is regular insulin with NPH insulin (70 units NPH and 30 units regular insulin per milliliter).

Insulin administration is the principal treatment for diabetes mellitus, but it is not a cure.

The different categories of insulins are:

➡ **Short-acting insulins:** regular insulin (crystalline zinc insulin), semilente insulin (prompt insulin zinc suspension), insulin lispro;

➡ **Intermediate-acting insulins:** NPH (isophane insulin suspension) and lente insulin (insulin zinc suspension);

➡ **Long-acting insulins:** PZI (protamine zinc insulin suspension) and ultralente insulin (extended insulin zinc suspension).

CLASSIFICATIONS

ANTIDIABETICS (cont'd)

Diabetic patients can monitor their glucose levels by using a glucometer, a simple device that can be used in the home. It requires a blood sample (a drop from a finger prick) and generally processes the sample within one minute.

Controlling glucose levels with insulin injections is a complex task since:

➡ Glucose concentrations fluctuate based on food ingestion.

➡ Cell sensitivity to insulin changes. Exercise increases sensitivity while stress, pregnancy, and some drugs decrease insulin sensitivity.

As a result, some diabetic patients take multiple injections of a short-acting insulin preparation to produce peaks in insulin concentrations and a long acting formulation to establish a baseline concentration. Variable rate infusion pumps are also used.

SULFONYLUREAS

Sulfonylureas are oral formulations used to treat Type 2 diabetes.

They promote insulin secretion, reducing the production of glucose by the liver, and increasing cell sensitivity to insulin. The sulfonylureas are divided into two groups: the first-generation drugs: acetohexamide, chlorpropamide, tolazamide, tolbutamide; and the second generation drugs: glyburide, glipizide, glimepiride.

BIGUINIDES

Biguanides decrease the absorption of glucose from the intestines and glucose output from the liver.

Metformin is the only biguanide available.

THIAZOLIDINEDIONES

Thiazolidinediones they lower blood glucose by increasing insulin sensitivity.

They are called "insulin sensitizers." They decrease hepatic glucose output but not insulin secretion. Troglitazone was approved in 1997 and is the first drug in this group.

MIGLITOL AND ACARBOSE

Miglitol and acarbose control the rise in blood glucose concentrations following meals by delaying the absorption of ingested carbohydrates. They do not increase insulin secretion or insulin sensitivity.

ANTIEMETICS

E mesis (vomiting) is a common adverse effect of chemotherapy given to cancer patients.

The vomiting center in the brain can be stimulated by conditions such as gastrointestinal irritation and motion sickness, or by a chemoreceptor trigger zone (CTZ) that responds to chemical stimulation from drugs, toxins, and uremia. Blocking dopamine receptors in the CTZ blocks its stimulation and emesis.

DOPAMINE ANTAGONISTS

Centrally acting dopamine antagonists are effective antiemetic agents. In addition to some phenothiazines (e.g., prochlorperazine, thiethylperazine, perphenazine, and promethazine), metoclopramide, haloperidol, and domperidone are effective. Cholinergic receptor antagonists such as cyclizine, meclizine, buclizine, diphenhydramine, and dimenhydrinate have also been used. Scopolamine is again available as a transdermal patch after being removed from the market for reformulation.

ANTIEMETICS (cont'd)

SEROTONIN ANTAGONISTS

Another neurotransmitter involved in emesis is serotonin.

High doses of metoclopramide were discovered to antagonize serotonin receptors in addition to dopamine receptors. The most effective agents are serotonin receptor antagonists. These include granisetron, ondansetron, and dolasetron.

One drug that came about by chance more than by design was dronabinol. This agent is the active ingredient in marijuana. Its efficacy in emetic control was discovered by observations that cancer patients who smoked marijuana had better emesis control than did those who did not. Controlled trials showed that dronabinol did indeed exert an antiemetic action but that it was not to be used as a first-line agent.

AGENTS FOR GOUT

Gout is a disorder in uric acid excretion that is characterized by hyperuricemia.

hyperuricemia
an abnormal concentration of uric acid in the blood.

Body fluids become supersaturated with uric acid and monosodium urate crystals accumulate in tissues and joints. Hyperuricemia can result from an overproduction of uric acid or a decrease in its excretion. Treatment generally involves:

➡ **Inhibiting inflammation:** Inflammation results from white blood cells (leukocytes) migrating to urate crystals. Colchicine prevents this migration and is a traditional treatment for gout. It relieves both pain and inflammation for gout sufferers. The non-steroidal anti-inflammatory drugs (NSAIDs) indomethacin and sulindac are also commonly used. Indomethacin has side effects in about half the patients taking it, so its usefulness on a long-term basis is quite limited.

➡ **Decreasing uric acid production:** Allopurinol was originally investigated as an antineoplastic agent, but was found to have significant activity in reducing the production of uric acid.

➡ **Increasing uric acid excretion:** Probenecid was originally used to decrease the renal excretion of penicillin and extend the supply of penicillin when it was scarce. It was also found to have anti-gout activity. Around 1960, sulfinpyrazone was found to be a significantly more effective agent in gout therapy.

ANTIHYPERLIPIDEMIC

Hyperlipidemia is known to cause atherosclerosis (a narrowing of the arteries) which is a major risk factor in heart attack and stroke.

endogenous
produced from within the body or within a cell.

Cholesterol is a primary factor in blocked arteries. It is an **endogenous** compound produced in cells and used in the construction of cell membranes. It may also, to a lesser extent, come from the diet. It circulates in the blood as a lipoprotein, a sphere with cholesterol and triglycerides in the center and phospholipids on the outside. It is measured as **total cholesterol, low-density lipoprotein (LDL)**, the so-called "bad" cholesterol, and **high-density lipoprotein (HDL)**, the "good" cholesterol.

CLASSIFICATIONS

ANTIHYPERLIPIDEMIC (cont'd)

There are a various antihyperlipidemic drugs, each with different effects in lowering cholesterol and triglycerides. The drugs can be classed as:

BILE ACID SEQUESTRANTS

The body uses cholesterol to produce the bile acids that are secreted into the intestine to assist in the absorption of fats.

These acids are normally reabsorbed back into the body. However, bile acid sequestrants in the intestine prevent them from being reabsorbed, causing bile acids to be lost, and increased cholesterol use to make new bile acids. This process leads to a decrease in LDL and total cholesterol. Cholestyramine and colestipol are the drugs in this class.

Antihyperlipidemics lower cholesterol and triglyceride levels.

HMG-CoA REDUCTASE INHIBITOR

Most of the body's cholesterol is made inside cells from fats.

The enzyme hydroxymethylglutaryl-coenzyme A (HMG-CoA) reductase is involved in the synthesis of cholesterol from fat. Therefore, HMG-CoA reductase inhibitors prevent cholesterol from being synthesized. These are the "**vastatin**" drugs and several are available. Lovastatin, fluvastatin, and atorvastatin have been found to lower cholesterol levels, but not triglyceride levels. Pravastatin and simvastatin reduce the risk of stroke or heart attack in patients who have normal cholesterol levels but who have had a heart attack.

"-vastatin" (or "-statin") drugs block the body's synthesis of cholesterol.

FIBRIC ACID DERIVATIVES

Fibric acid derivatives lower both cholesterol and triglyceride levels, though exactly how is not known.

They include clofibrate and gemfibrozil. Fenofibrate was approved in 1998 as adjunctive therapy for patients with very high triglyceride levels.

MISCELLANEOUS

Niacin (nicotinic acid) and probucol have different mechanisms for reducing cholesterol levels. Niacin is a vitamin that is involved in fat regulation in the body. Probucol inhibits cholesterol transport from the intestine and thus enhances the fecal excretion of cholesterol and bile acids.

ANTIHYPERTENSIVES

Hypertension (HTN) is an elevation of blood pressure above a normal range.

Blood pressure is the product of cardiac output and the total resistance to blood flow through the peripheral vascular system. It is measured as two values: systolic pressure and diastolic pressure. When blood is forced out of the heart, the increased pressure on the vascular system is called systolic. Diastolic pressure is the minimum pressure when the heart relaxes. When blood pressure is monitored, it is written (in mm Hg) as a relationship of systolic to diastolic pressures (e.g, 120/80). Normal pressure ranges differ according to gender and age. Men have higher pressures than women, and older people have higher pressures than younger people.

A sphygmomanometer is used to measure blood pressure.

ANTIHYPERTENSIVES (cont'd)

A systolic pressure of 120-140 and a diastolic pressure of 80-89 are normal for most adults, though this does vary somewhat by individual. Hypertensive ranges are as follows:

	SYSTOLIC	DIASTOLIC
Stage 1 (mild)	140-159	90-99
Stage 2 (moderate)	160-179	100-109
Stage 3 (severe)	180-209	110-119
Stage 4 (very severe)	≥ 210	≥ 120

Hypertension is a major risk factor for heart disease, diabetes, and other serious conditions.

In a small number of cases, hypertension has a known cause such as renal disease or endocrine tumors. However, for the vast majority of patients, the cause is unknown. This more common type of high blood pressure is called **essential hypertension.** It often has no symptoms but must be treated because the disease is a major risk factor for atherosclerosis, coronary artery disease, aortic aneurysm, congestive heart failure, and other serious conditions. Patients with recent-onset essential hypertension tend to have an elevated cardiac output. Patients with chronic sustained hypertension tend to have a normal or low cardiac output but an elevated vascular resistance. **Current antihypertensive medications lower blood pressure by decreasing either the cardiac output or the total peripheral resistance.**

Drugs that lower cardiac output do so by several mechanisms:
➡ decrease the force and rate of cardiac contraction
➡ decrease the blood volume (diuretics)
➡ decrease sympathetic outflow

Drugs that lower total peripheral resistance do so by these mechanisms:
➡ relax vascular smooth muscle
➡ decrease sympathetic outflow

In addition to such standard considerations as age, gender, race, etc., the presence of other medical conditions is also important in the selection of an antihypertensive drug for treatment. Many antihypertensive drugs have effects in other disease states such as an ACE inhibitor in heart failure or a calcium channel blocker in angina. As a result, one drug may be used to treat multiple disease states. Since once-daily dosing regimens improve patient compliance, drugs may also be selected on this basis. In the case of a transdermal formulation of clonidine, a single weekly dosing is possible.

β_1-BLOCKERS AND PERIPHERALLY ACTING α_1-BLOCKERS

β-blockers lower blood pressure by lowering cardiac output.

They block the action of certain nerves in cardiac muscle, lungs, and the smooth muscles of the blood vessels. β-blockers include metoprolol, acebutolol, esmolol, betaxolol, and atenolol.

The peripherally acting α_1-blockers are prazosin, terazosin, and doxazosin. Prazosin is the least used of the compounds due to its unwanted adverse reactions. Doxazosin and terazosin are the preferred drugs and can be administered either once or twice daily. Three other members of this class are guanadrel, guanethidine, and reserpine.

CLASSIFICATIONS

DIURETICS

Diuretics decrease blood pressure by decreasing blood volume.

They accomplish this by increasing the urinary excretion of salts and water (**diuresis**). As a result, they are popularly called "water pills." There are a number of classes of diuretics, each with a unique mechanism of action, affecting a different part of the kidney nephron:

Diuretics increase the elimination of salts and water through urination.

➡ **thiazides:** Thiazide diuretics increase the excretion of Na^+ and Cl^-. They include chlorothiazide, hydrochlorothiazide, chlorthalidone, metolazone, indapamide. Thiazides increase the excretion of other ions, and potassium loss caused by these diuretics may require potassium supplements.

➡ **loop:** Loop diuretics generate a larger elimination response than that of the thiazides. Furosemide, ethacrynic acid, bumetanide, and torsemide are the drugs in this class.

➡ **potassium-sparing:** Potassium sparing diuretics (spironolactone, triamterene, amiloride) are weak diuretics but are often used with other diuretics because of their potassium sparing effects, e.g., the combination diuretics Dyazide® (hydrochlorothiazide and triamterene) and Maxzide® (hydrochlorothiazide and triamterene).

➡ **carbonic anhydrase inhibitors:** Carbonic anhydrase inhibitors such as acetazolamide interfere with the action of carbonic anhydrase not only in the kidney but also in the eye. In fact, acetazolamide is used more often to reduce intraocular pressure in glaucoma than as a diuretic. Other inhibitors include methazolamide and dichlorphenamide.

osmosis
the natural force that propels a solvent in a higher concentration solution through a membrane to a lower concentration solution.

➡ **osmotic:** Osmotic diuretics have been available for decades. They are unique because they do not interact with receptors or directly block a renal transport mechanism. Their activity depends entirely on **osmosis**. Hypertonic solutions of glycerin, mannitol, isosorbide, and urea have all been employed as osmotic diuretics. Mannitol is the most commonly chosen when there is a need for a systemic osmotic agent.

ANGIOTENSIN-CONVERTING ENZYME INHIBITORS (ACE INHIBITORS)

Angiotensin II is a compound produced in the body that causes the constriction of blood vessels and the retention of sodium and water.

Blocking the angiotensin-converting enzyme (ACE) involved in the production of angiotensin II with an ACE inhibitor will result in the relaxation of blood vessels and the excretion of sodium and water.

ACE inhibitors are the "-pril" drugs. They produce their anti-hypertensive effects by relaxing the blood vessels

ACE inhibitors are the "**-pril**" drugs. Captopril was the first approved for clinical use. It has infrequent but severe adverse effects, many of which are attributed to the presence of a sulfhydryl group in captopril. Enalapril does not possess a sulfhydryl group nor the same adverse reactions. Additional ACE inhibitors have been developed, including lisinopril, benazepril, fosinopril, quinapril, ramipril, and trandolapril. All of these drugs possess a slower onset and a long duration of action relative to captopril and are all available for once-a-day therapy.

The "**-sartan**" drugs can be considered a subgroup of the ACE inhibitor class. Losartan, valsartan and eprosartan (approved in 1997), and irbesartan and candesartan (approved in 1998) are angiotensin II receptor (AT_1) antagonists, and provide the same type of therapy seen with the ACE inhibitors.

ANTIHYPERTENSIVES (cont'd)

Calcium channel blockers lower blood pressure by relaxing blood vessels.

CALCIUM CHANNEL BLOCKERS

Many cardiovascular diseases (including hypertension) are characterized by abnormally constricted blood vessels that result in increased vascular resistance.

This is often associated with an abnormally high calcium ion concentration in the vascular smooth muscles. Calcium channel blockers block the movement of calcium ions into cell membranes and cause the vascular smooth muscles to relax. Calcium channel blockers that are used for hypertension are verapamil, nifedipine, diltiazem, nicardipine, isradipine, felodipine, and amlodipine.

ORALLY ACTIVE DIRECT VASODILATORS

The orally active vasodilators hydralazine and minoxidil also lower blood pressure by relaxing the arterial smooth muscles. Their mechanism of action is different than that of the calcium channel blockers, and they have a greater selectivity (more specific in action) for arterial smooth muscles. They are used less frequently than diuretics, β-blockers, and ACE inhibitors.

selectivity
the characteristic in which a drug affects only certain specific receptors and tissues in the body.

CENTRALLY ACTING α-ADRENERGIC AGONISTS

Centrally acting α-adrenergic agonists are used with patients having moderate to severe hypertension.

They cause less **orthostatic hypotension** than drugs that act directly on the peripheral sympathetic neurons. Orthostatic hypotension is a light-headedness and dizziness that occurs when a person first stands and when severe, can cause the person to fall. Drugs in this class include clonidine, guanabenz, guanfacine, and methyldopa.

orthostatic hypertension
a drop in blood pressure upon standing up.

ANTI-INFECTIVES

Infection is a general term indicating that some type of microorganism is attacking the body.

The body has many microorganisms that live inside or on its surface. Infections involve either a superpopulation of an endogenous microorganism, or a microorganism that is not normally found in the body. Infections can involve microorganisms such as bacteria, viruses, fungi, protozoa, and amoebas, or larger organisms such as parasitic flukes and worms.

When anti-infective therapy is started, the organism responsible has often not been identified. This is called **empirical therapy**, and it is begun because it is often more important to start a therapy with a high probability of success than to wait until complete laboratory identification of the organism is made. **Definitive therapy** is used when the organism has been definitely identified. **Prophylactic or preventive therapy** with anti-infectives is given prior to surgery, to patients with weakened immune systems (cancer patients, AIDS patients), or to patients planning to travel abroad to areas having diseases that are not normally encountered at home.

CLASSIFICATIONS

ANTIBIOTICS

The term **antibiotic** traditionally refers to chemicals produced by microorganisms that suppress the growth of other microorganisms. The term **antimicrobial** refers to both synthetic agents and natural antibiotics. Many agents are originally isolated from microorganisms, but are later synthetically produced. Some agents are semi-synthetic. That is, the microorganism produces a key portion of the drug, and then various synthetic chemical modifications of that central part are made. This has effectively eliminated the distinction between the terms antibiotic and antimicrobial.

Antimicrobial agents can be **bactericidal** (bacteria killing) or **bacteriostatic** (bacteria growth retarding). Both bacteriostatic and bactericidal agents are effective as chemotherapeutic drugs, but both also rely on host defenses to aid in eliminating the pathogens. When host defenses are absent, bactericidal agents must be used.

Classes of antimicrobial agents can be grouped together based on their primary mechanism of action. The various groups interact at different cellular biochemical pathways or at different cellular structures to exert their effect. Four of the major points of interaction are:

➡ **Inhibition of synthesis or damage to the bacterial cell wall**
➡ **Inhibition or modification of protein synthesis**
➡ **Modification in energy metabolism**
➡ **Modification in synthesis or metabolism of nucleic acids (DNA)**

Inhibit Cell Wall Synthesis

There are many classes of antibiotics that produce their antibiotic effect by inhibiting cell wall synthesis. They may be differentiated by microorganism specificity and bacterial resistance. Two of the major classes are the penicillins and the cephalosporins.

Penicillins

Penicillin was discovered in 1928 and first used clinically in 1941. In 1941, penicillin G was a highly effective antibiotic. By 1947, it was not. The different penicillin derivatives have all been effective for a while, until resistant strains of bacteria develop, and new penicillins are needed. Drugs in the penicillin class can be identified by the "**-cillin**" in their names: methicillin, nafcillin, oxacillin, cloxacillin, dicloxacillin, amoxicillin, and ampicillin. Carbenicillin was approved in 1970 and was the first **semisynthetic** penicillin that was effective against a broad spectrum of microorganisms. This newer group of penicillins includes ticarcillin, piperacillin, and mezlocillin.

Imipenem is an extremely broad-spectrum penicillin antibiotic. An enzyme in the kidney rapidly metabolizes the drug, so cilastatin, a specific inhibitor of the kidney enzyme, is co-administered with imipenem. Primaxin® is the name of the combination product. Meropenem has a spectrum of activity similar to imipenem, but is not metabolized in the kidney and is administered alone.

Because many microorganisms produce **penicillinase**, the addition of a β-lactamase inhibitor such as sulbactam or clavulanic acid to a penicillin antibiotic produces a highly effective antianaerobic agent. Augmentin® (amoxicillin with clavulanic acid) administered orally, and Unasyn® (ampicillin with sulbactam) and Timentin® (ticarcillin with clavulanate potassium) administered parenterally are examples of an enzyme inhibitor combined with an antibiotic.

---

bactericidal
kills bacteria.

bacteriostatic
retards bacteria growth.

Penicillins and cepalosporins are the major classes of antibiotics that work by inhibiting cell wall synthesis in bacteria.

ANTI-INFECTIVES (cont'd)

Cephalosporins

In the 1970s, the "first generation" of cephalosporins included the orally administered cephalexin and the parenterally administered cephalothin and cephaloridine. In 1973, cefazolin became the first cephalosporin to bear the designation of "cef-" instead of "ceph-". Other agents are cephradine and cefadroxil. First generation cephalosporins are most active against gram-positive aerobes (bacteria that require air). **Gram** indicates a staining method for identifying microbes.

gram stain
a method for identifying microorganisms based on staining characteristics.

Cefamandole and cefoxitin are "second-generation" cephalosporins that show improved activity over first-generation agents. Cefuroxime was approved in 1983, and quickly replaced cefamandole. In 1985, cefotetan was approved and gradually replaced cefoxitin as the most effective cephalosporin against anaerobes (bacteria that do not require air). Other second-generation agents are cefonicid and cefmetazole.

"Third generation" cephalosporins arrived with the release of cefotaxime in 1981. These cephalosporins were active against serious aerobic gram-negative infections. Many were released in the span of three or four years: cefoperazone, ceftizoxime, ceftriaxone, and ceftazidime. Unfortunately, resistance developed rapidly to many of these drugs, in some cases within days of beginning antibiotic therapy. The more recent additions to this class are ceftibuten, cefpodoxime, and cefdinir.

Cefepime has activity against both gram-negative and gram-positive aerobes and is the first "fourth-generation" cephalosporin.

Other β-lactams

Aztreonam does not cause the same hypersensitivy reactions associated with the penicillins and cephalospoins.

Aztreonam is a parenteral synthetic antibiotic with a slightly different chemical structure than the penicillins and cephalosporins. This difference gives it substantial resistance to β-lactamases, which can destroy penicillins and cepaholsporins. In addition, aztreonam does not cause the hypersensitivity reactions commonly associated with the penicillins or cephalosporins.

Others

Vancomycin, teicoplanin, and bacitracin are cell wall inhibitors that are structurally quite different from the β-lactam penicillin and cephalosporin compounds and function by different mechanisms. Bacitracin is generally used topically and combined with other compounds such as neomycin or polymyxin.

Inhibition or Modification of Protein Synthesis

Some antimicrobial agents act by interfering with the microorganism's ability to synthesize proteins.

Aminoglycosides

Aminoglycosides, macrolides, and tetracyclines act by interfering with the microorganism's ability to synthesize proteins.

The aminoglycosides are bactericidal and effective against both gram-negative and gram-positive microorganisms. Streptomycin was the first aminoglycoside discovered (1944) and neomycin was isolated in 1949. The remainder of the class members are kanamycin, paromomycin, gentamicin, tobramycin, amikacin, and netilmicin. Spectinomycin has some of the structural characteristics of the aminoglycosides, but its overall activities are different from most aminoglycosides. In addition, spectinomycin is bacteriostatic.

CLASSIFICATIONS

ANTI-INFECTIVES (cont'd)

Possible side effects of aminoglycosides include deafness and renal failure.

Since their oral bioavailability is low, most aminoglycosides are parenterally administered. The aminoglycosides are quite similar in their actions, and they are also similar in their adverse reactions. Two well-known adverse reactions are **ototoxicity** (toxicity of the ear that might include deafness) and **nephrotoxicity** (kidney toxicity that might include renal failure).

Macrolides

Erythromycin, the first and still most widely used macrolide antibiotic, has been used since 1952. Until recently, erythromycin and troleandomycin were the only members of this class. Then azithromycin, clarithromycin, and dirithromycin (a pro-drug of erythromycylamine) were made available. Clarithromycin has been approved to treat the AIDS-related Mycobacterium *avium complex* (MAC).

Macrolides are effective against a wide range of microorganisms.

The macrolides are effective against a wide range of microorganisms and are primarily bacteriostatic. They have greater activity against gram-positive microorganisms than against gram-negative microorganisms. Erythromycin causes adverse gastrointestinal effects in many patients. Clarithromycin and azithromycin effect a smaller number of patients.

Tetracyclines

Tetracyclines are mainly bacteriostatic, but at high concentrations, can be bactericidal. They are effective against both gram-positive and gram-negative microorganisms. The first member of the class was chlortetracycline and was introduced in 1948. Other tetracycline drugs are now used and include tetracycline, doxycycline, minocycline, oxytetracycline, and demeclocycline.

Tetracyclines combine with metals such as iron, aluminum, calcium, and magnesium and should not be given with iron tablets, antacids, or milk products. This interaction is a major concern in children and pregnant women. Doxycycline interacts less with calcium but more with iron than the other tetracyclines.

Others

Chloramphenicol, clindamycin, and mupirocin interact with the same cellular sites as the macrolides.

Modification in Energy Metabolism

Sulfonamides

Sulfonamides are antibiotics that interfere with folic acid synthesis. They were the first bacterial agents. Their use began in the 1930s. Folic acid is essential for various processes in microorganisms. Sulfonamides used today include sulfacetamide, sulfisoxazole, sulfamethizole, sulfadiazine, sulfadoxine, sulfasalazine, and sulfamethoxazole. Trimethoprim and pyrimethamine inhibit folic acid synthesis in a different way and are used with the sulfonamides. The combination of sulfamethoxazole with trimethoprim is known as Co-trimoxazole (TMP/SMZ). Allergic reactions to sulfonamides are fairly common, but are generally not life-threatening. Sulfonamides are known to precipitate in the urinary tract, so patients are advised to drink plenty of water while taking them.

Sulfonamides should be taken with plenty of water.

ANTI-INFECTIVES (cont'd)

Modification in Synthesis or Metabolism of Nucleic Acids (DNA)

Quinolones

The quinolones inhibit an enzyme involved with DNA replication. Older quinolones, nalidixic acid, oxolinic acid, and cinoxacin are primarily used to treat urinary tract infections. The newer drugs in this class are called the fluoroquinolones because they have a fluorine atom in their structure. These newer drugs are effective against a wider spectrum of microorganisms.

The first fluoroquinolone was norfloxacin, approved in 1986. Other fluoroquinolones include ciprofloxacin, ofloxacin, enoxacin, lomefloxacin, levofloxacin, sparfloxacin, and grepafloxacin. All of the fluoroquinolones have fewer side effects and resistance generally develops slower than in the quinolone drugs.

Trovafloxacin and alatrofloxacin are related to the fluoroquinolone antibiotics. Trovafloxacin is the active drug and is the generic name for the oral tablets. Alatrofloxacin is a version of trovafloxacin and is the generic name of the intravenously administered product.

cation
a type of ion.

A major drug interaction can occur between the quinolones and certain cations (a type of ion). Antacids, iron supplements, and multivitamins with minerals that contain such cations as zinc and calcium can bind with the quinolones and decrease their oral bioavailability by as much as 90%. Staggering the administration times of the antibiotic and the antacids, etc., prevents the interaction.

ANTIMYCOBACTERIAL AGENTS

Mycobacteria are microorganisms that cause tuberculosis, leprosy, and Mycobacterium *avium complex* (MAC) disease in AIDS patients.

Tuberculosis and MAC disease are primarily respiratory tract infections. Leprosy initially effects the skin but ultimately involves the peripheral nervous system. All are chronic diseases requiring therapy for long periods of time.

Tuberculosis

Tuberculosis is an infectious disease which primarily affects the respiratory system.

Tuberculosis has been known for thousands of years, but the first effective drug, isoniazid (INH), wasn't used until 1952. The primary antituberculosis drugs include isoniazid, pyrazinamide, ethambutol, ethionamide, and rifampin. Isoniazid is the premier drug in this group. Secondary drugs include aminosalicylic acid, cycloserine, kanamycin, capreomycin, and amikacin. Rifapentine, approved in 1998, is the first new drug for tuberculosis in 25 years.

Therapy generally involves a combination of drugs. One reason is that each antituberculosis drug works by a different mechanism. Another is that resistance develops if only one agent is used. There are fixed-dose combinations such as Rifamate® (isoniazid with rifampin) and Rifater® (isoniazid, pyrazinamide, and rifampin).

CLASSIFICATIONS

Leprosy

The primary drug used to treat leprosy is dapsone, which is chemically similar to the sulfonamides. However, Mycobacterium *leprae*, the microorganism that causes leprosy, has become resistant to dapsone, and some infected populations have shown significant resistance. In light of this, the controversial drug thalidomide (Thalidomid®) has been approved for certain moderate to severe cases of erythema nodosum leprosum (ENL). Thalidomide is well known for its teratogenic effects and severe birth deformities. However, it has been considered the standard drug treatment for ENL by the World Health Organization since 1994, and has been under an investigational new drug application status sponsored by the US Public Health Service since the 1970s. The FDA has approved the marketing of thalidomide in the US under a comprehensive patient, physician, and pharmacist education and distribution mechanism called STEPS (System for Thalidomide Education and Prescribing Safety). Other drugs used to treat leprosy include clofazimine, rifampin, clarithromycin, and minocycline.

The controversial drug thalidomide has received new use in treating leprosy.

MAC

Mycobacterium *avium complex* disease is treated with a combination of clarithromycin or azithromycin and ethambutol. Other drugs that might be used in various combinations are rifabutin, clofazimine, ciprofloxacin, ofloxacin, or amikacin.

ANTIFUNGALS

Fungi have a more complex cell structure than bacteria or viruses, and antibacterial antibiotics are not effective against them.

For many years, amphotericin B was the most effective systemic antifungal drug available despite the variety of adverse reactions associated with its use. It is still used to treat the most serious fungal infections. Nystatin and griseofulvin are two other older antifungal drugs.

The "-azoles" work by changing the fungus cell membrane to cause it contents to leak out.

Miconazole was marketed in 1974 and was the first azole-type antifungal agent. Since then, ketoconazole, fluconazole, clotrimazole, econazole, and itraconazole have been approved. The "-azoles" change the cellular membrane so its contents leak out. The azole-type drugs have their own array of side effects, but they are less problematic than amphotericin B. There are several topically administered antifungals. This class of drugs include clioquinol, tolnaftate, undecylenic acid, naftifine, terbinafine, terconazole, and tioconazole. Most of these are available in cream formulations.

ANTI-PROTOZOAL AGENTS

Protozoa are single cell organisms that have infected humans for thousands of years. They are found throughout the world. In parts of Africa, Asia, and Central and South America, they are among the leading causes of disease and mortality. Protozoa are prevalent in developing areas where sanitation and public health measures are poor. Many different drugs having many different mechanisms of action are used to treat protozoal infections. Agents that inhibit folic acid synthesis include pyrimethamine, trimethoprim, sulfonamides, dapsone, and trimetrexate. Pyrimethamine, trimethoprim, and trimetrexate act on one enzyme involved in folic acid synthesis, and the sulfonamides and dapsone inhibit a different enzyme. A combination of pyrimethamine or trimethoprim with a sulfonamide can produce a greater effect.

ANTI-INFECTIVES (cont'd)

Several of the drugs used to treat protozoal infections are only available from the Centers for Disease Control and Prevention (CDC). These are supplied as investigational agents upon request:

- Bithionol
- Dehydroemetine
- Diloxanide
- Melarsoprol
- Nifurtimox
- Sodium antimony gluconate
- Sodium stibogluconate
- Suramin

The list below summarizes the major protozoal infections, the protozoa responsible and the common anti-protozoal drugs used in therapy.

- **Infection:** Malaria, caused by Plasmodium species
  Drugs: Chloroquine, primaquine, mefloquine, doxycycline, proguanil, quinine, pyrimethamine, sulfadiazine, quinidine

- **Infection:** Vaginitis, caused by Trichomonas *vaginalis*
  Drugs: Metronidazole, paramomycin, iodoquinol, diloxanide

- **Infection:** Chagas' disease caused by Trypanosoma *cruzi*
  Drugs: Nifurtimox, benznidazole, eflornithine, melarsoprol, suramin, pentamidine isethionate, sodium stibogluconate

- **Infection:** Sleeping Sickness, caused by Trypanosoma *brucei gambiense*, Trypanosoma *brucei rhodesiense*
  Drugs: Nifurtimox, benznidazole, eflornithine, melarsoprol, suramin, pentamidine isethionate, sodium stibogluconate

- **Infection:** Leishmania species
  Drugs: Nifurtimox, benznidazole, eflornithine, melarsoprol, suramin, pentamidine isethionate, sodium stibogluconate

- **Infection:** Mononucleosis-like syndrome, *in utero* infection, encephalitis, caused by Toxoplasma *gondii*
  Drugs: Pyrimethamine, sulfadiazine, spiramycin

- **Infection:** Diarrhea, giardiasis, enterocolitis, enteritis, caused by Entamoeba *histolytica*, Giardia *lamblia*, Cryptosporidium *parvum*, and Cyclospora species
  Drugs: Metronidazole, paramomycin, iodoquinol, diloxanide, furazolidone

With the rising incidence of acquired immune deficiency syndrome (AIDS), several protozoal infections have become more common. Infections due to Cyclospora *parvum*, Cryptosporidium, Toxoplasma *gondii*, Isospora *belli*, and Pneumocystis carinii are increasing in severity. Agents used to treat these infections include paromomycin, co-trimoxazole, pentamidine, dapsone, pyrimethamine, atovaquone, clindamycin, primaquine, trimetrexate, and sulfadiazine.

CLASSIFICATIONS

ANTI-INFECTIVES (cont'd)

ANTIMALARIALS

Malaria has been one of the most fatal diseases in human history from ancient times to the present.

It has been a major factor in a number of wars. As recently as the 19th century, it was widespread in Canada and the United States. Though it is now rare in the U.S., malaria is still a major problem in many tropical countries and for persons traveling to them.

Malaria is caused by the Plasmodium species of protozoa (specifically P. *vivax*, P. *ovale*, and P. *falciparum*). Sporozoites are introduced into the body through the "bite" of a female mosquito. The sporozoizites travel to the liver where they develop. When they have matured to merozoites, they are released into the blood stream (erythrocytic stage), and malaria symptoms appear. Drugs used against malaria act at the stage when the merozoites are released into the blood.

isomer
a variation of a drug that has the same molecular formula but a different arrangement of the atoms in the molecule.

Among the antimalarial agents, the quinoline derivatives are still the most important. Quinine was the first to be discovered in the 1600s, though it was not until 1820 that it was isolated and its structure identified. Its **isomer**, quinidine, is used primarily as an antiarrhythmic agent but is also used in cases of severe malaria. Quinacrine was the next drug approved for the treatment of malaria during World War II (1943). Chloroquine and hydroxychloroquine were also developed during WW II and were found to be less toxic than quinacrine. Primaquine was also developed during World War II. Mefloquine was developed during the Vietnam War in the search for an effective agent against the now resistant Plasmodium *falciparum*. Non-quinoline derivatives used in treating malaria today include pyrimethamine, sulfadiazine, tetracycline, clindamycin, and doxycycline. They are either used alone or more often in combination with quinoline derivatives. Halofantrine is given in cases of chloroquine or multi-drug resistant malaria.

ANTIHELMINTHIC AGENTS

Worms cause "helminthic" infections.

About thirty organisms that are common to man are often classified as intestinal or tissue nematodes (roundworms) and platyhelminths (flatworms). Flatworms are subdivided into the cestodes (tapeworms) and trematodes (flukes). Minor worm infections may show no symptoms, while major infections may be life threatening. Exceptions occur when a single worm or a limited number of worms gain access to a critical organ such as the brain or an eye, or when an adult worm migrates into and obstructs the common bile duct. Drug therapy is based on the infecting organism. The table below lists the drugs used for the major groups of helminthic infections. Ivermectin, suramin, and bithionol are available from the Centers for Disease Control upon request.

Infecting Organism	Drugs Available
Intestinal nematodes	Mebendazole, pyrantel, diethylcarbamazine, thiabendazole, albendazole
Tissue nematodes	Thiabendazole, albendazole, mebendazole, ivermectin, suramin, diethylcarbamazine
Cestodes	Praziquantel, albendazole
Trematodes	Praziquantel, bithionol, oxamniquine

ANTI-INFECTIVES (cont'd)

These drugs have various mechanisms of action. Albendazole, mebendazole, and thiabendazole appear to work by depleting the glucose stores in the worm. Pyrantel is a neuromuscular blocking agent. Praziquantel causes an influx of calcium that depolarizes the muscle cells in the worm, and leads to paralysis. Oxamniquine interferes with cell metabolism and growth.

URINARY TRACT ANTI-INFECTIVES

Urinary tract infections (UTIs) are treated with antiseptics and anti-infectives that inhibit bacterial proliferation in the urinary tract. Drugs that belong to this class include nalidixic acid, cinoxacin, fosfomycin, methenamine, and nitrofurantoin. Methenamine is not a true anti-infective. It is hydrolyzed to ammonia and formaldehyde in urine, and these are the active drugs of the compound. Many antibiotics with more general usefulness are also used in treating UTIs. These include cephalosporins, fluoroquinolones, penicillins, tetracyclines, and the trimethoprim-sulfamethoxazole combination.

ANTINEOPLASTICS

Cancer cells disregard the normal controls on cellular growth.

Chemotherapy involves using multiple drugs that act on cancer cells in different ways and have multiple side effects. It's given in cycles, with rest periods that allow the patient to recover.

They multiply out of control, have abnormal genetic content, and are generally nonfunctional. Tumors (also called **neoplasms** or cancers), and are either benign (nonprogressive) or malignant (spreading, growing worse). Over 100 different types of malignant neoplasms occur in man. In treating cancers, multiple drug therapy is used to take advantage of drugs that have different mechanisms of action. Because chemotherapy is more effective when cells are dividing rapidly, it is given in cycles that allow rest periods during which normal tissue is allowed to recover and tumor cells are allowed to re-enter a rapid division phase for the next cycle of chemotherapy.

ALKYLATING AGENTS

Alkylating agents act on nucleic acids (the building blocks of DNA) to interfere with cell metabolism and growth.

Alkylating agents interfere with cell metabolism and growth.

The first alkylating agents were developed from mustard gas used in World War I. Mechlorethamine (nitrogen mustard) was the first agent of this new class. Cyclophosphamide, chlorambucil, and melphalan are derivatives of nitrogen mustard. Melphalan and chlorambucil are no longer widely used. Another group of alkylating drugs is the nitrosoureas. Carmustine, lomustine, and streptozocin are used for very specific organ tumors such as brain, lung, and pancreas.

Other alkylating agents not related to the nitrogen mustards and nitrosoureas are procarbazine, dacarbazine, altretamine, thioTEPA, and busulfan. The platinum compounds, cisplatin and carboplatin, also are not related to the nitrogen mustards and nitrosoureas.

CLASSIFICATIONS

ANTINEOPLASTICS (cont'd)

ANTIMETABOLITES

Antimetabolites prevent cancer cell growth by becoming incorporated into its DNA and preventing it from functioning normally.

Antimetabolites prevent cancer cell growth by affecting its DNA.

Methotrexate (MTX) is one of the most versatile antineoplastics since it can be used in many malignancies. Methotrexate is the only anticancer drug for which an agent (calcium leucovorin) is available to reduce toxicity. Other antimetabolites include 5-fluorouracil (5-FU) and floxuridine. Cytarabine (Ara-C), mercaptopurine (6-MP), thioguanine (6-TG), and hydroxyurea are older members of this group while gemcitabine and fludarabine are newer agents. Capecitabine was approved in 1998.

ANTIBIOTICS

Some antibiotics are very effective in the treatment of certain tumors. These include bleomycin, pentostatin, idarubicin, doxorubicin, daunorubicin, actinomycin D (dactinomycin), mitomycin, mithramycin (its new name is plicamycin), and mitoxantrone. Their primary mechanism of action is to inhibit RNA synthesis.

HORMONAL AGENTS

A number of tumors depend upon hormones for their growth and development.

Hormonal anticancer drugs either block hormone production or block hormone action. Tamoxifen was the first hormonal antineoplastic agent and it blocks estrogen action in breast cancer cells. A chemical derivative of tamoxifen, toremifene also has antiestrogen activity and has been successful in treating selected tamoxifen failures.

Hormonal antineoplastics either block hormone production or hormone action.

Many hormonal anticancer drugs are available. They are often classed by the hormones they effect. For example, testolactone affects androgen, and bicalutamide, flutamide, and nilutamide are antiandrogen agents. Other drugs and the associated hormones (in parenthesis) are: megestrol and medroxyprogesterone (progestins), diethylstilbestrol (estrogen), estramustine (estrogen), and leuprolide and goserelin (gonadotropine-releasing hormone). Some drugs inhibit enzymes that are important for hormonal production: anastrozole, vorozole, and letrozole inhibit aromatase that is important in the conversion of androgens into estrogens.

PLANT ALKALOIDS

Plant alkaloids are antineoplastics derived from natural products or are semisynthetically created using natural products.

The periwinkle plant yields vincristine, vinblastine, and vinorelbine. The yew tree yields paclitaxel and docetaxel. Paclitaxel, docetaxel, vincristine, vinblastine, and vinorelbine all affect tubulin, a protein involved in cell division. The mayapple plant provides the starting material for the semisynthetic derivatives of etoposide and teniposide. These compounds are inhibitors of topoisomerase, an enzyme involved in with DNA replication.

MISCELLANEOUS

Many other antineoplastic agents are available. Some examples include aldesleukin, a synthetic version of interleukin-2 which helps white blood cells work, and Interferons Alfa-2a, Alfa-2b, and Alfa-n3 which interfere with RNA and protein synthesis.

ANTI-PARKINSON'S DISEASE

Parkinson's disease is a progressive disorder of the nervous system characterized by muscle tremors, weakness, and rigidity or stiffness of joints.

Parkinson's disease is associated with reduced dopamine levels in the brain, and Anti–Parkinson drugs are designed to increase dopamine levels.

The disease is age related, with the large majority of patients over 50 years of age. The tremor of Parkinson's disease occurs during periods of rest and is often reduced during voluntary movement. Patients may be unable to maintain a normal posture, which results in awkward movement and frequent falls. The disease may also be accompanied with severe impairments of thinking, memory, and language characteristic of dementia.

The disease is associated with a dramatic reduction in dopamine concentrations in the brain, and an increased concentration of acetylcholine. L-Dopa (levodopa, L-dihydroxyphenylalanine) is the most effective drug for treating Parkinson's disease. Levodopa is converted to dopamine by the enzyme L-aromatic amino acid decarboxylase, which is found in many tissues throughout the body. To assure the bioavailability of dopamine inside the brain (the site of action), a decarboxylase inhibitor, carbidopa, is often co-administered with levodopa.

Levodopa's effectiveness in a patient gradually diminishes after several years in most cases, so dopamine receptor agonists may be added to the treatment. Bromocriptine and pergolide are two available dopamine agonists, but they are not as effective as levodopa. Other dopamine receptor agonists include amantadine and selegiline. Pramipexole, a specific dopamine-D_3 receptor agonist, and ropinirole, a specific dopamine-D_2 receptor agonist, can be used alone in early therapy or in combination with levodopa/carbidopa in more advanced disease states.

Cholinergic receptor antagonists used in Parkinson's disease include benztropine, biperidin, procyclidine, trihexyphenidyl, ethopropazine, and diphenhydramine. These too are less effective than levodopa, but offer alternative or adjunctive therapy.

Tolcapone (approved in 1998) is an oral catechol-O-methyltransferase (COMT) inhibitor. COMT is responsible for the metabolism of dopa, dopamine, norepinephrine, epinephrine, and other similarly structured neurotransmitters. Tolcapone is used as an adjunct to levodopa/carbidopa treatment. Both tolcapone and a related drug, entacapone, prolong the activity of levodopa. However, tolcapone is more potent and longer acting than entacapone.

CLASSIFICATIONS

ANTIVIRALS

Viruses invade host cells and use the DNA or RNA of the host cell to copy or replicate themselves.

They cannot replicate themselves independently. Some viruses can invade cells and remain dormant for long periods of time. Therefore, the symptoms of viral infections may appear without an immediately identifiable exposure to the virus. Some illnesses caused by viruses are hepatitis B, genital herpes, warts, encephalitis, influenza, measles, AIDS, rabies, rubella, yellow fever, herpes zoster (shingles), and many upper respiratory tract and eye infections.

Many antiviral agents work by inhibiting a step in the viral replication process. They are considered **virustatic** because they do not destroy the virus but only block its replication. Many viral diseases require multiple drug therapy to effectively deal with viral mutations and resistance. Resistance to some antiviral agents has developed in as little as 3 months.

Uncoating Blockers & Inhibitors of RNA/DNA Synthesis

When a virus first enters the host cell, it removes its protective coating and introduces its genetic material into the cell.

Amantadine and rimantidine act at this step. Several antivirals block viral replication by blocking RNA and DNA synthesis. They are acyclovir, ganciclovir, foscarnet, ribavirin, and valacyclovir, penciclovir, and famciclovir. Additional antiviral agents are idoxuridine and trifluridine and fluorouracil.

Several drugs that inhibit **reverse transcriptase** (one of the enzymes involved in RNA and DNA synthesis) are used in treating human immunodeficiency virus (HIV) infections. The first of these drugs was zidovudine (AZT) which was initially tested as an antineoplastic drug but was not effective. Later, it was found to have activity against HIV. Other reverse transcriptase inhibitors include didanosine (ddl), zalcitabine (ddC), stavudine (d4T), lamivudine (3TC), nevirapine, and delavirdine. Fomivirsen is used for the treatment of refractory cytomegalovirus retinitis in AIDS patients. The combination of ribavirin and interferon alfa-2b (Rebetron®) is used for chronic hepatitis C.

Protease Inhibitors

After viral genetic material is produced by the host cell, it is converted into viral proteins.

A **protease** acts on these viral proteins to transform them into smaller subunits capable of infecting new cells. Blocking this protease prevents this process. Saquinavir became the first protease inhibitor in 1995. Indinavir, ritonavir and nelfinavir have subsequently been approved.

HPV Agents

Human papillomavirus (HPV) is responsible for genital warts.

One third of the sexually active population in the US is infected with HPV. Approximately 1 million new HPV infections occur annually in the US. Agents used to treat genial warts include trichloroacetic acid and topical fluorouracil. Imiquimod in a cream formulation has been approved for treating external genital and perianal warts.

Some antivirals act by blocking steps in the viral replication process.

CORTICOSTEROIDS

Cortisol (also called hydrocortisone) is the primary corticosteroid in humans.

It is synthesized in the adrenal glands. Cortisol produces a wide range of **glucocorticoid** effects that influence various metabolic pathways, modify the response of the immune system, and produce anti-inflammatory activity. It also has **mineralocorticoid** activity that alters electrolyte and fluid balance by influencing the kidney.

There are many corticosteroids in use today: hydrocortisone, cortisone, prednisone, methylprednisolone, prednisolone, dexamethasone, betamethasone, triamcinolone, flunisolide, beclomethasone, budesonide (Pulmicort® turbuhaler®), and fluticasone. Many have some mineralocorticoid activity, but they primarily have glucocorticoid activity. Hydrocortisone, prednisone, prednisolone, and methylprednisolone have significant anti-inflammatory activity. Dexamethasone, betamethasone, and triamcinolone have the maximal anti-inflammatory activity of the corticosteroids.

Corticosteroids are absorbed through the skin and into the vascular system, so careful application is needed to avoid systemic effects..

Glucocorticoids in creams, lotions, and ointments intended for cutaneous application are sometimes classed according to their potency. Clobetasol, diflorasone, halobetasol, and augmented betamethasone are considered **very high potency steroids. High potency steroids** include betamethasone dipropionate and valerate, desoximetasone, fluocinolone, fluocinonide, halcinonide, and triamcinolone. The **medium potency** drugs are betamethasone benzoate, hydrocortisone butyrate and valerate, and mometasone. The **low potency** topical glucocorticoids include desonide, dexamethasone, and hydrocortisone acetate. Some drugs are in more than one category depending on the dosage strength in the formulation or the salt form of the drug. Higher potency steroids should not be applied to large areas, the face, scrotum or areas with skin folds. **Systemic effects can occur if a significant amount of the corticosteroid is absorbed through the skin.**

Aldosterone is the major mineralocorticoid synthesized in the adrenal glands. There is only one drug that has a predominant mineralocorticoid activity and that is fludrocortisone.

DERMATOLOGICALS

The skin is the body's protective barrier against the environment.

Many different conditions or diseases are localized on or in the skin, requiring many different classes of drugs to be used in treatment. Conditions or diseases of the skin range from dermatitis caused by irritants or allergens to viral infections to severe burns. Product formulations used as dermatologicals also vary widely: ointments, creams, lotions, shampoos, sprays, bath additives, tapes, etc.

Dermatitis may be characterized by red, oozing, swelling, and/or scaling skin. Some causes of dermatitis may be easy to identify. For example, sunburn or poison ivy, drug reactions, reactions to food (hives), or insect bites are conditions where the

CLASSIFICATIONS

DERMATOLOGICALS (cont'd)

cause is easy to identify, and also easy to avoid (by sunscreen use, discontinuing drugs, avoidance of certain foods or insects). Products available for treating poison ivy contain many combinations of drugs:

➡ **astringents** (calamine, zinc oxide);
➡ **counterirritants** (camphor, methyl salicylate);
➡ **local anesthetics** (benzocaine, pramoxine, phenol);
➡ **antipruritics** (camphor, menthol).

Diaper rash is caused when skin is exposed to urine or feces. The exact cause is not known, but ammonia, bacteria, bacteria by-products, and pH may all be responsible. Methionine will produce ammonia free urine. Other products used for diaper rash include zinc oxide (drying agent), camphor (local anesthetic), kaolin (moisture absorbent), and the anti-infectives triclosan and eucalyptol to minimize bacteria proliferation.

Psoriasis is a chronic disease characterized by white scales over red patches on the skin. Most psoriatic lesions are found on the lower back, elbows, knees, scalp, and feet. Topical products containing coal tar, corticosteroids, and salicylic acid are often used. Additional agents include anthralin, calcipotriene, and ammoniated mercury. Methotrexate and etretinate are used systemically to treat psoriasis. Tazarotene, approved in 1997, is a topical retinoid prodrug for the treatment of psoriasis and acne vulgaris. Response to the drug may occur as early as 1 week and may be sustained as long as 12 weeks after discontinuation.

Dandruff (seborrhea) is characterized by epidermal flaking and scalp itching. The most commonly used antiseborrheic products contain the following active ingredients either alone or in combination: selenium sulfide, coal tar, pyrithione zinc, povidone-iodine, sulfacetamide, and chloroxine. These products are all available in shampoo formulations.

Topical anti-infectives include antivirals, antibiotics, and antifungals. The prescription drugs penciclovir and acyclovir are antivirals used to treat herpes labialis (cold sores) and herpes genitalis. Warts are also caused by viruses, but are generally treated topically with salicylic acid. Several antibiotics are used to treat minor cuts, wounds, and burns, where infections have been established. These antibiotics include bacitracin, neomycin, and polymyxin B. Erythromycin, tetracycline, and clindamycin are used to treat acne vulgaris; other acne drugs include adapalene, tretinoin (vitamin A), isotretinoin, azelaic acid, and sulfur. **In cases of second and third degree burns, bacterial infection is a serious complication to the healing process.** Nitrofurazone, mafenide, and silver sulfadiazine are given to both prevent and treat the sepsis that accompanies burns.

Common fungal infections include tinea pedis (athlete's foot), tinea cruris (jock itch), and tinea corporis (ringworm). Several drugs are used to treat these conditions: undecylenic acid, clioquinol, miconazole, econazole, ciclopirox, clotrimazole, triacetin, tolnaftate, nystatin, butenafine, ketoconazole, naftifine, and terbinafine.

GASTROINTESTINAL DRUGS

The gastrointestinal (GI) tract stores, digests, and absorbs nutrients and eliminates wastes.

The central nervous system and an variety of hormones regulate the GI tract organs. Treatable diseases include reflux esophagitis, peptic ulcer disease, delayed gastric emptying, gastroparesis, diarrhea, infections (e.g., Helicobacter *pylori* in peptic ulcer disease), and inflammation.

THERAPY ASSOCIATED WITH STOMACH ACID PRODUCTION

Secretion of stomach acid is regulated by histamine, acetylcholine, and other intestinal enzymes.

Peptic ulcers are benign lesions that occur from exposure to stomach acid and pepsin. Although the body has a mucosal "barrier" to stomach acid and pepsin, excesses of these agents or a defect in the mucosal barrier can cause the defense mechanism to fail and ulcers to form.

Antacids

Antacids neutralize existing stomach acid.

They do not reduce the secretion of acid. Antacids are generally composed of inorganic salts such as calcium carbonate, aluminum hydroxide, and magnesium hydroxide. Some antacids also contain simethicone, which is an "anti-gas" compound that reduces the bloating that sometimes accompanies gastric distress. Because of their short duration of action and because other agents are more effective, antacids are rarely used for treating peptic ulcer disease.

Gavison® is a combination of alginic acid, sodium bicarbonate, aluminum hydroxide, and magnesium trisilicate and is used to treat gastroesophageal reflux disease. Reflux esophagitis most often occurs when the lower esophageal sphincter allows stomach acid to flow into the esophagus. This produces painful irritation and inflammation of the esophageal mucosa.

Gastric Mucosal Agents

Sucralfate is an aluminum salt that acts with proteins at the ulcer site to form a protective layer.

It also binds pepsin and bile salts. Misoprostol exerts its action by inhibiting the secretion of stomach acid and enhancing the production of gastric mucus bicarbonate.

Histamine (H_2) Receptor Antagonists

H_2-receptor antagonists block the effects of histamine in stimulating gastric acid.

In 1977, the first H_2-receptor antagonist, cimetidine, was approved for use. Almost overnight, antacid therapy became outmoded. Tagamet® is probably one of the most prescribed drugs of all time. There are now additional H_2-receptor antagonists: ranitidine, famotidine, and nizatidine. These antisecretory agents have actions and adverse reactions similar to cimetidine, but are preferred because they do not have the drug interactions associated with cimetidine. Histamine produces a variety of physiological actions in tissues other than in the gastrointestinal tract, but H_2-receptor antagonists compete with histamine only in the gastrointestinal tract.

Antacid therapy was revolutionized by the introduction of cimetidine, a histamine receptor antagonist.

CLASSIFICATIONS

GASTROINTESTINAL DRUGS (cont'd)

Proton Pump Inhibitors

Omeprazole and lansoprazole also interfere with gastric acid secretion but by different means than the histamine receptor antagonists. They are also more potent in lowering the stomach's acid output.

PROKINETIC AGENTS

Prokinetic drugs increase the contractions of the smooth muscles in the GI tract and this increases the movement of material through the tract.

Prokinetic drugs increase the movement of material through the GI tract.

There are several mechanisms involved in the regulation of gastric emptying and movement, and each drug in this class affects a different mechanism. Prokinetic agents are used in a number of clinical situations such as gastroparesis, gastroesophageal reflux disease, gastrointestinal radiography, intestinal intubation, and for nausea and vomiting. Bethanechol and dexpanthenol are used in post-operative surgery.

Metoclopramide is a prokinetic agent and is also used as an antiemetic. However, it also produces sedation because of its dopamine receptor antagonism activity. Cisapride is used to treat gastroparesis and gastroesophageal reflux disease but has no antiemetic action.

ANTIDIARRHEALS

Diarrhea is an increased frequency of loose, watery stools and can be acute or chronic.
It is most often a symptom of bacterial or viral infection or some inflammatory or GI tract disease. Diarrhea results when the normal functioning of the large intestine is disrupted. This can be caused by a decreased absorption of water, an increased secretion of electrolytes into the intestinal contents, or an excessive amount of mucus production. The major concern with diarrhea is dehydration (loss of fluid and electrolytes).

Antiperistaltic Drugs

Antiperistaltic drugs inhibit the movement of the intestine.

Antiperistaltic drugs treat diarrhea by inhibiting the movements (peristalsis) of the intestine. Slowing the passage of intestinal contents through the GI tract allows more time for water and electrolytes to be absorbed. Diphenoxylate has been used for the treatment of diarrhea for decades. Loperamide, released in 1976, is more effective and has fewer side effects than diphenoxylate in acute or chronic diarrhea. In addition, loperamide offers a faster onset and longer duration than diphenoxylate.

Adsorbent Drugs

Adsorbent drugs work by attaching bacteria, toxins, and nutrients to their surface.

Adsorbent drugs such as charcoal, cholestyramine, attapulgite, polycarbophil, and kaolin-pectin (kaolin with pectin) work by adsorbing (attaching) bacteria, toxins, and nutrients to their surface. Polycarbophil adsorbs up to 60 times its original weight in water and is effective in decreasing diarrheal stools. Adsorbents are generally less effective than loperamide.

Secretion Inhibitors

Bismuth subsalicylate and octreotide inhibit intestinal secretions by distinctly different mechanisms. Bismuth subsalicylate prevents microorganisms from attaching to the intestinal mucosa, and appears to inactivate toxins that are produced by the microorganisms. Bismuth can turn the stool a dark black and this can be mistaken for blood. Octreotide inhibits serotonin secretion and is generally used in severe cases.

GASTROINTESTINAL DRUGS (cont'd)

Antibiotics

Antibiotics have both positive and negative effects in treating diarrhea. Some antibiotics kill the naturally occurring bacterial flora of the intestinal tract, and this can lead to diarrhea. In these cases, oral preparations of lactobacillus that replenish the intestinal bacteria are generally effective. In some instances, there is an overgrowth of a resistant microorganism such as Clostridium *difficile* that will lead to diarrhea. In these cases, antibiotics such as metronidazole and vancomycin are given. Prevention and treatment of traveler's diarrhea would include bismuth subsalicylate, loperamide, and perhaps antibiotics such as doxycycline and trimethoprim-sulfamethoxazole (Co-trimoxazole).

LAXATIVES AND STOOL SOFTENERS

The colon plays a significant role in fluid balance and excretion.

colon
the large intestine

Roughly one and one-half liters of fluid are absorbed back into the body from the large intestine daily. Constipation occurs when the fecal material in the colon becomes dehydrated. Non-drug therapy for constipation increases the dietary intake of fiber and water, both of which assist colonic contractions.

Constipation occurs when fecal material in the colon becomes dehydrated.

Drugs used to treat constipation are referred to as laxatives, stool softeners, purgatives or cathartics. Purgatives and cathartics rapidly promote the evacuation of a watery stool. **Laxatives should not be used chronically as they may cause dependence.** Psyllium is a possible exception in that it mimics the actions of food elements and is relatively innocuous. Laxatives are also commonly used to empty the colon before various diagnostic procedures. Stool softeners relieve constipation by hydrating fecal contents, which assists their movement through the colon.

Bulk forming laxatives (psyllium, methylcellulose, and polycarbophil) swell as they mix with the fluid in the intestine. They also soften the intestinal contents. Both of these actions stimulate the movement of the intestine. These agents generally take 12 to 24 hours or longer to act.

Stimulant laxatives irritate the lining of the intestine or the nerves in the wall of the intestine producing their action within hours of administration. These drugs are cascara sagrada, phenolphthalein, senna, and bisacodyl. Phenolphthalein can discolor the urine pink. Senna can color the feces yellow. Senna and cascara, due to their potency, can cause considerable abdominal cramping. Senna has been used successfully to overcome opiate-induced constipation in patients requiring large quantities of opiates. Castor oil is no longer recommended because it can cause colic and its stimulatory actions are strong enough to affect uterine contractility.

Saline laxatives are properly referred to as cathartics due to their rapidity of onset and tendency to promote a watery stool. These salts draw water into the intestine and the increased pressure stimulates movement in the intestine generally with 30 minutes to several hours. Milk of magnesia, magnesium citrate, and sodium phosphates are examples of this class of drugs.

Osmotic laxatives include mineral oil (used primarily in retention enemas), glycerin suppositories, and lactulose. These drugs increase the water content of the stool via an osmotic effect. Sorbitol is another osmotic laxative, but has a very powerful osmotic action that can cause intestinal cramps.

CLASSIFICATIONS

Emollient laxatives (stool softeners) facilitate the mixing of fatty and watery substances in the intestine to soften the fecal contents. Some of these products may take up to 5 days to act. Docusate (in various salt forms) is the major stool softener used in clinical practice.

PANCREATIC ENZYMES (DIGESTANTS)

Pancreatic acids in the small intestine are involved with the absorption of the fats, proteins, and starch that come from foods.

steatorrhea
a condition of excess fat in the feces.

Normally, there is an excess of enzyme secreted. However, if not enough enzyme is present, absorption of nutrients is poor and steatorrhea (excess fat in the feces) occurs. Very large doses of pancreatin and pancrelipase partially correct absorption so that a major improvement in fat absorption can be seen. However, steatorrhea is generally not reversed, even with large doses. Cimetidine or antacids may be co-administered to reduce the presence of gastric acid that would destroy the enzymes.

HEART DRUGS

The heart is a pump which uses complex chemical and electrical processes to function.

These processes stimulate the heart muscle to contract and relax systematically, and in the process pump blood through the cardiovascular system. This contraction and relaxation is referred to as the cardiac cycle. Because of its central role in the body, it is essential to protect the health of the heart and maintain or restore its normal function.

ANGINA PECTORIS DRUGS (ANTIANGINALS)

Angina pectoris is a heart condition characterized by sharp chest pains of short duration.

Sometimes pain is also felt in the arm or neck of the left side of the body. It is caused by an imbalance between the amount of oxygen needed by cardiac muscle cells and the amount of oxygen supplied to those cells. Pain decreases as the demand for oxygen is met by the supply. Antianginal drugs accomplish this by increasing cardiac blood flow and therefore oxygen supply, and/or reducing the heart's workload, which decreases the demand for oxygen.

Nitrates

vasodilators
drugs that relax and expand the blood vessels.

Nitrates are **vasodilators,** drugs that relax and expand the blood vessels. They reduce the heart's workload by reducing the amount of blood supplied to it. This reduces the pressure on the heart. The first nitrate, nitroglycerin, is still considered the drug of choice. Short-acting nitroglycerin products include sublingual tablets, translingual spray, and intravenous injection. Other formulations of nitroglycerin include a topical ointment, transdermal patches, and sustained-release capsules. The lingual products act within 1 - 3 minutes and last for 10 - 30 minutes. These are particularly useful for treatment of acute chest pain and for prevention of exercise induced angina. Transdermal patches are preferred for patient convenience. There are several transdermal patches, and no one product appears to be better than another.

HEART DRUGS (cont'd)

The one serious disadvantage of nitroglycerin is that its duration of action is short (generally 10-20 minutes). Long-acting oral nitrates include isosorbide dinitrate (ISDN), isosorbide mononitrate, erythrityl tetranitrate, and pentaerythritol tetranitrate. All of these drugs have similar activity.

Patients develop tolerance to nitrates if the drugs are used continuously for more than 24 to 48 hours. Tolerance can be prevented by having a nitrate-free period of 8 to 12 hours every 24 hours. For example, transdermal nitroglycerin can be placed on the skin in the morning and removed at bedtime.

Beta-blockers

Beta-blockers reduce the oxygen demand of the heart's muscles.

myocardial infarction heart attack.

These are the β-adrenergic receptor antagonists, generally referred to as the "β-blockers." When these drugs are used to treat angina, they produce a reduction in myocardial oxygen demand. There is generally also a reduction in the number of anginal attacks and nitrate requirements. Another benefit of these drugs is that they limit the severity and recurrence of **myocardial infarctions** (heart attacks). The β-blockers have many non-cardiovascular applications. They are used to reduce essential tremor, prevent anxiety, treat migraine headaches, and treat glaucoma.

The first β-blocker was propranolol and it was marketed in 1967. There are many β-blockers today, and they can be divided into the following categories:

➡ Nonselective blockers: timolol, carteolol, nadolol, propranolol, penbutolol, sotalol, pindolol
➡ Cardioselective blockers: atenolol, betaxolol, bisoprolol, esmolol, metoprolol, acebutolol
➡ Combined α- and β-blockers: labetalol, carvedilol

Calcium Channel Blockers

Calcium channel blockers relax the heart by reducing conduction and contraction. They also help the heart by relaxing the blood vessels.

Calcium ions are essential for the excitation of the conduction cells in the heart, and for the contraction of the myocardial cells. Calcium channel blockers inhibit the flow of calcium ions into the cells, reducing conduction through the heart as well as contraction. They also relax blood vessels, which increases the supply of blood and oxygen to the heart while reducing its workload. As a result, calcium channel blockers are also beneficial in treating hypertension.

Verapamil was the first cardioselective calcium channel blocker. The two other "first-generation" calcium channel blockers are nifedipine and diltiazem. "Second generation" blockers include amlodipine, felodipine, isradipine, nicardipine, and nimodipine. Bepridil is chemically and pharmacologically unique among the calcium channel blockers because it inhibits both calcium and sodium channels. It is reserved for treating angina after other agents have failed.

ANTIARRHYTHMICS

Disturbances in the rate or rhythm of the heartbeat are called arrhythmias. Arrhythmias may cause too rapid (**tachycardia**), too slow (**bradycardia**), or unsynchronized heart muscle contractions (premature contractions). Most arrhythmias are thought to result from disorders of impulse formation or conduction within the heart. The result of any arrhythmia is a decrease in the volume of blood pumped by the heart. Antiarrhythmic drugs are classified according to their effects on the impulse conduction and their mechanism of action.

CLASSIFICATIONS

HEART DRUGS (cont'd)

Class I Antiarrhythmics

These drugs block myocardial sodium channels. They are grouped into three subcategories, Ia, Ib, and Ic.

- ➥ The class Ia agents (quinidine, procainamide and disopyramide) produce **moderate** effects on depolarization.
- ➥ The class Ib agents (lidocaine, mexiletine and tocainide) produce **minor** effects on depolarization.
- ➥ The class Ic agents (moricizine and propafenone) produce **major** effects on depolarization.

Class II Antiarrhythmics

These are the β-blockers described above. Generally speaking, the use of β-blockers as antiarrhythmics is reserved for patients who require only control of ventricular rate during atrial tachyarrhythmias or who have mildly symptomatic ventricular arrhythmias. Antiarrhythmics in this class of drugs include propranolol, metoprolol, nadolol, atenolol, acebutolol, pindolol, sotalol, and timolol.

Class III Antiarrhythmics

Class III antiarrhythmics block potassium ion channels and include amiodarone, bretylium, and sotalol. Amiodarone has multiple electrophysiological effects. However, its use is limited because of its adverse effects. Bretylium is effective in treating **ventricular fibrillation** (the irregular heart action seen in cardiac arrest patients) in conjunction with cardioversion (heart shocks). It lowers the fibrillation threshold. Sotalol possesses both class II and III effects. The class II activity comes from one **isomer** of the drug and the class III effects come from another isomer. The sotalol marketed in the US is a mixture of the two isomers, and so the drug produces both class II and class III effects.

Class IV Antiarrhythmics

Class IV antiarrhythmics are calcium channel blockers. They slow conduction and reduce contraction. Only verapamil and diltiazem are indicated as class IV antiarrhythmics.

HEART FAILURE

Heart failure is a condition in which the heart does not function adequately as a pump.

When the left side of the heart cannot pump all the blood presented to it, fluid backs up into the lungs, causing shortness of breath and coughing. Less blood is supplied to the kidneys causing them to retain water and sodium, which leads to weight gain and swelling in the legs and feet. **Inotropes** are drugs that increase the force of cardiac contraction. There are three classes:

Digitalis Glycosides

The digitalis glycosides (e.g., digoxin and digitoxin) have been known for hundreds of years, but it wasn't until the early 1800s that the cardiac effects and renal diuretic activity of digitalis were identified. The digitalis glycosides produce their effects by inhibiting the sodium or potassium pump in the myocardial cell membrane.

ventricular fibrillation
irregular heart action seen in cardiac arrest patients.

isomer
a variation of a drug that has the same molecular formula but a different arrangement of the atoms in the molecule.

inotrope
a drug that increases the force of cardiac contraction.

HEART DRUGS (cont'd)

Adrenergic Receptor Agonists

Dopamine and dobutamine are the adrenergic receptor agonists used as inotropes. Dopamine produces many of the same effects as norepinephrine and epinephrine. However, dopamine has different pharmacological effects depending on the dose. At low doses, dopamine dilates the vessels in the heart and brain increasing the blood flow to those organs. At moderate doses, dopamine adds the cardiac inotropic effect on top of its vasodilatory effect. At higher doses, there is an increase in peripheral vascular resistance. Dobutamine is a synthetic version of dopamine but has different properties than dopamine. It does not have peripheral vascular activity.

Phosphodiesterase Inhibitors

Phosphodiesterase is an enzyme involved with the energy production of cells. Amrinone and milrinone are two phosphodiesterase inhibitors that are specific for the phosphodiesterase found in cardiac cells. They increases the force of cardiac contraction but not the rate.

HEMATOLOGICAL AGENTS

Blood coagulation involves a complex interaction of platelets, proteins, and tissue materials.

Clotting factors exist in the blood in inactive form and must be converted to an active form before clotting can be accomplished. The first step is the formation of a platelet complex that is most responsible for stopping bleeding. The second complex occurs when thrombin is formed and converts fibrinogen to fibrin. This second complex is an insoluble fibrin clot. Red blood cells adhere to the fibrin clot and ultimately form the true blood clot (thrombus). The following are the various clotting factors:

I	Fibrinogen		X	Stuart factor
II	Prothrombin		XI	Plasma thromboplastin antecedent
III	Tissue thromboplastin, tissue factor		XII	Hageman factor
IV	Calcium		XIII	Fibrin stabilizing factor
V	Labile factor, proaccelerin		HMW-K	High molecular weight Kininogen, Fitzgerald factor
VII	Proconvertin			
VIII	Antihemophilic factor (AHF)		PK	Prekallikrein, Fletcher factor
IX	Christmas factor, plasma thrombo-plastin component			

COAGULATION ENHANCERS

Many clotting factors have been produced from human plasma.

They are available for patients with deficiencies in one or more of these factors. For example, patients with hemophilia A have a genetic deficiency in Factor VIII and Antihemophilic Factor (AHF) is available for them. Factor IX Concentrates are available for patients with hemophilia B or who are deficient in factor IX.

CLASSIFICATIONS

HEMATOLOGICAL AGENTS (cont'd)

Vitamin K promotes the hepatic synthesis of a number of clotting factors. Phytonadione (vitamin K_1) is a synthetic analog of natural vitamin K. It possesses essentially the same type and degree of activity as the naturally occurring vitamin K. Some patients exhibit a severe hypersensitivity when receiving vitamin K for the first time. Consequently, extreme caution must be taken with these patients, especially if intravenous administration being used.

HEMATOPOIETIC AGENTS

Hematopoietic drugs assist or stimulate the growth of blood cells.

anemia
a deficiency of red blood cells in blood.

Erythropoietin is produced in the kidney and acts in the bone marrow to stimulate red blood cell (RBC) production. Deficiencies in erythropoietin production are seen in patients with renal failure and cancer. Patients with renal failure are routinely given erythropoietin. Cancer patients may receive erythropoietin to treat anemia, a common adverse effect of chemotherapy.

Anemia is a common side effect of chemotherapy.

The body produces other proteins involved in hematopoietic production: granulocyte colony stimulating factor (G-CSF) and granulocyte macrophage colony stimulating factor (GM-CSF). Filgrastim is identical to G-CSF and stimulates the proliferation of neutrophils (a white blood cell). Sargramostim behaves similarly to its natural counterpart GM-CSF. It stimulates the growth and development of red blood cells and several types white blood cells. Both of these drugs have been used to raise the neutrophil count after chemotherapy or radiation therapy. But because of sargramostim's breadth of activity, it is the agent used to accelerate recovery from bone marrow transplantation.

Pentoxifylline improves blood flow by decreasing blood viscosity. Oprelvekin is a genetically engineered interleukin-11 that stimulates platelet production and is used with chemotherapy patients.

ANTICOAGULATION AGENTS

Abnormal blood clot formation within blood vessels can cause heart attack, stroke, or pulmonary embolism (a blood clot in the lung).

These are all potentially fatal conditions. Anticoagulants are used to prevent these clots from forming. Anticoagulants are commonly called "blood thinners." The main concern with any anticoagulant therapy is excessive bleeding since the drug will prevent a clot from forming. Blood tests (assays) are used to maintain a level of anticoagulation that should prevent clot formation but not allow excessive bleeding.

anticoagulants act against blood clot formation.

Heparins

Heparin is a polysaccharide that was discovered in 1916 and is commercially obtained from hog intestinal mucosa or beef lung. Heparin is administered only by intravenous injection or infusion, and subcutaneous injection. Its anticoagulant effect is monitored by clotting assays such as the Activated Partial Thromboplastin Time (APTT) or the Prothrombin Time (PT). The APTT is widely used because it is quick, easily, and reproducible. Dalteparin, ardeparin (approved in 1997), and enoxaparin (approved in 1998) are low molecular weight fragments of heparin and have the same mechanism of anticoagulation activity as heparin. Danaparoid is another low molecular weight heparinoid that has activity similar to heparin.

Coumarins

The coumarins (dicoumarol and warfarin) resemble vitamin K in structure and act by blocking the synthesis of the clotting factors that are vitamin K-dependent. There is a 3 to 5 day delay before the anticoagulant effect of the drugs is observed and heparin is often given during that time period. The effects of the coumarins can be reversed with vitamin K. Warfarin is the most widely used coumarin derivative.

Thrombin Inhibitors

Hirudin is a protein isolated from the salivary gland of the European leech. One molecule of hirudin selectively and irreversibly binds one molecule of thrombin, even thrombin trapped in clots. Thrombin is a factor in many steps of coagulation and hirudin inactivates it by itself, as compared to heparin, which requires antithrombin III. Lepirudin, approved in 1998, is a recombinant form of natural hirudin.

Antiplatelet Agents

Antiplatelet drugs are used to prevent clot formation.

Antiplatelet agents are used to prevent arterial clot formation. Antiplatelet agents include aspirin, dipyridamole, ticlopidine, and clopidogrel. Aspirin and ticlopidine are more effective than dipyridamole. Ticlopidine is for patients who are aspirin sensitive.

Anagrelide is a platelet reducing agent that decreases elevated platelet counts. Abciximab is an antigen binding fragment (Fab) that binds to specific platelet receptors to prevent clotting. Abciximab is intended for use in combination with aspirin and heparin in heart surgery. Eptifibatide is an intravenous antiplatelet agent derived from rattlesnake venom. It interferes with the final phase of clot formation. Tirofiban also interferes with this phase.

Thrombolytic Enzymes

Thrombolytic drugs assist in dissolving blood clots.

Fibrinolysis is the body's system for dissolving clots after they have been formed. Thrombolytic drugs stimulate this process by aiding in the conversion of plasminogen to plasmin, which dissolves the fibrin within a clot. These agents include streptokinase, alteplase, urokinase, and anistreplase. Alteplase is a "clot-specific" thrombolytic agent. It produces plasmin primarily at the site of the clot, instead of throughout the systemic circulation. Anistreplase is a plasminogen streptokinase complex that slowly transforms to streptokinase to avoid a systemic effect. However, high doses have to be used, so the systemic effect generally results. The major side effects of the thrombolytic agents include bleeding and allergy.

HEMOSTATIC AGENTS

Hemostatic drugs prevent excessive bleeding.

Hemostatic drugs are used to treat or prevent excessive bleeding. Systemic hemostatic agents include aminocaproic acid, tranexamic acid, and aprotinin. Aminocaproic acid inhibits fibrinolysis. Tranexamic acid is for short term use (2 to 8 days) in hemophilia patients to reduce or prevent hemorrhages during and following tooth extractions. Aprotinin is used in patients undergoing cardiopulmonary bypass to reduce perioperative blood loss. Several topical hemostatic drugs are available. Thrombin (topical) is available as a powder. Microfibrillar collagen hemostat, a gelatin sponge, and oxidized cellulose are absorbable preparations used for minor bleeding from small capillaries, veins, and arteries when sutures are not practical or effective.

CLASSIFICATIONS

HORMONE RELATED AGENTS

Thyroid hormones are involved in many of the body's essential processes, including growth, metabolism, and CNS development.

desiccated thyroid
a dried animal thyroid.

THYROID HORMONES

Thyroid hormones are produced in the thyroid gland.
They consist of several substances including triiodothyronine (T_3) and tetraiodothyronine, which is called thyroxine (T_4) and are involved in many of the life-long developmental processes of the body. These processes include growth, metabolism, and central nervous system development. When administered as drugs, thyroid hormones produce effects that include decreasing cholesterol concentrations, stimulating the heart, and increasing the metabolism of proteins and carbohydrates. Diseases of the thyroid gland include **hypothyroidism** (an underproduction of thyroid hormone) and **hyperthyroidism** (an overproduction of thyroid hormone).

Hypothyroidism is treated by the administration of thyroid hormone. Desiccated thyroid is dried animal thyroid gland that contains natural T_3 and T_4 in its natural ratio. These preparations are generally prescribed in grains, the apothecary weight unit. Effects of these products vary because the concentrations of T_3 and T_4 vary between preparations. However, if desiccated thyroid is selected, patients should consistently use the same product and not switch brands. Example products of desiccated thyroid include Proloid®, Thyrar®, and Thyroid USP. Synthetic hormones are available. Levothyroxine is synthetic T_4, and liothyronine is synthetic T3. Liotrix (Thyrolar®) is a combination of T_3 and T_4.

The treatment of hyperthyroidism is more complex. Hyperthyroidism is often caused by an immune system disorder such as Graves' disease. In Graves' disease, antibodies produced in the person are directed to thyroid receptors in the same person and stimulate the overproduction of thyroid hormone. Anti-thyroid drugs, radioactive iodine, or surgery are used to reduce the effects of the excess hormone.

Anti-thyroid drugs block the synthesis of the thyroid hormones. Methimazole and propylthiouracil are anti-thyroid drugs that have been used since the 1950s. These agents are used in patients under 40 years of age having their first episode of Graves' hyperthyroidism, and in patients that do not need to have their thyroid gland removed. Methimazole can be dosed once daily, while propylthiouracil requires several doses per day.

Excess iodide can also inhibit T_3 and T_4 synthesis. Iodides were used as anti-thyroid drugs for many years, but today are used for other purposes. Iodine solutions include Lugol's Solution (8 mg of iodide/drop) and Saturated Solution of Potassium Iodide (SSKI) (50 mg of iodide/drop). Both of these products are dosed in drops, not teaspoonfuls, and diluted in juice or other liquids before administration.

ORAL CONTRACEPTIVES AND OVULATION STIMULANTS

Oral Contraceptives

The female sex hormones estrogens and the progestins control the development of female secondary sex characteristics, the menstrual cycle, ovulation, pregnancy, and many metabolic processes.

There are three natural human estrogens: 17β-estradiol, estriol, and estrone. The important natural progestin is progesterone.

Oral contraceptives (popularly called "the pill") include two types of formulations, estrogen and progestin combinations and progestin-only preparations. The combi-

HORMONE RELATED AGENTS (cont'd)

nation tablets work largely by inhibiting ovulation. They also change the lining of the uterus, slow the movement of the egg through the fallopian tubes to the uterus, and thicken the cervical mucus so that it is more difficult for sperm to penetrate through it. These effects make fertilization of the egg and implantation of the fertilized egg less likely if ovulation occur. The progestin-only pills do not inhibit ovulation as reliably and are more reliant on the other methods to prevent pregnancy.

When oral contraceptives were first developed, they contained high doses of both estrogens and progestins. Since that time, the doses of both hormones have been greatly decreased, improving the safety of oral contraceptives and reducing the number of side effects. Oral contraceptives now contain ethinyl estradiol or mestranol as the estrogen component and norethindrone, norgestrel, or ethynodiol diacetate as the progestin component.

Three types of combination oral contraceptives are now available: monophasic, biphasic, and triphasic. Monophasic tablets contain the same amounts of estrogen and progestin in each of the 21 tablets taken per menstrual cycle. Biphasic tablets contain a different ratio of estrogen to progestin for the first 10 days and the last 11 days of the cycle. Triphasic tablets vary the amount of hormones three times during the 21 days. The biphasic and triphasic tablets are designed to closely mimic normal hormonal changes and have fewer side effects. Progestin-only oral contraceptives contain the same amount of progestin (norethindrone or norgestrel) in each tablet.

Several longer lasting formulations have been developed. Medroxyprogesterone acetate (Depo-Provera®) is given as an injection every 3 months. The Progestasert® system, a T-shaped intrauterine device (IUD) provides contraception protection for up to 1 year. Levonorgestrel is implanted under the upper arm skin (Norplant®) and provides contraception protection for 5 years with the 6-rod system, or three years with the 2-rod system. Transdermal patches containing estradiol are also available. These patches use about 1/20th the amount of the daily oral dose of estradiol to achieve a similar effect. The transdermal patch is available either for twice a week or once every 7 days administration.

Ovulation Stimulants

Ovulation stimulants, or so-called "fertility agents," are used to stimulate or assist the ovulation process in infertility.

Human chorionic gonadotropin (HCG) was the first agent used to treat infertility. Its action is virtually identical to the luteinizing hormone (LH) that triggers ovulation. It also has activity identical to follicle stimulating hormone (FSH). FSH recruits and selects follicles (eggs) during the early phases of reproduction. Both LH and FSH are involved in follicular growth and maturation.

Clomiphene increases the output of LH and FSH. Menotropins and urofollitropin are human gonadotropins (**gonadotropins** are sex gland stimulants) and are combined with other therapies to aid in ovulation and achieve pregnancy. Menotropins has both FSH and LH activities. Urofollitropin primarily has FSH activity. Urofollitropin is obtained from the urine of postmenopausal females as compared to recombinant versions of FSH such as follitropin alfa and follitropin beta. Follitropin alfa is only given by subcutaneous administration while follitropin beta is given by either subcutaneous or intramuscular administration.

Since their release, amounts of estrogen and progestin in oral contraceptives have been greatly reduced, resulting in fewer side effects.

gonadotropins
sex gland stimulants

CLASSIFICATIONS

HORMONE RELATED AGENTS (cont'd)

Gonadotropin releasing hormone (GnRH) agonists are also used to induce ovulation in women with a dysfunctional hypothalamus. They also stimulate the release of LH and FSH. Gonadorelin acetate (not the hydrochloride salt form), histrelin, goserelin, and leuprolide are GnRH agonists. Nafarelin is a synthetic version of the natural GnRH but is about 200 times more potent, and is administered intranasally.

Multiple births are common when using these fertility agents. Clomiphene increases the risk of multiple births to 6 times normal. The combination of HCG and urofollitropin or menotropins also produces frequent multiple births. Therapy with GnRH agonists can also result in multiple births.

OXYTOCIC AND TOCOLYTIC AGENTS

Oxytocic agents stimulate uterine contractions. Tocolytic agents cause uterine relaxation.

Stimulation of the uterus is used in abortion, induction of labor, or postpartum hemorrhage. Uterine relaxants are used to prevent or arrest preterm labor, reverse over stimulation by oxytocic agents, facilitate uterine manipulations, and relieve painful uterine contractions during menstruation.

Oxytocin is a hormone produced in the pituitary gland that is commonly used to induce or assist labor in late gestation. The prostaglandins carboprost and dinoprostone are oxytocic agents used to induce abortion in early pregnancy. Dinoprostone is also used topically in late pregnancy to stimulate the cervix. Some ergot alkaloids (ergonovine, methylergonovine) are generally used for postpartum hemorrhage and **adjuvants** to delivery.

Tocolytic drugs relax not only myometrial muscles but also other smooth muscles and blood vessels. The β-adrenergic receptor agonists ritodrine and terbutaline have been widely used to prevent preterm labor. Magnesium sulfate is also frequently used.

The effects of ergot alkaloids ingested during pregnancy have been known for thousands of years and ergot was used therapeutically as a uterine stimulant nearly 400 years ago. Ergonovine and methylergonovine are primarily used as uterine stimulants. Methylsergide, ergotamine and dihydroergotamine are used in treating vascular headaches. Ergoloid mesylates is indicated for treating dementia. Bromocriptine is used for postpartum breast engorgement and as an anti-Parkinson's drug.

ANDROGENS AND ANTIANDROGENS

The pharmacological activity of androgens is the basis of male sex characteristics.

It is responsible for the normal growth and development of the male sex organs and secondary sex characteristics such as hair distribution, vocal cord thickening, body musculature and fat distribution. In both males and females, androgens stimulate body hair growth, bone growth, muscle development, and red blood cell formation.

Testosterone, the most important androgen in males, is produced in the testis. Women also produce it but in much smaller amounts than men. Men who are testosterone deficient are given testosterone replacement therapy. By contrast, excess androgen is not a clinical problem in adult men, though it may be in preadolescent males and in women.

---

adjuvant
a drug added to a prescription to enhance the action of the primary drug ingredient.

myometrium
the muscluuar wall of the uterus.

androgens
male sex hormones.

Testosterone is the most important androgen in men.

HORMONE RELATED AGENTS (cont'd)

Natural testosterone taken orally or through intramuscular injection is eliminated rapidly through urination and is generally ineffective. Esterified testosterone in an oil suspension is used for IM injection. Esterification (combining an organic acid with an alcohol to form an ester) prolongs testosterone action. Testosterone propionate has a relatively short duration of action (1 to 2 days). The more commonly used enanthate or cypionate esters can be given by deep IM injection every 2 to 3 weeks.

Transdermal delivery methods have been developed to provide continuous drug concentrations. Testoderm® is a transdermal system applied to the scrotum, where absorption is greater than through the thicker epidermis found elsewhere in the body. Androderm® is another transdermal system that is not applied to the scrotum but is applied to the back, abdomen, upper arms, or thigh.

esterification
combining an organic acid with an alcohol to form an ester.

Fluoxymesterone and methyltestosterone are synthetic derivatives of testosterone that have minor androgenic activity. Danazol is a weak androgen that interacts with progesterone as well as androgen receptors. Leuprolide stops the production of testosterone in males and estrogens in females.

Compounds that inhibit or block androgens are called antiandrogens or androgen antagonists. **Antiandrogens act by blocking the synthesis of testosterone, whereas androgen antagonists block testosterone action.** Drugs such as leuprolide, nafarelin, goserelin, and ketoconazole are antiandrogens. Flutamide, nilutamide, bicalutamide, spironolactone, and cimetidine act as androgen antagonists.

Finasteride (Proscar®) is a synthetic steroid that is used to reduce the size of the prostate in benign prostatic hyperplasia (BPH). Finasteride (Propecia®) is the same drug but in a different dosage form. This product is indicated for male pattern baldness. Finasteride may cause abnormalities in a male fetus, and women who are or may become pregnant should not be exposed to this drug in any form, including contact with semen from a sexual partner taking finasteride. Whole tablets are film coated to protect against exposure to the drug. Tamsulosin is an $\alpha 1_A$-adrenergic receptor antagonist that is fairly specific for the prostate. It is also indicated for the treatment of benign prostatic hyperplasia (BPH).

Anabolic steroids are derived from or are closely related to the androgen testosterone. They have androgenic as well as anabolic activity. Anabolic steroids promote the body tissue building processes and reverse the catabolic or tissue depleting processes. Oxymetholone, stanozolol, oxandrolone, and nadrolone are available as anabolic steroids. **Because of the potential for abuse, the anabolic steroids are scheduled as C-III controlled substances.**

CLASSIFICATIONS

The immune system defends the body against attack by microorganisms and disease.

When functioning normally, the immune system fights infection and disease by eliminating most foreign molecules and cells as well as abnormal endogenous molecules and cells. In cancer and other conditions where an infection becomes established, drug therapy kills only a fraction of the invading organisms or neoplastic cells, and a functional immune system is required to eradicate the remaining organisms or cells.

Cells of the immune system are formed from stem cells in bone marrow. They include B lymphocytes, T lymphocytes, erythrocytes, polymorphonuclear leukocytes, monocytes, macrophages, and mast cells. Of these cells, lymphocytes and macrophages are the primary cell types involved in the immune system. Another component of the immune response is antibodies.

IMMUNOGLOBULINS, FABS, AND MONOCLONAL ANTIBODIES

Antibodies (immunoglobulins) are one of the primary components of the human immune system.

They are produced in response to an antigen and bind only to that antigen. There are five classes of immunoglobulins: IgA, IgD, IgG, IgE, and IgM. When they are used as drugs, they provide active or passive immunization to one or more infectious diseases when there is not time for the body to produce the antibodies itself. They are also used in patients that are immunodeficient.

Immunoglobulins are obtained from donor plasma. They provide rapid initial protection but are not long-lasting (up to several months). Immunoglobulins administered by the intravenous route are generally more convenient, less painful, and more rapid-acting than when administered by intramuscular injection. Immunoglobulins used in intramuscular administration contain about 16% of gamma globulin (IgG). Those administered intravenously contain approximately 5% of gamma globulin.

Immune Globulin Intravenous (IGIV) and Immune Globulin Intramuscular (IMIG) provide immunization against a large number of antigens. IGIV produces desired effects almost immediately. IMIG generally requires 2 to 5 days to be effective.

Genetic engineering has produced a new class of immunoglobulins: monoclonal antibodies. They are reactive to a single antigen and can be produced in almost unlimited supply. The extension "-mab" is used for monoclonal antibodies. Another extension in drug name terminology is "fab". These drugs are **antigen binding fragments** of an antibody. These are the fragments of the whole antibody where the antigen binds. For example, Digoxin Immune Fab is a fragment of the specific digoxin antibody produced in sheep. It is used to treat life-threatening digoxin overdose, and has also been successfully used to treat digitoxin overdose.

Rituximab (approved in 1997) is a Fab of a genetically engineered monoclonal antibody used for the treatment of B-cell non-Hodgkin's lymphoma (NHL). It is the first monoclonal antibody to be used as a chemotherapeutic agent. Circulating B-cells are generally depleted within the first three doses, and remain depleted for up to 9 months in most patients after the drug is discontinued.

Immunoglobulins provide immunization to one or more infectious diseases.

Genetically engineered monoclonal antibodies have the advantage of being able to be produced in an unlimited supply.

IMMUNOLOGICAL AGENTS (cont'd)

Several monoclonal antibodies were approved in 1998. Palivizumab is used to prevent lower respiratory tract disease in high-risk pediatric patients. It is easier to administer than Respiratory Syncytial Virus Immune Globulin Intravenous (RSV-IGIV) and far more potent. Infliximab is a monoclonal antibody used to treat resistant Crohn's disease. It is also under investigation for use in rheumatoid arthritis. Trastuzumab is a monoclonal antibody used in treating metastatic breast cancer. It can be used with Taxol® as a first line therapy, or used alone after other therapies have failed.

IMMUNOSUPPRESSIVES

Organ transplants have been done in humans since the 1960s. But since a transplanted organ is "foreign," immunosuppressive agents are used to prevent organ rejection. The drugs used in immunosuppressive therapy each target a specific cell type of the immune system, eradicating that specific cell type but not affecting others. The principal drugs currently used include corticosteroids, azathioprine, cyclosporine, cyclophosphamide, tacrolimus, and mycophenolate. Most are very effective in inhibiting the immune response, but their toxicity limits their usefulness. A combination of drugs allows lower doses to be used that minimizes side effects.

Antibodies used in immunosuppressive therapy act against specific cell-surface components. Muromonab-CD3 is a monoclonal antibody that blocks the function of a molecule (CD3) in the membrane of human T cells. Daclizumab (approved in 1997) and basiliximab (1998) are newer monoclonal antibodies that act as interleukin-2 receptor antagonists.

> Immunosuppressive agents are used in transplant surgery to prevent organ rejection.

MUSCLE AND BONE RELATED

NEUROMUSCULAR BLOCKERS

Surgical procedures can be performed more safely and rapidly if skeletal muscles are relaxed.

Naturally occurring acetylcholine acts on muscle neurons to stimulate skeletal muscle tone. Neuromuscular blockers block the action of acetylcholine, though different muscle groups respond differently to this. Side effects of neuromuscular blockers can be significant, especially at high doses. They have no analgesic or anesthetic properties and are not alternatives to anesthesia or analgesia.

Neuromuscular blocking agents are widely used as adjuncts to anesthesia in surgery. Non-surgical uses include reducing general muscle spasms, reducing spasticity in neurological diseases and multiple sclerosis, and preventing bone fractures during electroconvulsive therapy. These drugs are also used as diagnostic agents for myasthenia gravis.

CLASSIFICATIONS

MUSCLE AND BONE RELATED (cont'd)

Neuromuscular blockers relax muscles or produce muscle paralysis.

There are two classes of neuromuscular blockers: depolarizing and nondepolarizing. A nondepolarizing drug prevents acetylcholine from stimulating motor nerves, resulting in muscle paralysis. D-Tubocurarine is an example of such an agent. It is a plant extract that is the active ingredient of the drug curare. Curare was used as an arrowhead poison that killed by causing skeletal muscle paralysis. Other nondepolarizing drugs include pancuronium, pipecuronium, doxacurium, vecuronium, mivacurium, atracurium, metocurine, rocuronium, and gallamine.

Succinylcholine is a depolarizing agent that is two molecules of acetylcholine coupled together and its action is longer than that of acetylcholine. Drugs that increase neuromuscular acetylcholine concentrations can often reverse the effects of the nondepolarizing agents. Neostigmine, pyridostigmine, and edrophonium are acetylcholinesterase inhibitors and are used to reverse the effects of nondepolarizing neuromuscular blocking agents.

Succinylcholine and mivacurium are short acting, with effects lasting 10 to 20 minutes. Intermediate acting agents such as atracurium and vecuronium have effects for 30 to 60 minutes. The long acting agents, tubocurarine, metocurine, pancuronium, doxacurium, and pipecuronium, have effects that last from 60 to 90 minutes.

SKELETAL MUSCLE RELAXANTS

Skeletal muscle relaxants have sedative properties and often reduce pain rather than directly relaxing muscles.

Skeletal muscle relaxants differ in many ways from neuromuscular blockers.

They are used for muscle sprains, strains, or spasms. They are not used as adjuncts to anesthesia. They all have sedative properties and many have CNS depressant effects, and it appears that these properties reduce pain, rather than a direct relaxation of muscles. Carisoprodol, chlorphenesin, chlorzoxazone, cyclobenzaprine, metaxalone, methocarbamol, and orphenadrine are drugs in this class of compounds. Three other drugs (diazepam, baclofen, and dantrolene) are used mainly for muscle spasticity associated with cerebral palsy, multiple sclerosis, and stroke.

BONE DISORDERS

Osteoporosis is a disorder in which bone mass is reduced resulting in bone weakness and fractures.

The calcium and phosphorus salts that form bone are constantly being absorbed out of the bone into the blood (**resorption**) and deposited back into the bone again. Osteoporosis occurs when more salts are resorbed into the blood from bone than are deposited back into the bone.

resorption
absorption of bone elements into the blood.

Osteoporosis is classified as type I or type II. Type I, also called postmenopausal osteoporosis, occurs predominately in women. Type I is associated with diminished serum estrogen concentrations and increased bone resorption. Type II, called senile osteoporosis, is caused by age related decreases in bone formation. The bone loss in type I is faster than in type II. Sodium fluoride plus calcium citrate has been found to be effective in stimulating bone formation. Intermittent administration of parathyroid hormone (PTH) also stimulates bone formation.

Bone resorption is inhibited by estrogens (ethinyl estradiol, conjugated estrogens, raloxifene), bisphosphonates (etidronate, alendronate, pamidronate, tiludronate, and risedronate), and calcitonin. Raloxifene produces estrogen-like effects on bone and lipid metabolism, but blocks the effects of estrogen on mammary tissue.

MUSCLE AND BONE RELATED (cont'd)

Calcitonin is a hormone secreted by the thyroid gland in humans. Calcitonin derived from salmon (calcitonin-salmon) has the same pharmacological actions as human calcitonin, although the two substances differ structurally. Calcitonin-salmon is approximately 50 times more potent than an equal weight of human calcitonin, but has a loss of effectiveness with continued use. This is probably related to a cellular event within the bone itself, and the formation of antibodies to the hormone.

Paget's disease of bone is characterized by both excessive formation and resorption occurring in an irregular manner in one or more bones. The bisphosphonates and calcitonin are approved for treatment of the disease.

OPHTHALMIC DRUGS

There are a variety of drugs used to treat conditions or diseases of the eye.

The diseases could include bacterial, viral, or fungal infections, inflammation, dry eyes, or glaucoma. Some drugs are used to aid in eye examinations and surgery. Topical application is the most common route of administration of ophthalmic drugs. The advantages of topical administration include convenience, simplicity, and patient self-administration. But topical products must be correctly administered since the eye has so many unique characteristics that limit the effectiveness of drug formulations (limited volume size, rapid clearing due to tear drainage, etc.).

Because of the special requirements for ophthalmic formulations, many of the drugs included in a product are not the active drug. Preservatives, viscosity-increasing agents, antioxidants, wetting agents, buffers, and tonicity agents are also included in the formulations. These control such factors as sterility, pH, isotonicity, etc.

Packaging standards have been proposed to help reduce confusion in labeling and identification of various topical ocular medications. When fully implemented, the standard colors for drug labels and bottle caps will include the following:

Therapeutic Class	Proposed Color
β-blockers	Yellow, blue or both
Mydriatics and cycloplegics	Red
Miotics	Green
NSAIDs	Grey
Anti-infectives	Brown, tan

ANTIGLAUCOMA AGENTS

Antiglaucoma drugs work by lowering the pressure in the eye that is caused by glaucoma.

Glaucoma is characterized by high pressure inside the eyeball, called **intraocular pressure.** If left untreated, glaucoma damages the optic nerve and retina and results in blindness. Glaucoma is caused when the outflow of aqueous humor fluid from the eyeball is blocked and pressure builds in the eyeball. **Closed-angle glaucoma** is a medical emergency that is surgically corrected. Antiglaucoma agents are used to treat closed-angle glaucoma until surgery can be performed. **Open-angle glaucoma** is a chronic disease treated with cholinergic receptor agonists, acetylcholinesterase

CLASSIFICATIONS

inhibitors, carbonic anhydrase inhibitors, β-adrenergic receptor antagonists, and adrenergic receptor agonists. **Each class of drugs lowers intraocular pressure by a different mechanism of action but in general they either decrease the rate of aqueous humor production or increase the outflow of aqueous humor from the eyeball.**

Cholinergic Receptor Agonists

Cholinergic receptor agonists were the first drugs used in treating glaucoma. They are still used as adjunctive agents. Drugs include acetylcholine, pilocarpine, and carbachol. Pilocarpine's effects persist for 14-24 hours when administered as a solution or gel. Pilocarpine is also available as an ocular insert (Ocusert®) placed between the lower eyelid and the eye that continuously releases drug and is replaced every 7 days. Pilocarpine counteracts the mydriatic (pupil dilation) effects of atropine used in ophthalmologic examinations. Carbachol is used less frequently than pilocarpine because its duration of action is only 6 to 8 hours.

Acetylcholinesterase Inhibitors

Acetylcholinesterase inhibitors are more potent and longer acting than the cholinergic receptor agonists. They include both **reversible** (short acting) and **irreversible** (long-acting) agents. A reversible inhibitor is physostigmine. Demecarium and echothiophate are irreversible inhibitors. The irreversible inhibitors are more likely to cause adverse reactions than the reversible inhibitor, and are generally reserved for patients who have not responded adequately to the other agents.

Carbonic Anhydrase Inhibitors

Carbonic anhydrase inhibitors are given as an adjunct to therapy. Dichlorphenamide, acetazolamide, and methazolamide are orally administered agents. Dorzolamide was developed to be a topical carbonic anhydrase inhibitor, and in 1998 brinzolamide joined it as the second topical drug.

β-Adrenergic Receptor Antagonists

β-Adrenergic receptor antagonists are often used as the first line therapy because they are more effective than the cholinergic receptor agonists, and have a more favorable adverse effect profile. They do not affect pupil size or ability to focus. They lower intraocular pressure by decreasing the rate of aqueous humor production. Typical drugs of this class used for ophthalmic purposes are betaxolol, carteolol, levobunolol, metipranolol, and timolol.

Adrenergic receptor agonists

Adrenergic receptor agonists include epinephrine, apraclonidine, dipivefrin, brimonidine, and atropine. They lower intraocular pressure mainly by increasing outflow of aqueous humor from the eye. Dipivefrin is a **prodrug** that has the same activity as epinephrine but fewer side effects.

prodrug
an inactive drug that becomes active after it is transformed by the body.

OPHTHALMIC DRUGS (cont'd)

OPHTHALMIC MYDRIATICS

Mydiatics are drugs that dilate the pupil, often for eye examinations.

Vasoconstrictors

The adrenergic receptor agonists used in the treatment of glaucoma increase the outflow of aqueous humor. They have additional effects such as:

- Pupil dilation (mydriasis)
- Relax muscles in the eye
- Vasoconstriction (an α-adrenergic receptor effect)
- Decrease in the formation of aqueous humor (a β-adrenergic receptor effect)

mydriatics
drugs that dilate the pupil.

Phenylephrine (2.5% and 10%) and hydroxyamphetamine are two such drugs used as mydriatics. Weaker adrenergic receptor agonists such as phenylephrine in a 0.12% concentration, naphazoline, oxymetazoline, and tetrahydrozoline are used as ophthalmic decongestants for symptomatic relief of minor eye irritations. They produce their decongestant effect by constricting the blood vessels in the conjunctiva.

Cycloplegics

These compounds have the same activity as the vasoconstrictors but in addition, they paralyze the accommodation reflex which focuses the eyes. Drugs with this activity include atropine, homatropine, scopolamine, cyclopentolate, and tropicamide.

OTHER OPHTHALMIC CONDITIONS

Allergic Conjunctivitis

Allergies may cause conjunctivitis. Drugs that block the release of histamine are used to treat it, including Levocabastine (which is indicated only for the signs and symptoms of allergic conjunctivitis), olopatadine (used to prevent itching of the eye), and emedastine.

Inflammation

Eye inflammation is treated with corticosteroids and NSAIDs.

Inflammation is treated with two classes of drugs, corticosteroids and NSAIDs. The corticosteroids are used to treat inflammatory conditions such as allergic conjunctivitis, nonspecific superficial keratitis, herpes zoster keratitis, cyclitis, and the cornea after injury. Fluorometholone, medrysone, prednisolone, dexamethasone, rimexolone, and loteprednol (approved in 1998) are ophthalmic corticosteroids indicated for these purposes. Flurbiprofen, suprofen, diclofenac, and ketorolac are the NSAIDs available as ophthalmic formulations. All four drugs have analgesic, antipyretic, and anti-inflammatory activities. Ketorolac and flurbiprofen are often used following cataract extraction.

Anti-infectives

Conjunctivitis is caused when the conjunctiva of the eye becomes inflamed due to infection, allergy, or environmental factors. If the irritation is due to an infection, then an anti-infective agent would be recommended. Bacitracin, gramicidin, chloramphenicol, tetracycline, erythromycin, polymyxin B, and trimethoprim are some of the agents used. Of the aminoglycosides, gentamicin, neomycin, and tobramycin are available for ophthalmic administration. Sodium sulfacetamide and sulfisoxazole are the sulfonamides available, and norfloxacin, ciprofloxacin, and ofloxacin are the quinolones used. Some of the anti-infectives are formulated in combination with each other and with corticosteroids.

CLASSIFICATIONS

Antiviral Agents

The antiviral agents used in topical ophthalmics are effective against herpes simplex viruses and cytomegalovirus. Idoxuridine, vidarabine, and trifluridine are effective against the herpes simplex infections of the conjunctiva and cornea. Ganciclovir is used for cytomegalovirus retinitis and for the prevention of retinitis in transplant patients. Foscarnet is used for AIDS patients with cytomegalovirus retinitis.

Topical Anesthetics

Some ophthalmic treatments might require a topical anesthetic. There are two available, tetracaine and proparacaine. They have about the same potency.

Artificial Tears

Artificial tears are lubricating solutions that are isotonic, buffered, and pH adjusted and stay in contact with the eye for prolonged periods of time. All of these are available over-the-counter and are intended for the relief of dry eyes. One product, Lacrisert®, is an insert made of hydroxypropylcellulose and is available by prescription only.

PAIN RELATED AGENTS

ANALGESIC AGENTS

Analgesia exists when no pain is felt even though the condition to cause it is present. Drugs that produce analgesia are called analgesics and fall into three groups. Two groups of drugs are used for mild to moderate pain. They are the nonsteroidal anti-inflammatory drugs (NSAIDs) and the salicylates (aspirin being the best known example). Some of these drugs also have antipyretic (fever reducing) activity and anti-inflammatory activity. The third group, the opioids, is used in cases of more severe pain. This class of drugs is also called "narcotic analgesics" and have a very high abuse potential.

Nonsteroidal anti-inflammatory drugs (NSAIDs)

NSAIDs are used to relieve mild to moderate pain, reduce fever, and treat rheumatic conditions. They are generally more potent than salicylates. The major side effects of most of the NSAIDs are gastrointestinal effects such as nausea, ulceration, bleeding, and gastritis. Some of the newer NSAIDs (etodolac, nabumetone, and oxaprozin) have fewer overall gastrointestinal problems compared to the older agents (indomethacin and sulindac).

The effectiveness of NSAIDs varies significantly between patients. A particular NSAID may be highly effective in one patient but not in another, and predicting effectiveness prior to use is very difficult. NSAIDs are initially selected based on their effectiveness for a specific condition and the dose to be administered. Lower doses of NSAIDs are given to produce analgesia, but generally there is no anti-inflammatory action. Higher doses of NSAIDs are generally required to produce the desired anti-inflammatory activity. The commonly used drug acetaminophen (Tylenol®) is also a NSAID that is used to relieve pain and reduce fever. Acetaminophen has no anti-inflammatory activity. It is a useful alternative to aspirin in children with chicken pox, in patients with ulcers or conditions likely to cause bleeding, and in patients with aspirin allergies.

Analgesic drugs block or reduce the perception of pain but not its cause.

NSAIDs vary greatly between patients in their effectiveness.

PAIN RELATED AGENTS (cont'd)

The NSAIDs are categorized by chemical group. The groups and representative examples are:

- **acetic acids**: diclofenac, etodolac, indomethacin, ketorolac, sulindac, tolmetin
- **pyrazolones**: oxyphenbutazone, phenylbutazone
- **oxicans**: piroxicam
- **fenamic acids**: meclofenamate, mefenamic acid
- **propionic acids**: fenoprofen, flurbiprofen, ibuprofen, ketoprofen, naproxen, oxaprozin
- **alkanones**: nabumetone, which is actually a prodrug similar to naproxen in chemical structure

Salicylates

Salicin is an extract of willow bark and the precursor to salicylic acid, an effective analgesic that is extremely irritating to the gastrointestinal tract. Many derivatives of salicylic acid have been made in an effort to avoid its GI irritation. Aspirin is a product of salicylic acid, and is converted to salicylic acid in the body. Aspirin is the main salicylate used today. There are a number of different aspirin products, some containing buffers and others with special coatings. All of these additives and formulation modifications are to decrease the gastrointestinal irritation that even aspirin causes.

The other salicylate salts (choline, sodium, and magnesium) and salsalate have less GI irritating effects than aspirin. Salsalate is insoluble in gastric secretions and is not absorbed until it reaches the small intestine. GI effects can be reduced if the salicylate is taken with food or a full glass of water. CNS effects can occur in patients taking large doses of salicylate. Tinnitus (ringing in the ears), hearing loss, and vertigo are some of the characteristics of "salicylism". These symptoms are reversible when the dose is reduced.

Salicylates are used for the treatment of mild to moderate joint, muscle, and nerve pain. Many salicylate products have anti-rheumatic and anti-inflammatory activity. They also have an antipyretic effect and can be used to lower fever.

Opioids

Opium is the white milky exudate of the poppy plant. Opium contains more than 20 different alkaloids. Morphine and codeine are the best known. Opium alkaloids interact with three different types of receptors in the brain. Each receptor type has been identified to have specific pharmacological activities:

μ (mu): stimulation produces euphoria, respiratory depression, and physical dependence

κ (kappa): stimulation produces analgesia via spinal pathways

σ (sigma): stimulation produces dysphoria and hallucinations

The alkaloids also interact with other receptors outside of the CNS, and so this group of compounds has various pharmacological actions in the body. The principal therapeutic uses of opium alkaloids are:

- relief of moderate to severe pain without loss of consciousness
- symptomatic treatment of acute diarrhea
- cough suppression
- maintenance therapy in opiate addicts

Aspirin is the primary salicylate used today.

Aspirin and other salicylates should be taken with plenty of water.

Aspirin should not be used in treating children with viral infections since it is associated with the development of the potentially fatal **Reye's Syndrome**.

CLASSIFICATIONS

PAIN RELATED AGENTS (cont'd)

agonist-antagonist
a drug with agonist activity at some receptors but antagonist activity at others.

rheumatoid arthritis
a disease in which the body's immune system attacks joint tissue.

The opioid analgesics (sometimes called **narcotic analgesics**) are classed as agonists or agonist-antagonists depending on their interaction with the opioid receptors. **Agonist-antagonists** have agonist activity at some receptors but antagonist activity at other receptors. Butorphanol and buprenorphine are in this class. The morphine-like agonists produce a stuporous, sleeplike state. The major agonists include morphine, codeine, oxycodone, oxymorphone, hydromorphone, methadone, meperidine, fentanyl, and propoxyphene. They tend to be less predictable and less addicting. Dezocine, nalbuphine, and pentazocine are the drugs in this class.

Others

Two drugs approved in 1998 are leflunomide and celecoxib. Leflunomide is an immunosuppressive agent that is used in treating **rheumatoid arthritis,** an antoimmune disease where the body's own immune system attacks joint tissues, leading to pain and inflammation, and often permanent deformity and disability. Celecoxib inhibits the release of inflammatory prostaglandins in the body and is indicated for treating rheumatoid arthritis as well as other inflammatory diseases.

MIGRAINE HEADACHES

Headache may be caused by a variety of disorders, and there are several different types of headaches. Migraine headaches are characterized by recurrent headaches that vary widely in intensity, frequency, and duration. There are several "triggers" to migraine headaches such as alcohol, caffeine, certain foods or drugs, psychological stress, emotions, depression, strenuous exercise, sensory stimuli such as light glare, and poor ventilation. Migraine headaches may be accompanied by nausea, vomiting, sensitivity to light, sensitivity to sound, vertigo, and tremor.

Migraine headaches are classified on the basis of whether they are preceded by aura (visual and sensory changes). Visual symptoms may include hazy vision, flashes of light, shimmering heat waves, etc. Possible sensory symptoms include weakness, facial tingling, and uncoordinated speech. Most persons who suffer from migraine do not have aura symptoms.

The cause of migraine headaches is not known, but is thought to be caused by the dilation of blood vessels in the brain. It is also possible that various neuronal factors are involved. Several classes of drugs have been used to treat migraine headaches such as NSAIDs, opioid analgesics, ergot alkaloids (ergotamine and dihydroergotamine), and antiemetics. Recent evidence has suggested that serotonin plays in role in migraine headaches, and selective serotonin agonists have been effective in treating migraines. Sumatriptan and three newer compounds released in 1998 (zolmitriptan, naratriptan, and rizatriptan) are selective serotonin agonists.

ANESTHETICS

Local Anesthetics

Cocaine was used clinically as a local anesthetic in ophthalmology, dentistry, and surgery in the late 1880s. In 1905, the first synthetic local anesthetic, procaine, was made and became the prototypical compound for this class of drugs. The more common local anesthetics are lidocaine, bupivacaine, and tetracaine.

PAIN RELATED AGENTS (cont'd)

Local anesthetics are used to decrease pain, temperature, touch sensation, and skeletal muscle tone. The degree of these actions depends on the dose and concentration of the drug and the site of application. Local anesthetics are used in a variety of clinical situations from topical application to the skin to injectable agents used for peripheral, central, or spinal nerve block. Some agents are used for specific indications in preparations intended for anorectal or ophthalmic use.

Local anesthetics are grouped by their chemical structure:

- ➡ **Esters:** procaine, benzocaine, butamben, chloroprocaine, proparacaine, and tetracaine.
- ➡ **Amides:** lidocaine, bupivacaine, dibucaine, etidocaine, mepivacaine, prilocaine, and ropivacaine.
- ➡ **Others:** dyclonine and pramoxine; suitable for patients with allergies to amides or esters.

The duration of action of injectable local anesthetic agents influences their use in various procedures. Procaine and chloroprocaine are the shortest-acting agents (less than 1 hour), followed by lidocaine, mepivacaine, and prilocaine, which have slightly longer duration of action (1/2 to 2 hours). The longer-acting agents include tetracaine (2-3 hours), bupivacaine (2-4 hours), etidocaine (2-3 hours), and ropivacaine. Ropivacaine exhibits a duration of 8-13 hours when used for peripheral nerve block. When used as an epidurally administered analgesic, its duration of action is only 3-6 hours.

General Anesthetics

General anesthesia has four characteristics: unconsciousness, analgesia, muscle relaxation, and reflex depression. Surgical procedures would not be possible without general anesthetics. Ether was the first general anesthetic used, but is flammable and explosive. Cyclopropane is also flammable and explosive, but halothane did not have these characteristics and has been used since the 1950s. Most of the general anesthetics used today are chemical derivatives of halothane or ether.

The general anesthetics are classed according to their route of administration, inhalation or intravenous injection. The onset of anesthesia produced by intravenous administration is more rapid, smoother, and more pleasant than that of the inhaled anesthetics. However, a combination of various agents is used. Anesthetics used in combination are used in small doses to avoid side effects. The combination may well include both inhaled and intravenous anesthetics.

Inhalation anesthetics include desflurane, diethyl ether (ether), enflurane, halothane, isoflurane, methoxyflurane, nitrous oxide, and sevoflurane.

With intravenous anesthetics, barbiturates and benzodiazepines affect the GABA receptors, and opiates influence the μ and k-opioid receptors. Other agents affect these and other receptors in the central nervous system. These anesthetics are alfentanil, etomidate, methohexital, meperidine, propofol, droperidol, ketamine, thiopental, fentanyl, sufentanil, diazepam, midazolam, and remifentanil.

A combination of anesthetics that can include both inhaled and intravenous agents are used in general anesthesia to produce a balanced anesthetic effect. This is because different anesthetics affect different receptor and so have different effects.

CLASSIFICATIONS

PSYCHOTROPIC AGENTS

Psychotropic agents are drugs that affect behavior, psychotic state, and sleep.

They are used to treat schizophrenia, depression, mania, anxiety, and arousal. Agents are grouped into three categories: antidepressants, antipsychotics (major tranquilizers), and sedatives-hypnotics.

ANTIDEPRESSANTS

Patients with major depression but not mania are said to have a **"unipolar"** disorder. Patients with both mania and depression have a **"bipolar"** disorder. Symptoms of depression include loss of interest in daily life, reduced appetite, insomnia, fatigue, feelings of worthlessness, and preoccupation with death or suicide. Symptoms of mania, by contrast, include inflated self-esteem, decreased need for sleep, and hyperactivity. Four classes of drugs are used in the treatment of unipolar depression. They are:

➡ Monoamine oxidase inhibitors (MAOIs)
➡ Tricyclic antidepressants
➡ Selective serotonin reuptake inhibitors (SSRIs)
➡ Heterocyclic antidepressants

Bipolar disorders are treated with lithium, and the anticonvulsants carbamazepine and valproate (valproic acid).

Monoamine oxidase inhibitors (MAOIs)

Monoamine oxidase (MAO) is an enzyme that metabolizes neurotransmitters such as epinephrine, norepinephrine, and serotonin. The activity of the enzyme is inhibited by drugs such as phenelzine and tranylcypromine (MAO inhibitors, MAOIs). Since the neurotransmitters are not metabolized, their action is enhanced. Inhibition of MAO is achieved in the first few days of treatment, but the antidepressant effect is generally not realized for several weeks. Characteristic side effects of these drugs include orthostatic hypotension (a drop in blood pressure upon arising) and a serious food interaction with aged cheeses, sausages, and red wine that results in severe hypertension. When MAOI therapy is discontinued, new MAO must be synthesized by the body. This may take up to two weeks after phenelzine therapy but may only require 3 to 5 days after tranylcypromine.

Tricyclic Antidepressants

The tricyclic antidepressants have a similar chemical structure and are all related. Tertiary amine tricyclic antidepressants (amitriptyline, clomipramine, doxepin, imipramine, and trimipramine) tend to be more sedating and have greater cholinergic receptor antagonist effects. Secondary amines (desipramine and nortriptyline) are generally better tolerated than the tertiary amines. Other secondary amines are amoxapine and protriptyline.

Tricyclic antidepressants affect norepinephrine and serotonin, and produce side effects which include dry mouth, blurred vision, constipation, difficulty urinating, dizziness upon standing, sedation, and sexual dysfunction. Mood elevation from antidepressant therapy may require 2 to 4 weeks of therapy, but the adverse effects are generally seen within a few hours.

MAOIs have a potentially severe drug-diet interaction with aged cheeses, sausages, and red wine.

Tricyclic antidepressants have side effects that include dry mouth, blurred vision, constipation, sedation, and sexual dysfunction.

PSYCHOTROPIC AGENTS (cont'd)

Selective Serotonin Reuptake Inhibitors (SSRIs)

The SSRIs are better tolerated than tricyclic antidepressants and have been used treat a wide variety of disorders including major depression, alcohol dependence, anorexia nervosa, borderline personality disorder, bulimia nervosa, eating disorders, obesity, obsessive-compulsive disorder, and panic disorder. SSRIs produce their effects by blocking the reuptake of serotonin. This class of drugs began in 1987 with fluoxetine. Since then, sertraline, paroxetine, fluvoxamine, and citalopram (approved in 1998) have been released. The primary side effect associated with the SSRIs is nausea. It will usually subside after a few weeks, but may be severe enough to necessitate stopping the drug. The highest incidence of nausea is found with fluvoxamine.

> The primary side effect of SSRI use is nausea.

Heterocyclic Antidepressants

The heterocyclic antidepressants are a chemically diverse group of drugs. Each affects specific neurotransmitters. Many of the drugs in this class are now considered third or fourth line agents. They include bupropion, venlafaxine, nefazodone, mirtazapine, maprotiline, and trazodone. Their antidepressant activity profiles and side effects are similar to the tricyclic antidepressants.

ANTIPSYCHOTICS (NEUROLEPTICS, MAJOR TRANQUILIZERS)

The term "**neuroleptic**" refers to the effects this class of compounds produces. They decrease conditioned behavioral responses, cause a lack of initiative and interest, blunt emotions, and produce limited sedation. They are used to treat patients with various cognitive and psychological disorders.

Antipsychotics interact with many different receptors to produce their effects. For example, the histamine receptor antagonism of these agents results in sedation. The adrenergic receptor antagonism is responsible for orthostatic hypotension and increased heart rate. The cholinergic receptor antagonism causes urinary retention, and memory impairment. "Typical" antipsychotics (D_1 and D_2 receptor antagonists) also have side effects of muscle rigidity, motor restlessness, and neck and facial muscle spasms.

> Antipsychotics have various side effects, depending upon their action. These include rapid heart beat, difficulty urinating, memory impairment, and muscle spasms.

The major class of drugs used as antipsychotics is the phenothiazines. Chlorpromazine, prochlorperazine, thioridazine, trifluoperazine, perphenazine, fluphenazine, and thiothixene are members of this group of agents. Haloperidol and loxapine share many of the same side effects as the phenothiazines, though they are structurally different. Atypical agents (D_4 antagonists) include clozapine, risperidone, olanzapine, sertindole, pimozide, and quetiapine.

SEDATIVES - HYPNOTICS

Sedatives are used to reduce anxiety (anxiolytic) or produce a calming effect. Hypnotic drugs are used to produce sleep or drowsiness.

Anxiolytic Drugs

Anxiety is the most commonly observed symptom in patients suffering from mental illness, though it also occurs in normal people. Normal anxiety is usually brief and related to a specific cause. Pathological anxiety is general, prolonged, and interferes with a person's ability to function.

CLASSIFICATIONS

PSYCHOTROPIC AGENTS (cont'd)

The benzodiazepines, introduced in the 1960s, are the primary anxiolytic drugs. The benzodiazepines also have been used as muscle relaxants, sedatives, and anticonvulsants. They have also been used in alcohol withdrawal and light anesthesia. Benzodiazepines act in the central nervous system (CNS) on GABA receptors. The benzodiazepines used as anxiolytic drugs are alprazolam, chlordiazepoxide, clorazepate, diazepam, halazepam, lorazepam, and oxazepam.

Buspirone also has anxiolytic properties. However, it does not have the anticonvulsant or muscle relaxant properties of the benzodiazepines. Flumazenil, a GABA receptor antagonist, is used to counter the effects of benzodiazepines.

Hypnotics

Insomnia is a symptom for many disorders. Hypnotics are used for a short period of time while the cause of the insomnia is determined. Sleep disorders can be divided into four categories:

- ➡ insomnias, disorder of initiating and maintaining sleep
- ➡ hypersomnias, disorders of excessive sleep or sleepiness
- ➡ circadian rhythm alterations, disturbances in awake-sleep schedules caused by such as shift-work changes and jet lag
- ➡ parasomnias, dysfunctions associated with sleep or partial arousals.

There are many neurotransmitters involved in the sleep process, and so there are many different types of drugs used as hypnotics. Hypnotics are generally benzodiazepines or barbiturates, although some antihistamines are used. Benzodiazepines indicated for insomnia include flurazepam, triazolam, temazepam, quazepam, lorazepam, and estazolam. Barbiturates include pentobarbital, secobarbital, and amobarbital. The antihistamines include doxylamine and diphenhydramine. One newer compound, zolpidem, is not structurally related to the benzodiazepines but does act as a GABA receptor agonist similar to the benzodiazepines.

RESPIRATORY DRUGS

Asthma is characterized by the obstruction of the pulmonary airways.

The lungs of asthma patients are hypersensitive to common allergens.

Patients experience tightness in the chest, wheezing, shortness of breath, and/or coughing. Even when asthma patients have a normal airflow, their lungs are hypersensitive to a number of naturally occurring stimuli such as cold air, exercise, or chemical fumes. Patients with asthma are also hyperreactive to tests used to measure lung function. This is due to the inflammation of their bronchi. Inflammation can be caused by a variety of agents, but hypersensitivity to common allergens is usually the cause. These allergens as generally something like ragweed pollen, grass pollen, dust mites, cockroaches, and domestic animals. These allergens also cause the release of histamine, which can trigger bronchospasm, but antihistamines are not effective in treating asthma.

RESPIRATORY DRUGS (cont'd)

Treatment of asthma generally involves a multi-step strategy. Such an approach might include:

- → Avoidance of the causing factors when possible
- → Use of cromolyn and nedocromil to prevent histamine release
- → Use of anti-inflammatory drugs which include corticosteroids
- → Use of drugs that can reverse bronchoconstriction or inhibit its development
- → Use of drugs that reduce the frequency of recurrent attacks of bronchospasm
- → Use of bronchodilators

bronchodilators
a medication that decongests the bronchial tubes.

The inflammation associated with asthma is characterized by an **early phase** and a **late phase.** The early phase involves a histamine release that causes runny nose, sneezing, nasal congestion, mucus secretion, and itching and tearing of the eyes. Cromolyn and nedocromil are used to block the release of histamine, but this is largely preventive, since they are not bronchodilators, antihistamines, or vasoconstrictors, and are not useful in treating acute asthma attacks.

edema
swelling from abnormal retention of fluid.

Inhaled corticosteroids are a common treatment for asthma. Metered dose inhalers are generally used to deliver measured doses.

Late phase inflammation is caused by edema, mucous release, and the infiltration of eosinophil (a type of white blood cell) into the airways. **Corticosteroids (oral, parenteral, or inhaled) are given in asthma to decrease late phase inflammation.** In the mid-1970s, the first inhaled corticosteroid (beclomethasone) was made available. Administering corticosteroids by inhalation limits the adverse reactions that occur when they are administered orally or parenterally. **Long term use of inhaled corticosteroids in children is not recommended because the corticosteroids may suppress growth and suppress the adrenal glands' production of hormones.**

Beclomethasone, budesonide, dexamethasone, flunisolide, fluticasone, and triamcinolone are used as inhaled corticosteroids. They are administered by nasal inhalation or oral inhalation using nasal sprays or solutions. Most oral inhalation administration is by metered dose inhalers that deliver a fixed dosage each time the device is activated. These devices require that the patient coordinate inspiration with the action of the inhaler for optimal drug delivery. Administration of orally inhaled corticosteroids can be aided by the use of chambers or spacers.

Other anti-inflammatory agents include cyclosporine, zileuton, zafirlukast, and motelukast. Zafirlukast may also be effective in treating allergic rhinitis and in the prevention of exercise induced bronchoconstriction.

Drugs that can reverse bronchoconstriction or inhibit its development include epinephrine, which has good bronchodilatory properties, but has side effects on the heart and circulation. Other drugs used are isoproterenol, isoetharine, albuterol, salmeterol, terbutaline, pirbuterol, and bitolterol.

bronchospasm
a narrowing of the bronchi, accompanied by wheezing and coughing, i.e, an "asthma attack."

Xanthine derivatives are used to reduce the frequency of recurrent attacks of bronchospasm. Xanthine derivatives that are used in treating asthma include theophylline and dyphylline. Theophylline directly relaxes the bronchi and improves the body's ability to respond to **hypoxemia** (low oxygen levels in the blood). These compounds also inhibit histamine release. Theophylline is the most widely used oral xanthine derivative. Aminophylline is a form of theophylline and is the preferred parenteral preparation. Oxtriphylline is a choline salt of theophylline. Dyphylline is not a theophylline salt. It has about one-tenth the potency of theophylline.

CLASSIFICATIONS

hypoxemia
low oxygen levels in
the blood, which can
be caused by asthma.

Muscarinic receptor antagonists have been shown to be effective bronchodilators. They inhibit the effects of acetylcholine on the bronchi. Atropine and ipratropium are the two drugs with these actions that are used in treating asthma. They are administered by inhalation therapy. Ipratropium is the favored drug because of its very favorable side effect profile that is the result of its low systemic effect. Atropine has a higher systemic absorption, which produces more undesirable systemic side effects.

ANTIHISTAMINES

Histamine is primarily produced by the body in mast cells.

It is released from the mast cells in response to an allergen. Histamine appears to interact with at least three distinct receptors: H_1, H_2, and H_3. H_1-receptor activity causes bronchoconstriction, runny nose, sneezing, nasal congestion, mucus secretion, and itching and tearing of the eyes. H_2-receptors are involved in gastric acid secretion. H_3-receptors influence the release of neurotransmitters in the central nervous system (CNS) and the peripheral nervous system.

Antihistamines affect a
number of different
receptors, and as a
result have a variety of
effects. These include
dry mouth, sedation,
anti-itch, antiemetic,
and antitussive.

Antihistamines are H_1-receptor antagonists. Many of the antihistamines also antagonize various other receptors, which accounts for the array of additional effects seen with the antihistamines. These include dryness of the mouth, antipruritic (anti-itch), sedative, antiemetic, anti-motion sickness, antiparkinsonian, antitussive, and local anesthetic properties.

Patients develop tolerance to antihistamines and frequently a patient will need to switch to an agent in a different chemical class to restore the antihistaminic effect. The antihistamines are classed according to their chemical structure. The different chemical classes and agents are below:

Alkylamines
    Brompheniramine
    Chorpheniramine
    Triprolidine
Piperizines
    Cetirizine
    Cyclizine
    Hydroxyzine
    Meclizine
Phenothiazines
    Methdilazine
    Promethazine
    Trimeprazine

Piperidines
    Astemizole
    Cyproheptadine
    Fexofenadine
    Loratadine
    Phenindamine
Ethanolamines
    Clemastine
    Dimenhydrinate
    Diphenhydramine
Ethylenediamines
    Pyrilamine
    Tripelennamine

RESPIRATORY DRUGS (cont'd)

Decongestants

Decongestants increase drainage and reduce congestion by shrinking mucous membranes.

Decongestants produce vasoconstriction that causes the mucous membranes to shrink.

This helps drainage, which decreases the stuffiness in the nose. Decongestants are intranasally administered directly onto swollen membranes by means of nasal sprays or drops. Decongestants are also used systemically using oral administration. Intranasal administration is often preferred because it relieves congestion better. However, when intranasal decongestants wear off, the returning congestion is usually worse than before the decongestant was used. This "rebound congestion" does not occur when using oral decongestants.

vasoconstriction
a constriction of the blood vessels.

The decongestant drugs are grouped according to their chemical structure. The **arylalkylamines** include:

- ➡ Phenylpropanolamine
- ➡ Pseudoephedrine
- ➡ Phenylephrine
- ➡ Epinephrine
- ➡ Ephedrine

The **imidazolines** include:

- ➡ Naphazoline
- ➡ Oxymetazoline
- ➡ Tetrahydrozoline
- ➡ Xylometazoline

Antitussives

antitussive
a drug that acts against a cough.

Coughs can be classified as productive or nonproductive depending on whether or not phlegm is expectorated with the cough.

A productive cough is helpful if it removes phlegm from the airways. This type of cough should only be treated if the coughing is frequent enough to disturb sleep or is unbearable to the patient. A nonproductive cough without chest congestion can be treated with an antitussive (cough suppressant). A nonproductive cough with chest congestion can be treated with an expectorant to try to facilitate the expectoration of phlegm.

Antitussives can be divided into two groups: narcotics and non-narcotics. The narcotics codeine and hydrocodone have antitussive properties when used at a lower dose than required to produce analgesia. Non-narcotic antitussives decrease the cough reflex without inducing many of the common characteristics of narcotic preparations. Dextromethorphan, diphenhydramine, and benzonatate are members of this class.

Expectorants

Guaifenesin is the only expectorant recognized as safe and effective by the FDA.

Expectorants, in theory, decrease the thickness of phlegm from the lungs which aids in its expulsion.

However, there is little scientific evidence to show that they actually have those activities. Guaifenesin is the only drug recognized as safe and effective by the FDA. Potassium iodide may have expectorant properties, but terpin hydrate is no longer approved for use as an expectorant.

CLASSIFICATIONS

VASOPRESSORS

Shock occurs when there is not enough blood flow to deliver the necessary oxygen and nutrients to cells and tissues.

This interferes with normal cell function, and if severe enough, can result in death. Shock can occur even if blood pressure is normal. Shock produces many physiological responses. Early responses may be referred to as "warm" shock because the blood flow to the skin, arms, and legs is still maintained. If shock is not treated, however, there is a significant loss of blood flow to the vital organs, skin, and the extremities. This later stage shock is termed "cold" shock.

There are several types of shock. Hypovolemic shock occurs when the volume of the blood supply is reduced by hemorrhage, burns, or diarrhea. Cardiogenic shock occurs when the heart is unable to produce an adequate output. Septic shock occurs as a result of an overwhelming circulatory infection. Obstructive shock occurs when blood flow to the tissues is blocked.

The treatment of shock begins with the administration of fluids.

The treatment of shock starts with providing adequate fluids because attempts to increase the circulation with vasopressors will be unsuccessful if the volume of the blood supply is too low. Adrenergic agents are then used to increase heart contraction and to cause vasoconstriction. **The combination of increased heart contraction and vasoconstriction will increase blood pressure.**

Vasopressors increase blood pressure and stimulate circulation.

Epinephrine, norepinephrine, ephedrine, mephentermine, metaraminol, and dopamine tend to have both cardiac and vasoconstriction activities. Isoproterenol and dobutamine tend to have more cardiac activities while methoxamine and phenylephrine have more vasoconstriction activity with less influence on the heart.

MISCELLANEOUS NEW DRUGS

Sildenafil (Viagra®) is indicated for male erectile dysfunction and was approved in 1998. It is a phosphodiesterase (PDE5) inhibitor that was originally tested as an antianginal agent, but was found to be more effective to treat impotence. The drug is orally administered. Other agents for erectile dysfunction are administered by penal injection or urethral suppository. There have been many deaths worldwide of males taking sildenafil and nitrates.

Sibutramine (Meridia®) was approved in 1997 for the treatment of obesity. Sibutramine is rapidly metabolized when orally administered and the two primary metabolites are responsible for the therapeutic activity. These metabolites inhibit the reuptake of dopamine, serotonin, and norepinephrine.

Tolterodine, released in 1998, is the first new drug approved for urinary incontinence in 20 years. It is a muscarinic receptor antagonist that inhibits bladder contraction, decreases detrusor pressure and incomplete emptying of the bladder.

SOUNDALIKE DRUGS

It is important to recognize that a number of drugs have similar sounding or looking names, but very different properties.

Confusing such drugs can lead to terrible, sometimes fatal consequences. Therefore, it is critical to make certain that you have the name correct when involved in any aspect of the prescription process. Following is a list of drugs that can be mistaken for one another either by their sound or how they appear when written. There are many others, but this should illustrate the need for accuracy in drug names.

Acetazolamide	Acetohexamide	Halcinonide	Halcion®
Alfentanil	Fentanyl, Sufentanil	Hydralazine	Hydroxyzine
Amitriptyline	Aminophylline	Hydrochlorothiazide	Hydroflumethiazide
Atenolol	Albuterol	Hydrocortisone	Hydrocodone
Azathioprine	Azatadine	Kanamycin	Garamycin®,
Baclofen	Bactroban®,		Gentamicin
	Beclovent®	Lisinopril	Fosinopril
Bupropion	Buspirone	Magnesium Sulfate	Manganese Sulfate
Calcitonin	Calcitriol	Methicillin	Mezlocillin
Captopril	Capitrol®	Metolazone	Metaxalone
Cefamandole	Cefmetazole	Metoprolol	Metaproterenol
Cefonicid	Cefobid®	Nifedipine	Nicardipine
Cefotaxime	Ceftizoxime	Oxymorphone	Oxymetholone
Cefoxitin	Cefotaxime	Pancuronium	Pipecuronium
Ceftizoxime	Ceftazidime	Pentobarbital	Phenobarbital
Cephalexin	Cephalothin	Phenytoin	Mephenytoin
Chlorpropamide	Chlorpromazine	Pramoxine	Pralidoxime
Clomiphene	Clomipramine	Prazosin	Prednisone
Clonazepam	Clofazimine	Prednisone	Prednisolone
Clorazepate	Clofibrate	Primidone	Prednisone
Clotrimazole	Co-trimoxazole	Proparacaine	Propoxyphene
Cyclosporine	Cycloserine	Quazepam	Oxazepam
Dexamethasone	Desoximetasone	Reserpine	Risperidone
Digoxin	Digitoxin	Ribavirin	Riboflavin
Diphenhydramine	Dimenhydrinate	Ritodrine	Ranitidine
Dopamine	Dobutamine	Sucralfate	Salsalate
Doxazosin	Doxorubicin	Sulfadiazine	Sulfasalazine
Doxepin	Doxapram, Doxidan®	Sulfamethizole	Sulfamethoxazole
Dronabinol	Droperidol	Terbutaline	Tolbutamide
Dyclonine	Dicyclomine	Terconazole	Tioconazole
Encainide	Flecainide	Testoderm®	Estraderm®
Enflurane	Isoflurane	Thyrar®	Thyrolar®
Etidronate	Etretinate	Thyrolar®	Theolair®
Flunisolide	Fluocinonide	Timolol	Atenolol
Glyburide	Glipizide	Tolazamide	Tolbutamide
Guanadrel	Gonadorelin	Torsemide	Furosemide
Guanethidine	Guanidine	Tretinoin	Trientine
Guanfacine	Guaifenesin,	Triamterene	Trimipramine
	Guanidine	Vincristine	Vinblastine

GLOSSARY

abstracting services services that summarize information from various primary sources for quick reference.

active transport the movement of drug molecules across membranes by active means, rather than passive diffusion.

acute condition a sudden condition requiring immediate treatment.

acute viral hepatitis a virus caused systemic infection that causes inflammation of the liver.

additive effects the increase in effect when two drugs with similar pharmacological actions are taken.

adjuvant a drug added to a prescription to enhance the action of the primary drug ingredient.

admixture the resulting solution when a drug is added to a parenteral solution.

adverse effect an unintended side affect of a medication that is negative or in some way injurious to a patient's health.

agonist drugs that activate receptors to accelerate or slow normal cell function.

agonist-antagonist a drug with agonist activity at some receptors but antagonist activity at others.

aliquot a portion of a mixture.

alveolar sacs (alveoli) the small sacs of specialized tissue that transfer oxygen out of inspired air into the blood and carbon dioxide out of the blood and into the air for expiration.

ampules sealed glass containers with an elongated neck that must be snapped off.

anaphylactic shock a potentially fatal hypersensitivity reaction producing severe respiratory distress and cardiovascular collapse.

anhydrous without water molecules.

androgens male sex hormones.

anemia a deficiency of red blood cells in blood.

antagonist drugs that bind with receptors but do not activate them. They block receptor action by preventing other drugs or substances from activating them.

antibiotic a substance which harms or kills microorganisms like bacteria and fungi.

anticipatory compounding compounding in advance of expected need.

antidote a drug that antagonizes the toxic effect of another drug.

antihyperlipidemics drugs that lower cholesterol and triglyceride levels.

antitoxin a substance that acts against a toxin in the body; also, a vaccine containing antitoxins, used to fight disease.

antitussive a drug that acts against a cough.

arrest knob the knob on a balance that prevents any movement of the balance.

aseptic techniques that maintain the sterility of sterile items.

automated dispensing system a system in which medications are dispensed from an automated unit at the point of use upon confirmation of an order communicated by computer from a central system.

auxiliary labels labels regarding specific warnings, foods or medications to avoid, potential side effects, and so on.

bactericidal kills bacteria.

bacteriostatic retards bacteria growth.

bevel an angled surface, as with the tip of a needle.

bioavailability the relative amount of an administered dose that reaches the general circulation and the rate at which this occurs.

biocompatibility not irritating or infection or abscess causing to body tissue.

bioequivalence the comparison of bioavailability between two dosage forms.

biopharmaceutics the study of the factors associated with drug products and physiological processes, and the resulting systemic concentrations of the drugs.

blocker another term for an antagonist drug, because antagonists block the action of neurotranmitters.

body surface area a measure used for dosage that is calculated from the height and weight of a person and measured in square meters.

bronchodilators a medication that decongests the bronchial tubes.

bronchospasm a narrowing of the bronchi, accompanied by wheezing and coughing, i.e, an "asthma attack."

browser a software program that allows users to view Web sites on the World Wide Web.

buffer system ingredients in a formulation designed to control the pH.

calcium channel blockers drugs that lower blood pressure by relaxing blood vessels.

calibrate to set, mark, or check the graduations of a measuring device.

carcinogenicity the ability of a substance to cause cancer.

centralized pharmacy system a system in which all pharmacy activities in the hospital are conducted at one location, the inpatient pharmacy.

cation a type of ion.

certification a legal proof or document that an individual meets certain objective standards, usually provided by a neutral professional organization.

chronic condition a continuing condition that requires ongoing treatment for a prolonged period.

cirrhosis a chronic and potentially fatal liver disease causing loss of function and resistance to blood flow through the liver.

clean rooms areas designed for the preparation of sterile products.

co-insurance an agreement for cost-sharing between the insurer and the insured.

co-pay the portion of the price of medication that the patient is required to pay.

code carts a locked cart of medications designed for emergency use only.

colloids particles up to a hundred times smaller than that those in suspensions that are, however, likewise suspended in a solution.

colon the large intestine.

competent being qualified and capable.

complex when molecules of different chemicals attach to each other, as in protein binding.

compliance doing what is required.

compression molding a method of making suppositories in which the ingredients are compressed in a mold.

concentration the strength of a solution as measured by the weight-to-volume or volume-to-volume of the substance being measured.

confidentiality the requirement of health care providers to keep all patient information private among the patient, the patient's insurer, and the providers directly involved in the patient's care.

conjunctiva the eyelid lining.

consultant pharmacist develops and maintains an individual pharmaceutical plan for each long-term care patient.

contraceptive device or formulation designed to prevent pregnancy.

controlled substance mark the mark (CII-CV) which indicates the control category of a drug with a potential for abuse.

conversions the change of one unit of measure into another so that both amounts are equal.

coring when a needle damages the rubber closure of a parenteral container, causing fragments of the closure to fall into the container and contaminate its contents.

coring when a needle damages the rubber closure of a parenteral container, causing fragments of the closure to fall into the container and contaminate its contents.

GLOSSARY

counting tray a tray designed for counting pills.

database a collection of information structured so that specific information within it can easily be retrieved and used.

decentralized pharmacy system a system in which pharmacy activities occur in multiple locations within a hospital.

deductible a set amount that must be paid by the patient for each benefit period before the insurer will cover additional expenses.

denominator the bottom or right number in a fraction which is divided into the numerator to give the fraction's value.

depth filter a filter placed inside a needle hub that can filter solutions being drawn in or expelled, but not both.

desiccated thyroid a dried animal thyroid.

dialysis movement of particles in a solution through permeable membranes.

diluent a liquid that dilutes a substance or solution.

disposition a term sometimes used to refer to all of the ADME processes together.

distributive pharmacist makes sure long-term care patients receive the correct medications ordered.

diuretics drugs that increase the elimination of salts and water through urination.

drug-diet interactions when elements of ingested nutrients interact with a drug and this affects the disposition of the drug.

dual co-pay co-pays that have two prices: one for generic and one for brand medications.

dumbwaiter a small elevator that carries objects (but not people) between floors of a building.

edema swelling from abnormal retention of fluid.

emulsifier a stabilizing agent in emulsions.

emulsions mixture of two liquids that do not dissolve into each other in which one liquid is spread through the other by mixing and use of a stabilizer.

endogenous produced from within the body or within a cell.

enterohepatic cycling the transfer of drugs and their metabolites from the liver to the bile in the gall bladder and then into the intestine.

enzyme a complex protein that causes chemical reactions in other substances

enzyme induction the increase in enzyme activity that results in greater metabolism of drugs.

enzyme inhibition the decrease in enzyme activity that results in reduced metabolism of drugs.

equivalent weight a drug's molecular weight divided by its valence, a common measure of electrolytes.

esterification combining an organic acid with an alcohol to form an ester.

extemporaneous compounding the on-demand preparation of a drug product according to a physician's prescription, formula, or recipe.

final filter a filter that filters solution immediately before it enters a patient's vein.

finger cots protective coverings for fingers.

first pass metabolism the substantial degradation of a drug caused by enzyme metabolism in the liver before the drug reaches the systemic circulation.

flexor movement an expansion or outward movement by muscles.

flocculating agent electrolytes used in the preparation of suspensions.

floor stock stock (such as large volume parenterals) that does not require patient specific labeling.

flow rate the rate (in ml/hour or ml/minute) at which solution is administered to the patient.

formulary a list of medications that are approved for use.

fusion molding a suppository preparation method in which the active ingredients are dispersed in a melted suppository base.

gastric emptying time the time a drug will stay in the stomach before it is emptied into the small intestine.

gauge a measurement—with needles, the higher the gauge, the thinner the lumen.

geometric dilution a technique for mixing two powders of unequal size.

glomerular filtration the blood filtering process of the kidneys.

gonadotropins sex gland stimulants.

gram stain a method for identifying microorganisms based on staining characteristics.

hemorrhoid painful swollen veins in the anal/rectal area, generally caused by strained bowel movements from hard stools.

HEPA filter a high efficiency particulate air filter.

heparin lock an injection device which uses heparin to keep blood from clotting in the device.

hepatic disease liver disease.

hepato a prefix meaning "of the liver."

HMOs a network of providers for which costs are covered inside but not outside of the network.

home care agencies home nursing care businesses that provide a range of health care services, including infusion.

homeostasis the state of equilibrium of the body.

hormone chemicals produced by the body that regulate body functions and processes.

human genome the complete set of genetic material contained in a human cell.

hydrates absorbs water.

hyperuricemia an abnormal concentration of uric acid in the blood.

hypoxemia low oxygen levels in the blood, which can be caused by asthma.

hydrophilic capable of associating with or absorbing water.

hydrophilic emulsifier a stabilizing agent for water based dispersion mediums.

hydrophobic water repelling; cannot associate with water.

hypersensitivity an abnormal sensitivity generally resulting in an allergic reaction.

hyperthyroidism a condition in which thyroid hormone secretions are above normal, often referred to as an overactive thyroid.

hypertonic when a solution has a greater osmolality than that of blood.

hypothyroidism a condition in which thyroid hormone secretions are below normal, often referred to as an underactive thyroid.

hypotonic when a solution has a lesser osmolality than that of blood.

idiosyncrasy an unexpected reaction the first time a drug is taken, generally due to genetic causes.

immiscible cannot be mixed.

infusion the slow continuous introduction of a solution into the blood stream.

injunction a court order preventing a specific action, such as the distribution of a potentially dangerous drug.

inotrope a drug that increases the force of cardiac contraction.

inpatient pharmacy the hospital pharmacy in a centralized system.

inspiration breathing in.

Internet Service Provider (ISP) a company that provides access to the Internet.

interpersonal skills skills involving relationships between people.

inventory to make an accounting of items on hand; also, with people, to assess characteristics, skills, qualities, etc.

ion molecular particles that carry electric charges.

isomer a variation of a drug that has the same molecular formula but a different arrangement of the atoms in the molecule.

isotonic when a solution has an osmolality equivalent to that of blood.

GLOSSARY

IUD an intrauterine contraceptive device that is placed in the uterus for a prolonged period of time.

labeling important associated information that is not on the label of the drug product, but is provided with the product in the form of an insert, brochure, or other document.

lacrimal canalicula the tear ducts.

lacrimal gland the gland that produces tears for the eye.

laminar flow continuous movement at a stable rate in one direction.

legend drug any drug which requires a prescription and either of these "legends" on the label: "Caution: Federal law prohibits dispensing without a prescription," or "Rx only."

levigation triturating a powdered drug with a solvent in which it is insoluble to reduce its particle size.

lipoidal fat like substance.

lipophilic emulsifier a stabilizing agent for oil based dispersion mediums.

lumen the hollow center of a needle.

lymphocytes a white blood cell that helps the body defend itself against bacteria and diseased cells.

lyophilized freeze-dried.

maintenance medication a medication that is required on a continuing basis for the treatment of a chronic condition.

materia medica generally pharmacology, but also refers to the drugs in use (from the Latin materia, matter, and medica, medical).

material safety data sheets OSHA required notices on hazardous substances which provide hazard, handling, clean-up, and first aid information.

maximum allowable cost (MAC) the maximum price per tablet (or other dispensing unit) an insurer or PBM will pay for a given product.

Medicaid a federal-state program, administered by the states, providing health care for the needy.

Medicare a federal program providing health care to people with certain disabilities over age 65; it includes basic hospital insurance and voluntary medical insurance.

medication administration record (MAR) a form that tracks the medications administered to a patient.

membrane filter a filter that attaches to a syringe and filters solution through a membrane as the solution is expelled from the syringe.

meniscus the curved surface of a column of liquid.

metabolite substance resulting from the body's transformation of an administered drug.

milliequivalent (mEq) a unit of measure for electrolytes in a solution.

minimum effective concentration (MEC) the blood concentration needed of a drug to produce a response.

mimetic another term for an agonist, because agonists imitate or "mimic" the action of the neurotransmitter.

miscible capable of being mixed together.

modem computer hardware that enables a computer to communicate through telephone lines.

molecular weight the sum of the atomic weights of one molecule.

mucilage a wet, slimy preparation formed as an initial step in a wet emulsion preparation method.

mydriatics drugs that dilate the pupil.

myocardial infarction heart attack.

myometrium the musculuar wall of the uterus.

nasal cavity the cavity behind the nose and above the roof of the mouth that filters air and moves mucous and inhaled contaminants outward and away from the lungs.

nasal inhaler a device which contains a drug that is vaporized by inhalation.

nasal mucosa the cellular lining of the nose.

NDC (National Drug Code) number the number assigned by the manufacturer. The first five digits indicate the manufacturer. The next four indicate the medication, its strength, and dosage form. The last two indicate the package size.

necrosis the death of cells.

negligence failing to do something that should or must be done.

nephron the functional unit of the kidneys.

nephrotoxicity the ability of a substance to harm the kidneys.

nomenclature a system of names specific to a particular field.

nomogram a chart showing relationships between measurements.

numerator the top or left number in a fraction that indicates a portion of the denominator to be used.

obstructive jaundice an obstruction of the bile excretion process.

oil-in-water an emulsion in which oil is dispersed through a water base.

online adjudication the resolution of prescription coverage through the communication of the pharmacy computer with the third party computer.

onset of action the time MEC is reached and the response occurs.

ophthalmic related to the eye.

Orange Book the common name for the FDA's Approved Drugs Products.

orthostatic hypertension a drop in blood pressure upon standing up.

osmolality a characteristic of a solution determined by the number of dissolved particles in it.

osmosis the action in which a drug in a higher concentration solution passes through a permeable membrane to a lower concentration solution.

outpatient pharmacy a pharmacy attached to a hospital servicing patients who have left the hospital or who are visiting doctors in a hospital outpatient clinic.

panacea a cure-all (from the Greek panakeia, same meaning).

passive diffusion the movement of drugs from an area of higher concentration to lower concentration.

neurotransmitter chemicals released by nerves that interact with receptors to cause an effect.

patient assistance programs manufacturer sponsored prescription drug programs for the needy.

pediatric having to do with the treatment of children.

percutaneous the absorption of drugs through the skin, often for a systemic effect.

pH the pH scale measures the acidity or the opposite (alkalinity) of a substance. 7 is the neutral midpoint of the scale, values below which represent increasing acidity, and above which represent increasing alkalinity.

pharmaceutical alternative drug products that contain the same active ingredients, but not necessarily in the same amount or dosage form.

pharmaceutical equivalent drug products that contain identical amounts of the same active ingredients in the same dosage form.

pharmaceutical of or about drugs; also, a drug product.

pharmacology the study of drugs—their properties, uses, application, and effects (from the Greek pharmakon: drug, and logos: word or thought).

pharmacopeia an authoritative listing of drugs and issues related to their use.

pharmacy benefits managers companies that administer drug benefit programs

piggybacks small volume solution added to an LVP.

placebo an inactive substance given in place of a medication.

pneumatic tube a system which shuttles objects through a tube using compressed air as the force.

GLOSSARY

point of sale system (POS) an inventory system in which the item is deducted from inventory as it is sold or dispensed.

policy and procedure manual documentation of required policies, procedures, and disciplinary actions in a hospital.

positional notation the position of the number carries a mathematical significance or value.

POSs a network of providers where the patient's primary care physician must be a member and costs outside the network may be partially reimbursed.

PPOs a network of providers where costs outside the network may be partially reimbursed and the patient's primary care physician need not be a member.

prefix a modifying component of a term located before the other components of the term.

prescription drug benefit cards cards that contain third party billing information for prescription drug purchases.

primary emulsion the initial emulsion formed in a preparation to which ingredients are added to create the final volume.

primary literature original reports of clinical and other types of research projects and studies.

PRN order an order for medication to be administered only on an as needed basis.

prodrug an inactive drug that becomes active after it is transformed by the body.

protein binding the attachment of a drug molecule to a plasma or tissue protein, effectively making the drug inactive, but also keeping it within the body.

punch method a method for filling capsules by repeatedly pushing or "punching" the capsule into an amount of drug powder.

pyrogens chemicals produced by microorganisms that can cause pyretic (fever) reactions in patients.

qsad the quantity needed to make a prescribed amount.

Qualified Medicare Beneficiaries Medicare patients who may at times qualify for prescription drug coverage through a state administered program.

recall the action taken to remove a drug from the market and have it returned to the manufacturer.

reorder points minimum and maximum stock levels which determine when a reorder is placed and for how much.

resorption absorption of bone elements into the blood.

rheumatoid arthritis a disease in which the body's immune system attacks joint tissue.

root word the base component of a term which gives it a meaning that may be modified by other components.

satellites pharmacy locations in a decentralized sytems that operate outside the central pharmacy.

saturated solution a solution containing the maximum amount of drug it can contain at room temperature.

search engine software that searches the web for information related to criteria entered by the user.

secondary literature general reference works based upon primary literature sources.

selective (action) the characteristic of a drug that makes its action specific to certain receptors and the tissues they affect.

sharps needles, jagged glass or metal objects, or any items that might puncture or cut the skin.

signa the directions for use on the prescription that must be printed on the prescription label.

signature log a book in which patients sign for the prescriptions they receive, for legal and insurance purposes.

site of action the location where an administered drug produces an effect.

sonication exposure to high frequency sound waves.

sphygmomanometer a device used to measure blood pressure.

stability the chemical and physical integrity of the dosage unit, and when appropriate, its ability to withstand microbiological contamination.

standing order a standard medication order for patients to receive medication at scheduled intervals.

STAT order an order for medication to be administered immediately.

steatorrhea a condition of excess fat in the feces.

sterile a sterile condition is one which is free of all microorganisms, both harmful and harmless.

suffix a modifying component of a term located after the other components of the term.

supersaturated solution a solution containing a larger amount of drug than it normally contains at room temperature.

suspending agent a thickening agent used in the preparation of suspensions.

synergism when two drugs with different sites or mechanisms of action produce greater effects when taken together than when taken alone.

synthetic with chemicals, combining simpler chemicals into more complex compounds, creating a new chemical not found in nature as a result.

Syrup USP 850 grams of sucrose and 450 ml of water per liter.

tertiary literature condensed works based on primary literature, such as textbooks, monographs, etc.

therapeutic equivalent pharmaceutical equivalents that produce the same effects in patients.

therapeutic serving to cure or heal.

therapeutic window a drug's blood concentration range between its minimum effective concentration and minimum toxic concentration.

topical applied for local effect, usually to the skin.

total parenteral nutrition administration of all nutrients intravenously.

transcorneal transport drug transfer into the eye.

trituration the fine grinding of a powder.

turnover the rate at which inventory is used, generally expressed in number of days.

tuberculosis an infectious disease which primarily affects the respiratory system.

U&C or UCR usual and customary—the maximum amount of payment for a given prescription, determined by the insurer to be a usual and customary (and reasonable) price.

unit dose a package containing the amount of a drug required for one dose.

universal claim form a standard claim form accepted by many insurers.

URL(uniform resource locator) a web address.

valence the number of positive or negative charges on an ion.

vasoconstriction a constriction of the blood vessels.

vasodilators drugs that relax and expand the blood vessels.

variable an unknown value in a mathematical equation.

ventricular fibrillation irregular heart action seen in cardiac arrest patients.

vial a small glass or plastic container with a rubber closure sealing the contents in the container.

viscosity the thickness of a liquid.

volumetric measures volume.

water soluble the property of a substance being able to dissolve in water.

water-in-oil an emulsion in which water is dispersed through an oil base.

waters of hydration water molecules that attach to drug molecules.

wheal a raised blister-like area on the skin, as caused by an intradermal injection.

workers' compensation an employer compensation program for employees accidentally injured on the job.

World Wide Web a collection of electronic documents at Internet addresses called Web sites.

QUICK INDEX